SHEN

For Churchill Livingstone

Publishing Manager: Karen Morley
Development Editor: Louise Allsop, Kerry McGechie
Project Manager: Elouise Ball
Design Direction: Andrew Chapman
Illustrator: Oxford Illustrations
Illustration Buyer: Gillian Richards

SHEN

Psycho-Emotional Aspects of Chinese Medicine

Elisa Rossi MD PhD BA

Acupuncturist, Psychotherapist and Private Practitioner
in Chinese Medicine, Milan, Italy.

Laura Caretto

Teacher and Translator in MediCina, School of Chinese,
Medicine and Acupuncture, Milan, Italy.

Foreword by
Volker Scheid PhD FRCHM MBAcC
Practitioner of Chinese Medicine and Lecturer, UK

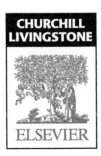

CHURCHILL LIVINGSTONE

ELSEVIER

CHURCHILL
LIVINGSTONE
ELSEVIER

An imprint of Elsevier Limited

First published 2002

ISBN 9780443101816

British Library Cataloguing in Publication Data
A catalogue record for this book is available from the British Library

Library of Congress Cataloging in Publication Data
A catalog record for this book is available from the Library of Congress

---

Notice

Knowledge and best practice in this field are constantly changing. As new research and experience broaden our knowledge, changes in practice, treatment and drug therapy may become necessary or appropriate. Readers are advised to check the most current information provided (i) on procedures featured or (ii) by the manufacturer of each product to be administered, to verify the recommended dose or formula, the method and duration of administration, and contraindications. It is the responsibility of the practitioner, relying on their own experience and knowledge of the patient, to make diagnoses, to determine dosages and the best treatment for each individual patient, and to take all appropriate safety precautions. To the fullest extent of the law, neither the publisher nor the editor assumes any liability for any injury and/or damage.

 ELSEVIER your source for books, journals and multimedia in the health sciences

www.elsevierhealth.com

Working together to grow
libraries in developing countries

www.elsevier.com | www.bookaid.org | www.sabre.org

ELSEVIER   BOOK AID International   Sabre Foundation

The Publisher's policy is to use paper manufactured from sustainable forests

Printed and bound in the United Kingdom
Transferred to Digital Print 2011

Contents

Foreword *by Volker Scheid*   ix
Acknowledgements   xiii
Introduction   xv
    Structure of the text   xvi
    Questions of terminology and nosography   xix

SECTION I – CLINICAL FOUNDATIONS OF *SHEN*

1. **Following the *dao* and nourishing life   3**
    Emotions and classical thought   4
    Non-action and the way   4
    Without memory or desire   6
    Internal practices   9
    Medical tradition   10
    Qigong   12
    Principal texts on the practices of meditation, nourishment of life and internal alchemy   13

2. **Emotions and the movement of *qi*   17**
    Terminology   17
    Emotions and classical thought   19
    Emotions as causes of illness   20
    Emotions, movement of *qi* and organs   23
    The 'Benshen' Chapter of the *Lingshu*   26
    Pathogenic processes   28
    Relationship among emotions and the five elements – *wuxing*   30
    Clinical notes   32
    Notes on the gall bladder and determination   39

3. **The psychic souls: *shen*, *hun*, *po*, *yi* and *zhi*   47**
    Shen   47
    Hun and *po*   52
    Yi and *zhi*   63

SECTION II – CLASSICAL ASPECTS OF PATHOGENS, SYMPTOMS AND SYNDROMES

4. **Constraint-*yu*   73**
    The term *yu*   74
    Spreading and draining – the *shuxie* function of the liver   74

Emotions and *yu*   76
External and internal factors   78
Yu syndrome, phlegm and blood stasis   79

5. **Emotions and heat   85**
    Liu Wansu and the theory of heat   85
    Li Dongyuan and *yin* fire   86
    Zhu Danxi and ministerial fire   88
    Zhang Jiebin, constitution and consumption of *yin*   90

6. **Agitation and restlessness – *fanzao*   97**
    Aetiology   98

7. **Insomnia   103**
    Description   104
    Aetiology according to the classical texts   105
    Evaluation according to the modality of presentation   106
    Notes on treatment   109
    Treatment according to some contemporary authors   110

8. **Mental health conditions – *diankuang*   125**
    Description   127
    Aetiology   129
    Treatment   134

9. **Classic syndromes: *zangzao*, *bentunqi*, *baihebing*, *meiheqi*   141**
    Zangzao   141
    Bentunqi   145
    Baibebing   151
    Meibeqi   154

SECTION III – THERAPEUTIC APPROACHES

10. **Principal patterns of Fullness – *shi*   171**
    Stagnation of liver *qi*   171
    Heart fire   179
    Liver fire and stomach fire   183
    Obstruction by phlegm-*tan*   185
    Stasis of blood-*xue*   189

11. **Principal patterns of emptiness-*xu* 203**
Emptiness of heart and spleen 204
Emptiness of heart *yin*, with empty fire 215

12. **Stimulation methods 233**
Acupuncture 233
Complementary techniques 235

13. **Points with diverse applications 247**
Principal points of the *ren mai* and *du mai*
in relation to *shen* disorders 247
Back *shu* points and corresponding points
of the lateral branch of the bladder channel 255
Heart and pericardium points 255

14. **Treatment with emotions in classical texts 261**
The physician as a guide 262
'Alter the emotions and change the nature' 263
Going around the obstacle 264
Control of emotions through emotions 266
Obsessive thoughts and anger 268

15. **The space shared by the patient
and the acupuncturist 271**
Regulate the *shen* 273
Stumbling blocks, traps and spider webs 274
The needle, this strange object 276
Setting and time of therapy 278
Dynamics of the therapeutic relationship 282
Abstention, empathy and neutrality 284
The patient inside of me 287

16. **Events related to acupuncture 293**
Immediate effects 293
Unexpected effects 294
Requests in psychological conditions
and chronic illness 297

**SECTION IV – CONTEMPORARY CLINICAL
CONTRIBUTIONS**

17. **Tongue and *shen* 307**
Barbara Kirchbaum
Introduction 307
Tongue diagnosis and *shen* 307
Summary of the key signs regarding *shen* 309

18. **Stress disorders: considerations
and clinical notes 313**
Qiao Wenlei
Introduction 313
Stress syndrome 314
Clinical manifestations 316
Objective examination 318
Treatment 318
Clinical cases 322
'Whiplash' 325

19. **Use of points in severe psychiatric
pathology 331**
Zhang Mingjiu
Introduction 331
Serious *shen* disorder and the choice of points 332
Shen 333
Po 338
Hun 341
Yi 344
Zhi 345
Comments 346
Syndromes 347

20. **Clinic for mental disorders 351**
Jin Shubai (*notes drawn from the text 'Acupuncture
and Moxibustion in the Treatment of Mental Disorders'*)
Introduction 351
Diankuang 352
Yuzheng 362

21. **Alterations of the *qi* and their somatic
manifestations 371**
Zhang Shijie
Introduction 371
Analysis and synthesis in the diagnostic process 373
The importance of channels in the interpretation
of pathology 375

22. **Hyperactivity and attention deficit
disorder 385**
Julian Scott (*reproduced from a book by Julian Scott
entitled 'Acupuncture in the Treatment of Children'*)
Introduction 385
Aetiology and pathogenesis 387
Patterns and symptoms 389
Treatment 391

23. Anxiety disorder: protocol applied in a public health unit   397
Introduction   397
Traditional Chinese Medicine in the treatment of Generalised Anxiety Disorders   398
Collecting the initial data   401

SECTION V – APPENDICES

A. The pulse   409
B. Notes on diagnostic framing in conventional psychiatry   419
C. TCM on the internet   425
D. Basic chronology   427
E. Glossary   429
F. Bibliography   433
G. List of points mentioned   441

Index   443

Foreword

by Volker Scheid

Chinese medicine in China is referred to as 'Chinese medicine' (*zhongyi*). Transferred to the West it changes into 'Traditional Chinese Medicine' (TCM). Whence this emphasis on tradition, we might ask? The immediate historical events surrounding this choice are easy to trace and take us to China in the 1950s. Charged with promoting their medicine abroad also once it had been declared a national treasure a group of Chinese translators felt this might be more easily achieved if the adjective 'traditional' was prefixed to the indigenous designation. The label was accepted – in the main uncritically – and proved to be a potent force in the promotion of Chinese medicine.

The more important second question is what this judicious assessment of Western sensibilities says about ourselves and our relationship to Chinese medicine. I believe that the label 'TCM' has been so successful because by offering a double negation it holds out a treble promise. TCM offers itself up to be non-Western *and* non-modern at the same time but also, and this is the crucial point, as somehow universal and therefore more easily acquired by ourselves. What could be more appealing to Westerners searching for alternatives to their own way of running the world who do not, when all is said and done, want to give up their own identity?

In the long run, however, one cannot have one's cake and eat it. Just as the rest of the world needed to westernise in order to utilise Western biomedicine, we will only ever become meaningful participants of the Chinese medical community by becoming more Chinese. The first step in this direction would be to let go of the 'T' in TCM, to consider it not as an asset but as a problem. And there are, indeed, many problems associated with being traditional.

Western critics of Chinese medicine, for instance, point out that unlike science, imagined as progressive and open to positive change, traditional knowledge is closed, impervious to critique and therefore, of necessity, inferior. Within the Chinese medicine community we face the problem of tradition in other ways. As we become more familiar with what we assumed to be one tradition, we discover that it is, in fact, made up of many different traditions, schools of thought, and lineages of transmission. How should we relate to this plurality? How do we know what is important and what is not, what to develop and from where to start?

But how to take this step considering that we have invested so much of our identity in the 'T' in TCM? The best place, I suggest, is to accept that tradition is, in fact, a problem and not a solution, or more precisely a *problematique*. A *problematique* is what the sinologist and historian Benjamin Schwarz refers to as recurring issues in human history and culture. It is what the modern Chinese, drawing on Marx, Lenin and Mao Zedong, call a contradiction (*maodun*) and diagnose in every patient and situation. It is to apply the tools of our trade – *yin* and *yang* and the knowledge of ongoing transformation and an awareness of permanent change – not only to our patients but to ourselves and to what we do.

Chinese physicians themselves have long been aware of the *problematique* at the bottom of their tradition, the contradiction at the heart of their medicine. On the one hand, the medical classics were the foundation of all medical practice. On the other, the myriad manifestations of illness, newly emergent diseases, and the changing nature of humans and society forever seemed to go beyond what the classics had to offer. The manner in which physicians reacted to this *problematique* has been as varied and diverse as the illnesses and disorders they sought to cure. Some believed that the problem was insufficient understanding of the classics by moderns, others that it was the insufficiency of the classics in relation to the modern. Some argued for more scholarly discourse, others for the primacy of empiricism. Gradually, a number of rhetorical formulas emerged around which a medical community could define itself in spite of continued diversity of opinion on almost all concrete issues: 'Study the ancients without getting stuck in the old' (*shi gu er bu ni gu*); or 'Medicine is opinion/intention' (*yi zhe yi ye*).

I believe it is this shared orientation to commonly experienced problems rather than an insistence on specific ideas or techniques on which any living tradition (with a small 't') is founded. If for biomedicine this shared orientation implies getting rid of the old to make way for the new, for practitioners of Chinese medicine it has always meant to reinterpret the old so as to fit it more effectively to the contexts of our lives. This attitude is rooted in empiricism and sensitivity to the present as much as in scholarship and respect for the past. And it is this attitude that has for many centuries allowed for the development of tradition without the danger of ever losing it.

If we in the West wish to contribute to this process, to become a true part of the tradition we so visibly claim to represent, we need to accept that innovation and development, whether on the level of individual practice of Chinese medicine as a whole, must proceed from the ancients before it can leave them behind.

Elisa Rossi and Laura Caretto show us in exemplary fashion how this might be done. First, they restore time and plurality to tradition by providing us with detailed expositions about the development of disease concepts and therapeutic approaches drawn from a wide reading of classical sources. Unlike modern textbooks, who flatten this diversity by citing from these texts as if they had all been written at the same time by authors who all shared the same ideas, readers are thereby drawn into the *problematiques* of psycho-spiritual disorders viewed from the perspectives of Chinese medicine. They gain a profound understanding of the actual depth of our tradition but also of its debates and unresolved issues as different authors disagree with each other about fundamental points. We are thus forced to make up our own minds in order to decide what is best for our own patients.

Here, too, Rossi and Caretto provide guidance but do not press us into accepting their views. Treatment protocols and point selections are presented as hypotheses rather than as being set in stone or delivered to us from on up high. Drawing on their own clinical experience and that of others the authors draw readers into a process of reflection that requires of them ultimately to make their own choices.

Finally, once more most unusual in a contemporary Chinese medicine text, Rossi and Caretto provide space for other contemporary authors, specialists in their own fields, to supplement the main text through additional essays. Again, the reader is informed but not presented with a single and singular system of ideas.

'Shen' is therefore more than an acupuncture textbook or a clinical manual for the treatment of psycho-spiritual disorders. By relating their personal clinical experience to a profound engagement with the medical archive of Chinese medicine, the authors have created a model for how to develop Chinese medicine in the West. This is an important achievement.

Acknowledgements

This book exists thanks to many different, but all very precious, contributions.

Of great importance have been the kindness and support of friends, the passionate and fascinating stories of patients, the generosity and attention of masters, the reflections of colleagues, the faith of the editor, and the existence of the association MediCina as a place for the construction of knowledge.

An essential contribution has been that of Laura Caretto, whose knowledge of the language, familiarity with the texts and expertise in Chinese medicine allowed critical and timely links to be made with classical and contemporary sources.

I am particularly grateful to Mireille Degouville, Salvo Inglese, Margherita Majno, Stefano Rossi and Grazia Rotolo for the revision of the text and for the suggestions on elements of Chinese linguistics, psychiatric references, medical elaborations, and the shape and clarity of the work.

Introduction

'All acupuncture methods must find their root in the *shen*'.[1] This is the opening of the first Chinese text dedicated to acupuncture.

Those who treat the ill and in particular those who use non-conventional medicines are well aware of the importance of certain psychic aspects in the disorders told by patients. Some patients speak directly of anxiety, depression, insomnia and agitation, expressing an emotional and mental discomfort; others describe this 'feeling unwell' through sensations such as pain, weight, swelling, knots.

There are times when the 'emotional illness' shows itself clearly, and others in which it insinuates gradually, with the most alarming expressions. In both cases it is clear that a psychic part permeates our everyday practice. On these occasions Chinese medicine is quite useful because it considers the person as a whole; it addresses the 'ill',[2] which in Latin is '*malatus*' from '*male habitu (m)*' – someone who is not in a good state.

Acupuncture has attracted many of us precisely because it is a medicine that considers the person as a whole. Moreover it seems to produce substantial effects even on the subtlest aspects, in spite of its apparent focus on the body. It is always fascinating to see how important is the connection between psychic and physical disorders in the 'Chinese' mode of interpreting signs in patients. It is also of great comfort to see how our work is facilitated by not having to separate emotional, mental and somatic layers.[3]

The effectiveness of acupuncture is also confirmed by clinical practice and by research studies. It is a discipline that stands in a consistent theoretical universe, with a well-documented tradition of experience and clinical reflection. Furthermore it is a flexible tool that can be adapted to different sociocultural situations.

---

[1] Hangfu Mi, *Zhenjiu Jiayijing* ('The systematic classic of acupuncture and moxibustion', AD259), Chapter 1. These words echo the first sentence of Chapter 8 of the *Lingshu*.

[2] NB: in Italian 'ill' is 'malato'. We also remind the readers that in Italy acupuncture can be practised only by MDs.

[3] Moreover the distinction between mental and somatic illness has disappeared even from a conventional psychiatry text such as the DSM, the most used institutional manual. In it we read: 'Although this volume is titled *Diagnostic and Statistic Manual of Mental Disorders*, the term *mental disorder* unfortunately implies a distinction between 'mental' and 'physical' disorders, that is a reductionist anachronism of mind/body dualism. A compelling literature documents that there is much 'physical' in 'mental' disorders and much 'mental' in 'physical' disorders.' In: DSM-IV, 1996, Introduction, p. xxi.

The following work aims at reviewing, connecting and deepening those aspects of Chinese medicine in which the psychic component is recognised to be particularly relevant.

The frequently entangled set of signs and symptoms presented by the patient can often prevent the diagnostic framework from being immediately evident and one can feel disoriented when considering the suggested treatments. To facilitate the processes of thought and operative practice, this book proposes a systematisation, from the point of view of Chinese medicine, of different patterns, and describes in detail the progress of a treatment in a series of clinical cases.

The clinical sections are presented in both their theoretical and practical aspects. They are especially useful as 'nets' that can be used to connect the thoughts and considerations that develop when attending a patient.

The origin of this book is based on the interest engendered by references to *shen* and emotions in classical literature. I shared this curiosity with Laura Caretto, who graduated in Traditional Chinese Medicine in Beijing and in Oriental Languages in Venice with a thesis on emotions in medical literature.

A specific section stemmed from the study of those elements of texts that refer to certain pathogenetic processes and symptoms recurring in the alteration of emotions. This section examines various elements that are essential not only for the psychic illness but also for Chinese medicine in its totality.

It may be that certain theoretical subtleties of the classics are of greater interest to those who have a wide clinical experience, but awareness of the complexity of the subject is important at all levels of interaction with Chinese medicine.

The section on contemporary contributions stems from an interest in the way 'emotional illnesses' are treated nowadays. Here I have gathered together works with very different approaches, but all sharing a connection with the theme of this book and the fact that they are the outputs of practitioners who have long worked, observed and reflected. The selection is not based on a judgmental comparison with other works; it is simply based on personal relationships with the authors and the desire to share with my colleagues a number of undoubtedly interesting theoretical and practical elaborations.

Although the book is primarily designed for those who already know about and use acupuncture, some parts may also be useful during a first phase of study. Moreover some issues may also appeal to those who work from an angle different from that of Chinese medicine, but who are nevertheless engaged in researching the way people have thought and dealt with psychic disorders and mental illnesses.

STRUCTURE OF THE TEXT

The text is based first of all on the research and translation of what has been passed down to us by classical works.

The choice of consulting the texts in their original language stems from a need to discover the roots of a thought that has always given great importance to the written text, with a focus on continuous quotes, commentaries, re-editions and compilations. These classical and contemporary comments have been of great significance for the translation of the quotes in Italian and English. This statement is confirmed as soon as we think of how easily text fragments coming from an unknown cultural model may create decontextualised explanations or strengthen *a priori* opinions.

This is the work of Laura Caretto: her knowledge of medical literature allowed the retrieval of traces and signs scattered in every crevice of the existing enormous medical corpus. The precision and attention in her examination of the sources and comments safeguards the quality of the translation. Her continuous collaboration with Chinese medical doctors guarantees a connection between words and the practical reality of medicine.

In the more theoretical sections we have decided to reproduce a large number of quotes *verbatim*, on account of both the evocative power they possess and of their explanatory sharpness. Likewise we have chosen a very faithful translation so as to preserve the syntactic flow of the text, relatively far removed from Italian and English sentence constructions, but for this very reason even more evocative. With a similar intention we have kept punctuation to a minimum, considering how it is traditionally absent from classic texts.

In order to limit the inaccuracy intrinsic to every translation, the book starts with some notes clarifying terminology and with some specifications about the definition and classification of psychic illnesses.

Reading Notes

The presentation of the material is aimed at those who have a basic knowledge of Chinese medicine and it is articulated on various levels.

- The first section, fundamental in every clinical discourse, is of more general interest: it opens with a chapter which recalls the bases of the Chinese thought and the practices for the 'nourishment of life', followed by a discourse on emotions and movements of the *qi*, and by a revision of the concept of *shen* (see Chapters 1, 2 and 3).
- The discussion differentiating the various pathological patterns with their connected aetiopathogenesis, symptomatologies and treatment hypothesis is developed in the later chapters relating to clinical systematisation. These chapters possess a certain autonomy within the text and can be used as a reference guide when in front of the patient (see Chapters 7, 10 and 11).
- The clinical systematisation and several of the case discussions refer to information contained in the chapters on stimulation methods and revision of certain points with diverse use (see Chapters 12 and 13).

- Specific consideration is given to elements that are common in everyday practice: the space in which patient and acupuncturist meet, certain problems that are rooted in the dynamic of the therapeutic relationship, and the psychic action of acupuncture (see Chapters 15, 16 and many of the comments on clinical cases).

- Of more theoretical relevance are the chapters developing ideas about pathogenic processes (see Chapters 2 and 5), aspects of symptomatology (see Chapters 6 and 7) and syndrome definitions (see Chapters 8 and 9). These topics permeate the entire history of medical thought, but they often remain unexpressed in the basic study of acupuncture and in its modern use. Along with these discussions we present a number of classic examples of cases treated 'with emotions' (see Chapter 14).

- Another level, which is developed mostly in the footnotes, focuses on certain questions of terminology, recalls some of the issues that are still under debate and guarantees the possibility of accessing Chinese and Western sources.

- Furthermore throughout the work is found a number of 'clinical notes, always distinguished from the text to which they refer. Such annotations focus on aspects derived from practical experiences and from personal considerations. This gives them a practical twist and allows them to take into consideration those difficulties encountered personally, those discussed with students and those debated with colleagues.

- Analysis of treatment using traditional pharmacology, internal practices working with the *qi*, and *tuina* manipulation techniques is beyond the intentions of this text. For the same reason I do not discuss the nosological, epidemiological, diagnostic and therapeutic aspects relative to the Western biomedical viewpoint.

Clinical Cases

Clinical cases are taken from a personal experience. Biographical data have been modified to ensure anonymity, whilst retaining those features necessary for the understanding of the case.

Case studies at the end of the chapters focus on their central issue, but because they are actual complex situations some aspects often revisit issues discussed elsewhere in the text.

I have used a common structure to illustrate the symptoms, diagnostic hypothesis and course of the therapy. However, a number of cases are discussed in relation to specific elements on which I wanted to focus, so that case history, diagnosis and treatment are only outlined.

In presenting cases I have used an informal style of communication, rather than choosing more formal medical language. This has allowed me to retain the words used by patients and to reproduce better the nuances of the therapeutic experience.

Reflection on the elements that have led to a specific diagnosis and on the associated therapeutic principles is left for the most part to the reader, who can find all suggestions for this kind of practice in the clinical section. The investigation is considered to be complete so if a symptom is not mentioned it means it was not present. On the other hand, the treatment employed is described with greater detail: I discuss the reasons for my choice of points and I specify the timing of the therapy in order to allow the reader to follow its course closely.

As in order to evaluate a therapy it is necessary to know about its trend, I have added some follow-up notes.

Cases are basically presented as suggestions for thought: as often happens among colleagues, clinical stories are often an occasion for talking about acupuncture in general. Such an attitude is reflected in the comments to clinical stories, which consist of notes encompassing disparate elements that were often the very reason for presenting the case: discrepancies in the clinical pattern, a particularly difficult diagnosis, details about therapeutic choices, problems linked to the relationship with the patient, reflections on mistakes, thoughts on specific points or stimulations, and considerations of the patient's response – notes that actually concern the practice of acupuncture as a whole.

QUESTIONS OF TERMINOLOGY AND NOSOGRAPHY

Human suffering takes various forms, its symptoms are varied and have many shapes; illness has many different names.

The 'giving of a name' is a fundamental feature of human thought and of its expression: it implies the recognition of the named object and its positioning in a system of categories. This organisation of human experience takes place within a specific culture that models its forms and relations.

The naming of medicine is also an expression of society and culture, and therefore it has various and specific aspects. The way in which we interpret a sign and define a diagnosis stems from specific cultural features: diagnosis is a semiotic act, whereby the symptoms experienced by the patient are interpreted as a sign of a particular illness. These interpretations have a meaning only in relation to specific categories and criteria.[4]

---

[4] The role of cultural differences in the definition of illnesses is also recognised in the fourth revision of the DSM, which takes into consideration culturally characterised syndromes. Works on transcultural psychiatry, which must face the problem of comparing different medical systems, highlight the fact that 'culture is a factor which can guarantee organisation or offer a particular order to forms of disorder'. This means that the ways of falling ill are also selected and dictated by cultures. 'The main problem stemming from the comparativist methodology is the interpretation of the diagnostic process as a cultural construction descending from a set of knowledge and techniques (clinical method) deeply rooted in the cognitive logics of a certain culture.' In: S. Inglese and C. Peccarisi, 'Psichiatria oltre frontiera. Viaggio intorno alle sindromi culturalmente ordinate', 1997, p. 11, UTET, Milan.

An attempt to assimilate Chinese patterns to biomedical ones (that is, to conventional Western medicine patterns) would be a forced interpretation. The two medicines not only have different ways of treating but also differ in their defining of the diagnosis. In fact they have different frameworks of physiology and pathology, and interpretation processes utilise dissimilar concepts.

Clarification of Terminology

The construction of a text on psychic, emotional and mental illnesses based on works that are foreign to us involves a number of complicated issues in relation to accurate use of specific terminologies and adequate categories. The nosological difficulties surrounding the definition of illnesses are a part of all medical thoughts, but in the case of Chinese medicine the problems are enlarged by the difficulties of the language and in particular the literary Chinese of different time periods.

Because of the relevance of the text reconstruction to its very meaning, translation of the fundamental works has been carried out in consultation with commentaries of various periods. All quoted passages have been retranslated with the intention of providing a version that would follow the same interpretative guidelines and guarantee the homogeneity of the terms.[5]

The translation reflects very closely the original structure of classical Chinese, often articulated in characteristic forms such as: sentences built with four characters, more coordinates than subordinates, and a syntax which uses subject and object in a circular form. The resulting prose is quite different from our common modes of expression but it brings us closer to the original discourse.

For all the Chinese terms we use the *pinyin* system, which is the official phonetic translation used in China, recognised by the WHO and almost universally widespread. We use italic for all Chinese words.

The transcription has a syllabic base, as suggested by current Sinological conventions.[6]

There are few terms that have been kept in Chinese, but certain specific characters have been maintained whenever they could be of use to those readers who know the language.

The criteria determining translation choices within the vocabulary on emotions are specified here or in the following chapters. For each case we have

---

[5] Where it is not otherwise indicated the original Italian translations are by Laura Caretto. The original Italian translation of European languages is the author's.
[6] We remind the reader that until the late sixties the concept of character was preferred to that of word. This is the reason why we still find in many texts a monosyllabic transcription of titles, names and sentences.

kept a fixed correspondence between the Chinese terms and the [Italian and] English ones indicated in the Glossary.

In the abbreviations of classical and extra points, to aid the reader we have integrated the classical quotes by putting the abbreviation of the point next to its name.

Since we always refer to organs in their Chinese sense, we never use capital letters.

In order not to create a dichotomy between abstract/symbolic and concrete/material, which is completely unknown to the Chinese thought, we never use capital letters, not even for terms such as 'fire', 'earth', or 'path'.

We maintain the abbreviation TCM (*Traditional Chinese Medicine*) since it defines a specific systematisation of Chinese medicine, discussed further on.

We use the term 'classic' in a non-specific way, with reference to all literature prior to TCM. We nevertheless recall that the expression 'Classical China' corresponds to the period from 500 to 200BC.

Quotes and bibliographic references follow common rules. The completeness of the bibliographic references in the footnotes varies depending on the needs of the discussion, but all books can be found listed in the Bibliography.

Emotional Illnesses

Illnesses with a major psychic component – which we variously define as mental disorder, psychiatric pathologies, emotional alterations, etc – are called 'emotional illnesses' *qingzhi jibing* 情 志 疾 病 or *qingzhi bing* 情志病, which is a classical expression still in use.

This definition does not have precise categorical boundaries, as is also the case for the designation of mental illnesses or psychic pathologies in conventional psychiatry.[7]

The term 'emotions' is the translation of *zhi* 志, *qing* 清 and *qingzhi* 清志 and involves the whole sphere of sentiments and passions, the whole of the internal mental, emotional and affective movements – namely the world which we now call 'psychic/psychological'.

Since it is impossible to outline a precise difference between the three terms, in order to link each of them to a different European word, every time the term 'emotions' appears we quote the original character.

---

[7] 'In DSM-IV each of the mental disorders is conceptualised as a clinically significant behavioural or psychological syndrome or pattern. That occurs in an individual and that is associated with present distress (e.g. a painful symptom) or disability (i.e., impairment in one or more important areas of functioning) or with a significantly increased risk of suffering death, pain, disability, or an important loss of freedom.' In: DSM-IV, 1996, Introduction, p. xxi. Also in general medicine many illnesses are defined according to different levels of abstraction: for example with an anatomopathological description (duodenal ulcer), a presentation of the symptoms (migraine), a deviation from a physical norm (arterial hypertension), or an aetiological definition (hepatitis C).

For a more articulated discussion refer to the specific chapter. Here we mention that the five emotions are: *nu* 怒 rage, *xi* 喜 euphoria, *si* 思; thought, *bei* 悲 sadness and *kong* 恐 fear.

When there is a reference to *qiqing* 七 情, the seven emotions, they include *you* 忧 anguish and *jing* 惊 fright.

The choice of using the terms 'euphoria' and 'thought' needs to be briefly clarified.

Xi, often translated in English texts as 'excessive joy', can actually be well translated as 'euphoria' since *xi* corresponds to the feeling of euphoric happiness during popular feasts, rich in food, wine and music. It is thus a joy very close to the agitation of fire, while the other character used in the classics – *le* 乐 – is well represented by the term 'joy' since it expresses a more intimate feeling, connected with rituals and ceremonies, in reference to a state of peace and harmony.[8]

Si is often translated in medicine texts as 'excessive thought', possibly because the Greek–Judaic tradition looks at thought as a very positive action, recognising a pathological twist only in its excess. We have chosen to maintain the literal translation, that is simply 'thought', because in the Daoist conception thought substitutes for the ability to respond immediately; it is a mediation lacking the harmony of a spontaneous response.[9] Also in the Buddhist tradition thought can be an obstacle in the search for a state of 'emptiness of the mind'.

Other Terms Concerning Psychic Aspects

See the Glossary for the specific terms recurring in the text.

Certain terms, which appear with unspecific meanings in classical texts, have been rediscovered by the literature in the 1980s, as part of a process of revaluation of the psychic/psychological aspects of Chinese medicine, for example *yiliao* 医 疗 'thought-therapy' or *jingshen liaofa* 精 神 疗 法 'psychic therapeutic method'.[10]

---

[8] Already the classics before Han made this distinction: ' *le* 乐 has singing and dance [of the rites], *xi* 喜 has charity [of the feasts]', in: *Zuozhuan*, chap. 'Zhaogong ershiwu nian'. The character *xi* is composed of 'mouth' and 'tambourine', that is 'to play the drums and sing' (Wieger 167b, Karlgren 129), while the complex form of *le* (the same homograph *yue* indicates 'music') depicts bells on the sides of a ceremonial drum on a wooden stand (Wieger 88c, Karlgren 568).

[9] For a discussion on thought-*si* 思 as an artificial-*wei* 伪 element that opposes natural-*xing* 性, within the concepts of resonance and spontaneity, see the introductive chapter (Chapter 1).

[10] We find this term both in contemporary authors such as Wang Miqu, 1985, and classical texts 'If in the heart there is an accumulation of heat, medicines will not be able to reach it and we will use *yiliao*.' In: Fang Jizhuan, *Liaoshi* ('History of the Liao dynasty', 905–1125). As an example we recall that the term *zhexue* 'philosophy' does not belong to the tradition: it was introduced in China from Japan, where it was created at the end of the nineteenth century under Western influence.

All the terms translating words and concepts belonging to contemporary Western disciplines have obviously been created recently. They use characters that have always been related to the psychic field, but – as all substantives in modern Chinese – they have two or three syllables.

They mostly contain the terms *xin* 心, *shen* 神, *jing* 惊, *zhi* 志 and *yi* 意. For more information refer to the specific chapter (Chapter 3).

Xin, the heart, is considered the organ of knowledge, which enables us to know, to think, to assess and to feel. The radical 'heart' is quite common in terms referring to thought or feelings. From this term comes *xinli* 心理, which is similar to our prefix 'psycho' (*xin* is 'heart' in the psychic sense, *li* is the natural principle of things), and words such as: *xinlixue* 心理学 – psychology, *xinli zhiliao* 心理治疗 – psychotherapy and *xinli fenxi* 心理分析 – psychoanalysis.

Shen 神, the subtlest aspect of *qi*, is discussed in a specific chapter. We recall here that nowadays in China it is translated as 'mind'. *Shenzhi* 神志 is currently used with the meaning of 'mind', but the two characters appear together also in classical texts. In such cases we have kept the Chinese form.

Jingshen 惊神 is the modern translation of the Western term 'mental, psychic' (but it is also used in an unspecific way to say 'spirit', in the sense of 'liveliness', or in constructions such as 'spirit of self-sacrifice', 'spirit of the age'). From it derive, as examples, *jingshen bing* 精神病 mental illness, *jingshen bingxue* 精神病学; psychiatry and *jingshen yiyuzheng* 精神抑郁证 mental depression.

TCM – Traditional Chinese Medicine

In the study and application of Chinese medicine, the aspects of denomination and classification of pathologies have a number of different problems. The first is with regard to modern Chinese medicine, which results from a stratification and integration of over two thousand years of clinical and theoretical work.[11] Recognising the complexity of such a structure may be useful in finding some landmarks which can help guide practitioners theoretically and in practice: this text bases clinical framing and treatment on the syndrome differentiation according to TCM.[12]

The systematisation titled 'Traditional Chinese Medicine – TCM' began under the People's Republic. This type of research occurred substantially at

---

[11] With regard to the heterogeneity and plurality of Chinese medicine see also Unschuld, particularly the introduction to *Medicine in China*, 1985; Sivin, 1995; Kaptchuk et al and the concept of 'herbalisation of acupuncture' (*The Journal of Chinese Medicine*, no. 17, 1985); the discussion by Deadman and Flaws (*The Journal of Chinese Medicine*, n.38, 1992); and the debate in *The European Journal of Oriental Medicine* (vol. 1 nos 1 and 2, 1993, vol. 1 nos 3 and 4, 1994, and vol. 2 no. 1, 1996), among which are the contributions by Garvey, Blackwell, Diebschlag, Scheid and Bensky. See also the annotations by Zhang Shijie on the methodology of the diagnostic process (Chapter 21).
[12] As already specified we have decided to keep the abbreviation TCM as it defines this very system.

the end of the 1950s when Mao Zedong started a process of re-evaluation of traditional medicine, which the intellectual and progressive community had until then considered a dated and superstitious belief, labelling it as part of the remains of the old feudal system.

The elaboration of a diagnostic and intervention method based on a clear and consistent structure had to integrate different traditions, based on a direct transmission and on a logical procedure unsuited to being positioned in a definitive scheme. This process has marginalised certain aspects of the medical discourse. On the other hand it has made it recognisable in diverse situations, has guaranteed the possibility of transmitting it and has allowed its use within controlled methodologies.

Now TCM is the prevailing theoretical model in China and in the world and it is the reference point for contemporary didactic, literature and research.

The consistency of this system allowed Chinese medicine to resist the impact and confrontation with the Western biomedical model, now predominant with respect to other traditional medicines in the world.

Globalisation does not exclude the enduring efficacy of traditional medicines, but their validity is usually limited to a specific cultural community. In contrast, traditional Chinese medicine is characterised by a generalised practice in a complex society such as the Chinese one, and by a precise institutional position in a politically and numerically important nation. It also recognises a transcultural application since it is now widespread in many culturally distant countries: from economically advanced ones to developing countries such as African states and Cuba. Lastly it is a non-conventional medical system that is recognised by the 'official' scientific community.

Definitions and Classifications

Contemporary Chinese texts – and thus many TCM texts in English – use classifications that can overlap in their general guidelines but which are definitely not univocal.

The present classification criteria take into consideration those illnesses traditionally recognised to have a significant psychic component. At the same time they use many terms borrowed from Western psychiatry but often considered antiquated by the Western scientific community.

Attention to the task of classifying medicine and emotional illnesses can already be found in the history of Chinese medicine, particularly in the Ming period. We relate a couple of examples that highlight the fundamental structure on which modern classifications are still based.

The *Leijing* has 29 chapters on emotional illnesses, *qingzhibing*, among which are discussions on 'constriction' pathologies such as *yuzheng*, madness *diankuang*, mental exhaustion *neishanglao*, insomnia *bumei*, dementia *chidai* and fictitious illness *zhabing*.[13] A slightly later text has a section entitled *shenzhi* in which there are discussions on illnesses such as madness, restlessness and agitation, restlessness from emptiness, pain, delirium, involuntary movements, continual laughter and crying, rage, sadness, fright, palpitations, fear, loss of memory, and being possessed.[14]

Contemporary Nosology

The issue of illness classification is extremely important for the understanding of medical thought, but in this occasion we only give some hints that may be used for guiding those who can only consult translated texts.

The more specialised clinical texts usually discuss psychiatry and neurology together.

The more general manuals often list psychiatric disorders within the section 'internal diseases', including for example respiratory, gastroenterological and neurological illnesses.

In clinical records there are often two diagnoses: the biomedical one and the Chinese; it is a sign of how different medical traditions attempt to integrate elements of different cultures, an effort to combine references from different perspectives, but it can produce frequent overlaps in terminology and nosography.[15]

The pathologies considered usually embrace 'classical' illnesses such as *diankuang* (sometimes translated as 'manic–depressive disorder' or 'schizophrenia'), *yuzheng* (variously translated as 'depression', 'melancholy', or 'hysteria'), *zangzao* (translated as 'visceral agitation' or 'hysteria'), *meiheqi* ('plum-stone qi'), *baihebing* ('*baihe* syndrome', but also 'neurasthenia') and *bentunqi* ('running piglet *qi*').

On other occasions the framework is based on Western terminology (for example 'neurosis', 'hysteria', 'schizophrenia' and 'hyperactivity of childhood') and discusses the correspondences in traditional Chinese medicine, so that we read for example: 'Schizophrenia. In traditional Chinese medicine this illness is included in the categories of *yuzheng* (melancholia), *dian* (depressive psychosis), *kuang* (mania), etc.'[16]

---

[13] Zhang Jiebin, *Leijing* ('The Classic of Categories', 1624), Book 21. It is interesting to observe how the last chapter, '*Yangxinglun*' ('Nourishing the nature') is dedicated to internal practices of 'nourishment of life'.

[14] Zhang Luyu, *Zhangshi yitong* ('Medical Compendium of Master Zhang', 1695), Book 6. 'As being possessed' is the translation of *rumo zouhuo*.

[15] For a discussion about the relationship between Chinese medicine and conventional/dominant medicine and about integration and assimilation see also the article by Scheid and Bensky 'Medicine as Signification', The European Journal of Oriental Medicine, vol. 2, no. 6, 1998, and the following debate.

[16] Hou Jinglun ed., *Traditional Chinese Treatment for Psychogenic and Neurological Diseases*, 1996, p. 143.

Furthermore there is usually a list of:

- illnesses whose aetiology is strongly linked with emotions, for example insomnia, sleepiness, lack of memory (*jianwang*, often translated as 'amnesia'), palpitations, tiredness, etc.;
- illnesses which refer to patterns directly related to emotional dynamics, for example excessive rage, easy sadness, easy fear, easy preoccupation, easy fright;
- neurological illnesses such as epilepsy, migraines, vertigo;
- illnesses with psychic symptoms and organic origin such as trauma, poisoning, infections, postnatal syndromes;
- child illnesses such as crying and night fright, 'the five delays and the five weaknesses';
- illnesses that are framed as signs of emotional disturbances, for example too many dreams, sexual impotence, seminal losses.[17]

The use of Western terms is not univocal; for example *yuzheng* is often nowadays translated as 'depression', but in a recent manual is otherwise translated 'melancholia' and it is a symptom of hysteria: 'Melancholia (*yuzheng*) is a general term for an illness resulting from an emotional depression and from *qi* stagnation. A disorder in the circulation of the *qi* can alter the blood system and produce many pathologic consequences. In this section we will discuss only hysteria. To treat migraine, insomnia, palpitations, seminal losses and plum-stone syndrome one can refer to the specific chapters.'[18] Here there is no adaptation to the psychiatric classification used today, but there is a reference to 'hysteria', to which are often connected syndromes such as *zangzao, baihebing, bentunqi, meiheqi* (although *meiheqi* can be found among the 'eye, nose, mouth and throat illnesses').

Anxiousness or panic attacks are recognised as a specific disorder.

Food disorders as such are absent: the term 'anorexia' is only used to indicate a symptom, that is, in the sense of lack of appetite.

We recall that the culturally characterised syndromes reported in the DSM-IV do not appear in Chinese classics nor in modern TCM texts: these illnesses usually belong to cultural systems that are an expression of simpler contexts, in which individuals share the same political, economic and religious reality. China is a complex society that has developed just as complex and articulated medical systems.[19]

---

[17] 'Seminal losses' correspond to *yijing*, often translated as 'spermatorrhoea'. There is a female equivalent, *mengjiao*, which is the dreaming of sexual activity: 'The pathogenesis of this illness is the same as that of men's nocturnal pollutions. This illness belongs to the category of mental illnesses.' In: Liu Gongwang ed., *Clinical Acupuncture and Moxibustion*, Tianjin, 1996, p. 250.

[18] Liu Gongwang ed., 1996, p. 234.

[19] These syndromes, listed in Appendix I of the fourth edition of the DSM, are part of a specific cultural context. Different syndromes refer to the Far East, but only *Shenkui* is specific to Taiwan and China. It means 'loss of kidney', a popular term describing a set of somatic and psychic anxiety symptoms linked to a loss of *jing*, seminal fluid and at the same time 'life energy'. There is also a reference to a psychotic reaction to *qigong*, which is also included in the 'Chinese Classification of Mental Disorders, Second Edition – CCMD-2', consisting in an acute episode that occurs in vulnerable subjects performing *qigong* incorrectly.

SECTION I

CLINICAL FOUNDATIONS OF *SHEN*

CHAPTER 1 FOLLOWING THE *DAO* AND NOURISHING LIFE

Illness and treatment are always linked to the way in which the world is thought and organised. To practice Chinese medicine one must have some knowledge of how its reference universe is conceived, as well as being familiar with the way one should move within it.

This complex issue is impossible to summarise in a small number of pages, but it is important to keep in mind that the paths and solutions applied by Chinese medicine in the prevention and treatment of psychic disorders are strongly connected to the practices for 'nourishing life'. Chapter 1, where I refer to these practices and to the underlying Chinese classical thought, focuses on the extent of the concept of treatment.

Internal practices, which accompany the whole history of Chinese thought and which represent an essential part of the therapeutic work, are mainly an experiential nucleus and their core belongs to the work conducted with different masters. And for this heart we often lack appropriate words.

CHAPTER 2 EMOTIONS AND THE MOVEMENT OF *QI*

CHAPTER 3 THE PSYCHIC SOULS – *SHEN*, *HUN*, *PO*, *YI* AND *ZHI*

More plainly, Chapters 2 and 3 analyse closely certain elaborations that are fundamental for the discussion on what belongs to the psychic world, that is the concepts of emotions and *shen*.

References to *shen* in its multiple appearances and to emotions in relation to the *qi* and pathology are extremely fragmented, scattered in various works, and often difficult to interpret. This was an even more valid reason for gathering together their traces spread among the enormous Chinese medical corpus, up to this day vary rarely translated, and proposing a critical revision.

Knowing better this complexity, and the importance of these concepts, means having the possibility to handle more easily their relationships and implications. It allows us to use them in the clinical work with greater consistency and, at the same time, with more confidence and spontaneity.

These chapters also aim at proposing some possibilities for the revision of the concepts of *shen* and emotional illnesses, starting in any case from a base that has been verified with great care and precision.

Following the *Dao* and Nourishing Life

1

> In our times, people continuously request help from diviners and offer prayers for health and healing, yet illnesses are on the rise. It is as though during an archery contest the archer failed to hit the target and asked for a different one to substitute for it – how can this substitution possibly help him to hit the centre of the target? If you want a pot of soup to stop boiling, you must remove it from the fire. In their references to all these doctors and healers with their medicines and potions aimed at expelling sickness, alleviating it and controlling it, the sages of the past had very little respect for them, since in their opinion they were taking care of the branches and not the roots.[1]

The respect that we as doctors have for our treatments varies, but certainly as acupuncturists we know that the course of health and illness is based on the state of *qi* and it is upon the *qi* that we act when we treat a patient.

In the clinic, we should always keep in mind that the treatment of emotions is a therapy in the most complete sense of the term: the practitioner treats the patient, but patients also take charge of their own lives and take responsibility for it.

Illness can present with more psychological or more somatic manifestations, but in both cases: 'The sage does not treat when there is already illness, but when the illness does not yet exist; he does not treat when there is already disorder-*luan* (乱). Waiting to treat until after the illness has already developed or bringing order after disorder has already developed is comparable to digging a well when one is thirsty, and casting a knife after the battle has already been engaged.'[2]

It is therefore the work on *qi* – those internal practices for cultivating life about whose necessity classical philosophers and doctors of all schools agree – that really constitutes the most profound, lasting and significant intervention.

---

[1] *Lushi chunqiu*, Chapter 12, quoted in: Needham, 1982, p. 93. The *Lushi chunqiu* ('Annuals of spring and autumn by master Lu) is one of the six Confucian classics, dated around the 3rd century BC.
[2] *Suwen*, Chapter 2.

EMOTIONS AND CLASSICAL THOUGHT

Discussion of emotions and their pathologies belongs to a much broader and deeper territory than that inherent in medicine in the strictest sense, and any investigation of *shen*, emotions and psychologically related illnesses must presume some knowledge of the ways in which Chinese thought conceived of this reality.

A formal and detailed elaboration of this subject is beyond the scope of this text, but a few brief notes are necessary in order to distinguish the terms used and will also serve to direct the reader.

Among the various works on Chinese thought we will refer here principally to Graham's studies, whose foreword to the Italian edition well underlined the difficulties that present themselves to those who take their cue from a totally different world view: 'the study of that thought implicates a constant involvement on our part in crucial questions of moral philosophy, such as the relationship between philosophy and the history of science, the deconstruction of pre-established conceptual formats, the problems with relating thought to language structure and thought correlated to logic.'[3]

Although unable here to treat the subject exhaustively, we will nevertheless mention some background elements such as the correlative order underlying Chinese cognitive thought in comparison to the analytical method of Western philosophy and science. This is the feature that also distinguishes its medical model, with regards not only to the deciphering of signs (and symptoms), but also physiological and individual pathological processes.

It is often remarked that, whereas Western philosophers ask 'What is Truth?', Chinese masters ask about 'the Way', expressing themselves rather through aphorisms, examples, parables and paradoxical anecdotes.[4]

NON-ACTING AND THE WAY

A recurring motif in traditional Chinese wisdom is *wuwei* (无为), which means 'non-acting' or 'non-doing'.[5] This term dates back to the Analects of

---

[3] Maurizio Scarpari, in A. C. Graham, 1999, p. XX. The linguist and philolopist A. C. Graham has translated and reconstructed ancient Chinese texts of great value, and his work *'Disputers of Tao: Philosophical Argument in Ancient China'* (1989) is recognised as one of the most accurate and complete texts on the history of classical Chinese thought.

[4] See also H. Fingarette, 1972, who argues that the language of classical Chinese is performative rather than descriptive: the pronunciation of the word is the actual act, just like the 'guilty' of the judge or the 'yes' in a wedding. These words do not describe or evoke an action; they are the action itself.

[5] *Wu* 无 is a negative particle; *wei* 为, represented by a pictogram of an elephant conducted by a hand, means: 1. 'do, accomplish', 2. 'act, serve as', 3. 'be, become', 4. 'govern' (Wieger 1915, p. 49h; Karlgren 1940, p. 1313).

Confucius and finds full development in the Daoist texts *Laozi* and *Zhuangzi*, which express themselves as follows: 'The ancients who cultivated the *dao* nourished their understanding with stillness, understanding being born they did not use it to do (*wei*), and this is called 'nourishing understanding with stillness'[6] and '*Wei* indicates the ordinary and deliberate action of the man who pursues a goal, in contrast to the spontaneous processes of nature that are as they are.'[7]

In fact, *wuwei* is an idea that is tied to the pair of concepts *dao* (道) 'way' and *de* (德) 'power', in which real power manifests itself without the strain of having to act but rather coincides with the natural unfolding of things. Strictly speaking, *de* indicates power in the sense of the possession of specific properties and intrinsic strengths, such that one is able to express one's own nature in a spontaneous way. This pertains to both people and things: the classic Confucian *Liji* speaks of the *de* of wood, fire, earth, metal and water; in the Daoist text *Zhuangzi* it says that the preparation of a fighting cock is finished when its *de* is complete; the *de* of a person is the potential of acting in accordance with *dao*.[8]

This ability to act in accordance with *dao* also implies an external resonance: the possibility of drawing others to yourself through this power so that, for example, it is possible to govern without resorting to force and coercion. Rituals and ceremonies are in this sense ritualistic acts that operate by spreading influence; people with *de* possess an aptitude and natural abilities such that by adhering to *dao* they influence the surroundings and improve them even without acting/doing.

Dao, the Way, is the unfolding of *de*; it is made up of the flow of things in which each is brought to completion; in human endeavours it consists of actions that favour the maturation of both individuals and things in conformity with their respective natures.[9] The concept of *dao* has been used over time in various ways; it can indicate variously the correct course of human life, or

---

[6] *Zhuangzi*, Chapter 16. For the term 'knowledge' *zhi* see the discussion on *yi* and *zhi* (Chapter 3); here 'stillness' is the translation of *tian*, which means 'calmness, to be without worries' (other terms which are often used are *an* 安 'peace' and *jing* 静 'calm'). The 'Dialogues' or 'Selected quotes' (*Lunyu*) by Confucius are a 5th century BC selection of quotes and short stories from Confucius' and some of his disciples' lives. The two texts are named after two great Daoist masters. The *Zhuangzi* is made up of different parts, dating from the 4th to the 2nd century BC. The *Laozi* (also known as *Daodejing* or *Tao te Ching*, 'The book of the path and the virtue') appears around the 3rd century BC and is named after Laozi who we presume lived at the time of Confucius. According to Graham the two works are quite different in thought, the two names were not associated and the 'Daoist school' *daojia* is a later creation of the historian Sima Tan, who died in 110BC. (A. C. Graham, 1999, p. 231–2).
[7] A. C. Graham, 1999, p. 316.
[8] *Liji*, Chapter 6; *Zhuangzi*, Chapter 19. The term *de* 德, with its character containing the radical 'heart', 'footprints', 'correct', has often been translated as 'virtue', but in this case the term must be interpreted in its most literary sense of 'faculty, power'.
[9] The character *dao* 道 is composed of 'head' and 'to go' (Karlgren p. 978). For more information on the relation between the concept of *dao* and the psychoanalytic work as one who aims at knowing and developing its nature rather than giving specific indications see also the article by E. Rossi, 'Il corpo, la mente e noi' (The body, the mind, and ourselves), 1994.

the proper form of governance, or then again those things happening outside of the human sphere.[10]

Man coincides with *dao* – which omits nothing because it does not make choices – at the moment he stops making distinctions and follows the impulse of heaven. Desire and aversion derive from separation and classification, whereas the sage's way of acting stems from an impulse that is neither desire nor aversion. The sage does not make choices because there is only one way to act: when situations are perceived with perfect clarity there is only one possible answer. In this way, one follows spontaneously and at the same time acquiesces in the inevitable.[11]

In this context there is no dichotomy or contradiction between the concepts of spontaneous and inevitable: inevitable is not the opposite of 'freedom' (liberty), but rather refers to that universe to which, for example, the stroke of a painter or the pause in a melody belong, since they are the only possible/proper things in that moment.

This position is not only seen in the Daoist tradition:

> It seems in any case that Confucius did not normally give alternatives. According to him, you can follow the Way if you have sufficient vision to see it and enough strength to remain in it; otherwise all you do is fall out of it due to blindness and weakness (….) In particular, Confucius doesn't think in terms of choices between *ends*. He is not concerned about 'desires' (*yu* 欲) and especially not about 'intent'.[12]

Even for the first Confucians like Xunzi (3rd century AD), 'good' is what the sage prefers spontaneously, but you can arrive at this point only by 'transforming your own nature' – in other words by bringing order out of contrasting desires, which by nature are anarchic and bearers of internal and external conflicts. Through this transformation of (his) nature, the sage can reach and follow that which his heart desires; according to Xunzi, this ability of the sage produces morality, just as the vase is produced by the potter starting from the clay.

WITHOUT MEMORY OR DESIRE

To develop *de* and conform to *dao* one has to remain free (open) in one's responses, move fluidly like water, be as still as a mirror and respond with

---

[10] See also Needham, 1982, p.73: 'The first Daoists, dealing as protoscientists with their 'natural magic' were extremely practical men. They always acted in a framework of thought which considered the *dao* as essentially imminent, as the actual Order of Nature.'

[11] Spontaneity is the translation of *ziran* 自 È , which literally means 'as it is in itself'; 'inevitable' is the translation of 不得 已 *bu de yi*, literally 'not possible in any other way'. 'To choose is to exclude', in *Zhuangzi*, Chapter 33.

[12] A. C. Graham, 1999, p. 28. Graham's text specifies that 'intent' in this case is the translation of 志 *zhi*, which is close to *zhi* 'to go', with the addition of the radical 'heart'.

immediacy, like an echo. This non-mediated response combines spontaneity and necessity; it is a way of acting that has the qualities of resonance, and it requires an empty heart. 'The heart, like a mirror, does not accompany the things that go, it does not welcome the things that arrive; it answers, but does not preserve.[13]

To avoid interference by that which is already stored (in the heart) with that which he is about to receive, the sage empties his heart through stillness. This emptiness not only allows the person to receive, but it is the stillness itself that initiates movement and significant actions: 'In stillness there is emptiness, emptiness then is filled, what fills it finds its place by itself, emptying itself it is tranquil, stillness then moves, when it moves it is efficient.'[14]

Even a medical text like the *Neijing* starts by expressing this same basic concept: 'If one is calm, serene, empty-*xi*, and without-*wu*, true *qi* follows. If *jing* and *shen* are protected inside, from where can illnesses come?' If *zhi* is idle and there are few desires the heart is at peace and there is no fear.'[15]

The text recognises that 'in man, worry and anguish, thoughts and apprehensions injure the heart', nevertheless, it is also aware that common reality is different from a desirable but mythical state of consonance (harmony) with nature. It explicitly identifies the presence of internal worries and bodily suffering and specifies that in illnesses it is necessary to use needles and medicines, because those words and gestures that act directly on altering *qi* and *jing* do not possess sufficient healing powers. To the Yellow Emperor's question:

> I would like to ask why in olden times to treat diseases it was possible to transform the essence-*jing* and change the *qi* with spells and the people were healed, but instead, today to treat disease one treats the interior with poisonous medicines and treats the exterior with needles, and sometimes the patients are healed and sometimes the patients are not healed. How is this possible?

Qi Bo responds:

> In ancient times man lived among birds and wild animals, he moved around to defend himself from the cold, he stayed inside in order to avoid the summer

---

[13] *Zhuangzi*, Chapter 7. The references to water, mirror and echo can be found in Chapter 33 dedicated to the schools of thought, in which we find a quote from the Bodhisattva Avalokitesvara Guan Yin.

[14] *Zhuangzi*, Chapter 13. In the first chapter of the most known version of the *Daodejing* it is said that one must not constantly have desires and at the same time that one must constantly have desires (through these two modes one sees two different realities). Bion maintains that in front of a patient the psychoanalyst must be 'without memory and desire'. This because 'The patient can feel that the psychoanalyst has not deliberately undressed his memory and desire and can consequently feel dominated by the state of mind of the psychoanalyst, or rather by the state of mind represented by the term "desire" and therefore feel represented in it'. In *Attenzione e interpretazione*, 1973, p. 59. See also the discussion on empathy and abstention in Chapter 15.

[15] *Suwen*, Chapter 1. For a discussion on the term *zhi* 志 (1. 'will', 2. 'mind', 3. 'emotion', 4. 'memory') see Chapter 3. The relationship between emotions and illness is examined in Chapter 4. 'Idleness' is the translation of *xian* 閑, with its ancient character showing a door through which we can see the moon, it means 'idle, unoccupied, unutilised, free time' (Karlgren 609, 571), close to our term 're-creation'.

heat, he did not have an accumulation of profuse complications internally, and externally he did not have to make a career as a functionary, it was a simple world and pathogens could not penetrate internally, therefore the interior was not treated with poisonous medicines, the exterior was not treated with needles, but one was healed by the spells to move *jing* and transform *qi*. Modern man, however, is different; worries dwell inside of him, bodily suffering damages him on the exterior, he has lost the adaptation to the seasons, he goes against the proper principles of cold and heat, malevolent winds penetrate in abundance, empty and perverse penetrate the bones and the five organs in the interior, on the outside they damage the orifices and the skin, therefore light diseases become serious and important diseases cause death, and spells cannot remedy them.[16]

The indication to conform to the *dao* remains in any case fundamental to the answer to Huang Di's question about the methods of resolving illness with acupuncture, since man is 'born from the *qi* of heaven and earth, that which is most precious among all that exists between the heaven which covers and the earth which supports', 'kings, princes, and common men, all desire to remain healthy, while diseases continue to worsen and internally there is worry'. Qi Bo, in fact, responds by affirming that, although specific knowledge of acupuncture is obviously necessary, the nucleus of knowledge and action are *dao* and the regulation of *shen*:

> ... the five elements and reciprocal control-*ke,* the five attentions in performing acupuncture, disperse fullness and tonify emptiness, this everyone knows, but he who conforms to the laws of heaven and earth moves in response-*ying*, harmonises like an echo, follows like a shadow; the *dao* has neither demons nor ghosts, it comes and goes autonomously. ... Then I desire to know what is this *dao*. ... For those who needle, the real needling-*zhen* is first of all to regulate the *shen*. There are five requisites for a good acupuncturist, though many ignore them, The first is to regulate the *shen*, the second is to know how to nourish life, the third is to know the properties of the substances, the fourth is to know how to prepare stone points of various dimensions, the fifth is to know the diagnosis of organs, blood and *qi*.[17]

---

[16] *Suwen*, Chapters 73 and 13. 'Spells' is the translation of *zhuyou* 祝 由. The *zhu* were men who possessed the art of prediction, diviners, those who could communicate with the heavens, and the *shen*. The ideogram, which today means 'to wish', also contains the character 'mouth' and 'man' following the radical *shen* (Karlgren p. 163). According to the *Shuowen*, the etymological dictionary of the Han period, the *zhu* were similar to the *wu*, 'shamans', whose ancient pictogram shows a dancing person holding some feathers (Needham, 1982, vol. 1, p. 107) while the modern character shows two people, the radical 'work' and, according to Wieger, indicates two magicians dancing to obtain the rain (Wieger p. 27e, Karlgren p. 1282).

[17] *Suwen*, Chapter 25. The terms used are those of the philosophical texts from the 3rd century BC, in which we first find the words *gan* 感 'waken, stimulate' and *ying* 应 'reaction, immediate response' to indicate that sort of action which occurs without meditation, like an immediate resonance, an echo. It is likely that the allusion to the *dao* was more of a thought on how the study of natural laws had surpassed the more ancient shamanic medicine rather than a reference to *guishen* 鬼神 spirits and ghosts.

INTERNAL PRACTICES

This knowledge of how to 'nourish life', or *yangsheng* (养 生), refers to certain meditative or internal practices found throughout Chinese cultural history that are tightly interwoven with any discussion of emotions, from their role as a cause of illness to their pathological manifestations and their cure. Even a minimally accurate review, however, is beyond the scope of these notes, which are limited to a brief excursion into the tradition of *yangsheng* practice.[18]

Yangsheng, or 'nourishment of life', is a term used both in the classics and in modern language. It is interesting to note that in the non-simplified form of the *yang* ideogram the character for 'food' is present, suggesting the idea of substance (*yang* is the same term used in 'nourishing *yin*') and the ancient pictogram for *sheng* represents a growing plant.[19] In phrases referring to the cultivation or the maintenance of nature/life one sometimes finds the character *xing* (性) 'nature' used instead of *sheng* (生), from which it differs only in the addition of the 'heart' radical. However, we should also remember that the word 'nature' comes from the Latin *nascor* 'to be born'.

These practices of cultivating life are an integral part of the worldview and teachings of all Chinese masters, quite apart from specific philosophical traditions. We have already underlined how the mechanism leading to understanding, and the pathway through which the process of resonance influences the exterior, is one of internal experiences that enable the person to hear and respond with immediacy, rather than rational debate.

The most ancient historical documents already show the development of internal practices with the aim of stabilising the heart through *de*, so that the emotions would not disturb the *shen* and the *qi* can correspond with *dao*. In *Guanzi*, probably the most ancient 'mystical' text, we read:

> The heart is calm on the inside, the eyes are limpid, the ears clear, the four limbs are stable and strong, then *jing* has a residence. [...] *Shen* in man comes and goes, no one can imagine it, if one loses it there is disorder, if one grasps it there is order.
>
> Caring for the residence with attention causes the *jing* to arrive. [...] Worry or sadness, euphoria or anger, the *dao* has nowhere to reside, one must tranquillise love and desire, rectify recklessness and disorder. Do not pull or push, good luck comes by itself, the *dao* comes by itself, to favour and direct. In stillness, one can grasp it, in agitation, one loses it, the *shen* of the heart comes

---

[18] A comprehensive overview of *yangsheng* practices can be found in the selection of articles edited by L. Kohn, *Taoist Meditation and Longevity Techniques*, Center for Chinese Studies: University of Michigan, 1989. There are important reference texts by Maspero, 1971; Despeaux, 1979; Robinet, 1993; Pregadio, 1987; Esposito, 1997.

[19] The different meanings of the character *yang* 养 are: 1. 'nourish, increase', 2. 'maintain, care for', 3. 'give birth', 4. 'form, cultivate', 5. 'rest, recover' (Karlgren p. 211); those of the character *sheng* 生 are: 1. 'give birth', 2. 'originate', 3. 'grow something', 4. 'exist', 5. 'live, liveliness', 6. 'student', 7. 'alive', 8. 'immature', 9. 'raw', 10. 'unrefined', 11. 'strange' (Wieger p. 79f, Karlgren p. 874).

and goes, so small that it has nothing smaller inside, so big that there is nothing bigger outside of it. Stricken by nervousness we lose it, if the heart is calm there is *dao*.[20]

An inscription on jade that dates from the period of the Warring States (BC 475–221) speaks explicitly of breathing and internal circulation of *qi*:

> Make *qi* flow deeply, it will then accumulate, if it accumulates it will expand, if it expands it will sink, if it sinks it will settle, if it settles it will consolidate, if it consolidates it will germinate, if it germinates it will grow, if it grows it will return, if it returns it will reunite with heaven. If heaven is above, the earth is below; if you follow this you will live, if you go against this, you will die.[21]

'Deep breathing' possesses qualities that surpass the normal pulmonary functions: *Zhuangzi* speaks of 'breath that comes from the heels, while normal men breath from the throat' and 'inhale and exhale, expel the old and introduce the new, contract yourself like a bear and extend yourself like a bird, all this prolongs life.'[22]

These *yangsheng* practices emerge from a culture that is focused on personal development, even though they are discussed in Mencius as a method of serving heaven and the meditative techniques described in *Guanzi* also fulfil a social function: 'the cultivation of breathing and the imitation of the movements of birds and animals in the *Zhuangzi* are part of conforming oneself to the universal way without reference to a moral or social loom'.[23]

MEDICAL TRADITION

Daoyin (导 引) practices were used by the various Daoist, Buddhist, Confucian and martial schools, but they were also an integral part of the medical art.[24] They consist of techniques to conduct *qi* internally or of exercises aimed at eliminating pathogens and unblocking emotions.

Medical texts on silk and bamboo tablets were found in the Zhangjiashan and Mawangdui tombs from the Han period (but preceding the *Neijing*) describ-

---

[20] *Guanzi*, Chapter 2. The *Guanzi* is a collection of texts of which the most ancient is the chapter on the 'Inner discipline' (4th century BC).

[21] Here we can already find the basic concepts on which the internal practices work: accumulate-*chu* 储, stabilise-*ding* 定, consolidate-*gu* 固, lower-*xia* 下 , and go back-*tui* 退 to rejoin the anterior heaven.

[22] *Zhuangzi*, Chapter 6.

[23] On this subject see the work of Vivienne Lo, 'The Influence of Western Han *Nurturing Life* Literature on the Development of Acumoxa Therapy', presented at the Needham Research Institute conference in March 1995. It also offers a deep examination of the origin and development of the term *yangsheng*.

[24] *Daoyin* is a term used by Daoists. *Dao* is composed by *dao* 'path' and the radical 'hand' and it means 'to conduct, guide, transmit, direct' (Karlgren p. 978). *Yin* is formed by *gong* 'bow' and a line representing the string, which means 'to pull, guide, conduct' (Wieger p. 87a, Karlgren p. 271).

ing breathing and *qi* enhancement and circulation exercises together with 44 drawings of movements with men and women of various ages.[25]

The 'five animal game', or *wuqin zhiuxi*, is attributed to the figure of Hua Tuo, a doctor of the 2nd century AD who was famous both for his knowledge of acupuncture (from which the name of the paravertebral points *huatuojiaji*) and for his surgical skills and the use of the first anaesthetics. In his biography, Hua Tuo introduces this exercise explaining that 'the body needs moderate movements: moving and balancing it to the right and to the left, the *qi* of food will be distributed, the blood will circulate well, illnesses cannot be generated, the body becomes like the hinges of a door that never rust. Therefore the ancient sages practised the movements of *daoyin*: move the head like a bear, look behind you without turning the neck'.[26] This exercise of the five animals has been continuously revisited over time by the various traditions and, even today, masters will include their own version in their practice.[27]

The 'king of medicine' Sun Simiao concerned himself deeply with these arts, which he defined as *yangxing* (养 性), ('nourishing nature') and to which he dedicated a section of his principal text.[28] Profoundly influenced by the Daoist doctors Ge Hong and Tao Hongjing, experts in pharmacy and alchemical research, Sun Simiao used the internal techniques for producing and conducting *qi* to heal sickness: 'Lightly close your eyes and concentrate on internal vision, make your heart produce fire, think of the place where you are sick and then attack it with this fire. In this way the illness is cured.'[29]

The reader is directed to the end of this chapter for the various schools and principal works regarding *yangsheng*, meditative practices, *daoyin*, internal alchemy, etc.[30]

---

[25] In Mawangdui's tomb dating to 168 BC some medical texts were found. They had been written between the 3rd and 2nd century but the contents are much more ancient (for a discussion on this topic see also Giulia Boschi, 1997, p. 62–70).

[26] *Sanguozhi* ('Stories of the three reigns'), Chapter 29, Qiu Peiran (ed), *Zhongguo yixue dacheng*, Yueli shushe, Shanghai, 1994.

[27] For example the text *Ancient Way to Keep Fit*, published in China in 1990, shows the three versions: the first from the text of the Song period (960–1279) *Yunji qiqian*; the second from a copy on brocade owned by the Shen Shou family (prov. Zhejiang) since the 10th century; and the third from the *Yimen guangdu* encyclopaedia composed by the Daoist Zhou Lujing in the 17th century.

[28] Sun Simiao, *Qianjin yaofang* ('Remedies worth a thousand golden pieces for emergencies', 625). This section is Book 27, *Yangxing*, made up of various chapters among which are: *'Daolin yangxing'* ('Nourishing nature for Daoists'), *'Juchufa'* ('Rules for living'), *'Anmofa'* ('Methods for massage', which describes some still used methods for self-massage), *'Tiaoqifa'* ('Methods for regulating the *qi'*, presenting various exercises including the 'six sounds'), and *'Fangzhong buyi'*, ('Tonification in the bedroom', that is sexual techniques).

[29] Quoted in *Daoshu*. Ge Hong, 281–341, wrote the text *Baopuzi* ('The master who embraces simplicity') and Tao Hongjing, 452–536, wrote the *Yangxing yanminglu* ('Nourishing nature and lengthening life'), in which we read: 'If one wants to eliminate illnesses by letting the *qi* flow, he must concentrate on the place where the illnesses shows: if there is head ache on the head, if there is foot ache on the foot, harmonise the *qi* to attack the illness'.

[30] Respectively: *daoyin* 导 引, *yunqi* 运 气, *tuna* 吐 纳, *jingzuo* 静 坐 (in the Daoist tradition) or *zuochuan* 坐 禅 (in the Buddhist tradition). *Gong* implies a deliberate and constant effort. It can be translated as: 1. 'ability', 2. 'result', 3. 'effort' (Karlgren p. 469). I sincerely thank master Li Xiaoming, for the introduction in Italy of a *qigong* practice at high level and I am grateful to him for his teachings in Milano in March 1990.

QIGONG

Today we term the above group of internal practices *qigong* (气 功), a name that groups together exercises that in different regions and periods had various names such as 'conducting', 'circulating *qi*', 'inhaling and exhaling', 'sitting in stillness', etc. *Qigong* is therefore an expression of recent origin, translatable as 'qi practices', in which the character *gong* is composed of the radicals for 'work'-*gong* and 'power'-*li*.

The first institute of *qigong* was founded at Tangshan (Hebei province) in 1955, where clinical activities were carried out together with a therapeutic evaluation study. During the Cultural Revolution *qigong* practice was considered an expression of abasing spiritualism and was discouraged and even prohibited. Those who already practised it, however, often continued to do so, for example 'during the long assemblies, standing still, practising internal *qigong*'.[31]

At the end of the 1970s its therapeutic value was recognised anew and it is once more used in public hospitals and in clinics the emission of *qi* is studied, in particular to evaluate the effect on the immune system, using biomedical methods and instruments.[32]

In general it is said that practising *qigong* regulates movement, breathing and the mind; however, there are many types. It is possible, for example, to find practices of *qi* nourishment and guidance, which are more internal, external exercises in which greater attention is given to muscular and joint work, and exercises for the elimination of pathogens. *Qi* may furthermore be directed on to another person for therapeutic goals. The exercises, which can be either static or moving, may utilise the emission of sounds, visualisations, silent recitations, self-massage, static postures or specific types of stepping.

Qigong has many functions – to circulate *qi*, enrich pure *qi* and expel impure *qi*, reinforce the internal organs and to harmonise man with the universe. These generally involve nourishing the *dantian* (丹 田): '*Dantian* is an area where true *qi* accumulates and is preserved: 'Concentrate the mind on the *dantian*' generally refers to the lower *dantian* – the starting point of the circulation of *qi* in the *Ren, Du* and *Chong Mai*, the cardinal point of the rising, descending, opening and closing of true *qi*, the progenitor of life, the root of the five organs and the six bowels, the origin of the twelve meridians, the reunion of *yin* and *yang*, the door of breathing, the place of the reunion of fire and water, and also

---

[31] From a story by Lu Guanjun (director of the *qigong* and tuina department in the Guanganmen hospital in Beijing, with whom we have worked in August–September 1992) who remembered how, at the time of the 'Great Leap Forward', during the famine at the beginning of the 1950s, *qigong* was diffused to help bear the hunger.

[32] A good overview of the state of research on the effects of the emission of the *qi waiqi* 外气 can be found in Boschi, 1997, Chapter 12.

the place in which the reproductive essence of man is preserved and where women nourish the fetus.'[33]

The practices of regulation, conservation and guidance of *qi* have an intrinsic overall therapeutic value, but exercises can also be selected according to the type of imbalance present so as to focus on specific therapeutic interventions.

The work of accumulation, guidance and transformation of one's own *qi* belongs to the internal alchemical techniques of *neidan* (内丹) from the Daoist tradition; the best known exercises used in this sense are the small and large heavenly circulations, *Xiao/Da Zhoutian* (小/大周天), in which *qi* is conducted to the extremities and to the surface (to the body hairs-*maofa*), or only along the midline *Ren* and *Du* channels respectively.[34]

The Buddhist masters recognise as priorities the elements of stability-*ding* 定, stillness-*jing* 静, emptiness-*xu* 虚; and spirit-*ling* 灵; in order to not be at the mercy of the emotions, one must be stable and still, in such a way that the heart is empty and one can reach the spirit.[35] In fact, the cultivation of a basic attitude that permits one to maintain a distance from that which destabilises the heart remains fundamentally important, as we read in Li Dongyuan, who dedicates the three final chapters of *Piweilun* to this: 'Be tranquil in neutrality, look little, diminish desires, speak little, save words, all this to nourish *qi*, don't tire yourself inconsiderately in order to nourish form, empty the heart to protect the *shen*, conciliate with numbers the length of life, profits and losses.'[36]

PRINCIPAL TEXTS ON THE PRACTICES OF MEDITATION, NOURISHMENT OF LIFE, AND INTERNAL ALCHEMY

Taking into account that the output of texts on this subject is practically as extensive as the literature on acupuncture and herbs, we will note here

---

[33] *Chinese qigong*, 1988, p.33. On the localisation of the *dantian* see Chapter 13. A very interesting study on the female traditions can be found in C. Despeaux, 'Le immortali dell'Antica Cina' ('The immortals of Ancient China'), 1991.

[34] Along the path there are three areas of very difficult passage: 'On the back there are three passages (*sanguan*): *weilu, jiaji, yuzhen*', which are usually referred respectively to the area of the perineum or coccyx, to the backbone particularly at the level of T7 *Zhiyang* Du-9 or of L2 *Mingmen* Du-4, and to the occipital level corresponding with *Yuzhen* BL-9. Quoted in: Zhao Taichang, *Dacheng jieyao* ('Great compendium of the highest results').

[35] From the *qigong* master Liu Dong, who adds: 'When the heart is empty it is not us who practise the *qigong*, but it is the *qigong* that practises us: something can arrive from the outside only if we are ready on the inside, cleaned from the poisons that cloud the Buddha within us'. (Seminar in January 2001, MediCina, Milano). For a discussion on the term *ling* see Chapter 3.

[36] Li Dongyuan, *Piweilun* ('Treatise on spleen and stomach', 1249), Chapter 'Yuanyu'. The term 'neutral' is the translation of *danbo* 淡泊, also 'bland, tasteless' and 'thin'; 'the numbers' means the natural rules. And closely: 'love and hate do not influence emotions-*qing*, anguish and thoughts do not stay in the *yi*, if one is peaceful and with no anxieties the body and the *qi* are in harmony and in peace, so that the shape and the *shen* are one and the outside and inside communicate'. In: Wang Huaiyin (ed.), *Taiping shenghui fang* ('Wise prescriptions from the Taiping period', 992). For a discussion on the term *yi* 意 (1. 'idea, meaning', 2. 'desire, intention', 4. 'to think, expect', 5. 'attention') see Chapter 3.

only the principle works. We use the classification generally used by Chinese commentaries in presenting works.[37]

Most Ancient Works

Yijing (also called *Zhouyi*, 'The book of changes').
Laozi (also called *Daodejing*, 'The book of the way and its virtue').
Zhuangzi (it takes its name from the Daoist master).
Baopuzi ('The master who embraces simplicity'), by Ge Hong (281–341)
Heguanzi ('The master with the pheasant-feathered cap'), which goes back to
    the 2nd–3rd century BC in its most ancient parts, while the modern form is
    datable to the 3rd or 4th century AD.

Most Ancient Medical Texts

Suwen ('Essential questions'), in particular Chapters 1, 2, 5, 8, 41, 60.
Lingshu ('Spiritual pivot'), in particular Chapters 8, 10, 11, 17.
Yangxing yanminglu ('Recordings of the art of health and life preservation'), by
    Tao Hongjing (452–536).
Qianjin yaofang ('Thousand golden pieces', 625), by Sun Simiao.

Nei Guan (Internal Vision)

During the Tang Dynasty (618–906) a tendency to mysticism developed in Daoism; Buddhist elements were introduced, but translated in such a way that the contemplation of the divinity of the body seen as a microcosm was central. The works were inspired by the *Neiguanjing* ('Classic of contemplation/internal vision'), a brief treatise of unknown dating.

The principal texts are by Sima Chengzen, patriarch of the Shang Qing ('Supreme purity') Daoist school, which appeared at the end of the 4th century, including *Zuowanglun* ('Treatise on sitting and forgetting'); *Tianyinzi yangshengshu* ('The art of *yangshen* by Tianyinzi') and *Fuqi jingyilun* ('Treatise on the essential meaning of absorbing *qi*').

There are also later works, for example from the Qing Dynasty is *Dacheng jieyao* ('Essence of great results') by Zhao Taiching.

Daoyin

Mawangdui Daoyintu ('Illustrations of Daoyin in the Mawangdui tombs', Western Han Dynasty period, 202BC–AD24), but also containing previous material.

Taiqing Daoyin Yangshengjing ('Daoyin classic of great purity for nourishing life'), by unknown author, who gathered various ancient texts on *daoyin* and had a major influence on later periods.

Wuqinxi ('The five animals game'), attributed to Hua Tao (Eastern Han Dynasty period, 24–220).

Yijinjing ('Classic on transforming the tendons'), originally by Da Mo (Northern Wei Dynasty period, 368–534).

Laozi Anmofa ('Massage methods of Laozi'), by Sun Simiao.

Tianlanguo Anmofa ('Massage methods of the heavenly reign'), by Sun Simiao.

Yangshengfang Daoyinfa ('Prescriptions for nourishing life and *daoyin* methods'), by Chao Yuanfang (found in the *Zhubing Yuanhoulun*, 610). This text refers to another lost work, *Yangshengjing* ('Classic for nourishing life'), also referred to by Sun Simiao and later by Wang Shou in *Waitai Miyao*. The application of *daoyin* exercises in the medical field for the treatment of various pathologies is mentioned.

Chifengsui ('Marrow of the red phoenix', 1578), by Zhou Lujing.

Zunshen Bajian ('Eight explanations for harmonising life', 1591), by Gao Lian, a general work that contains indications on various aspects of life: exercise, diet, habits, hobbies. It is also famous in foreign countries thanks to J. Dudgeon's translation in 1895.

Cheng Xiyi Ershisiqi Daoyin Zuogong Tushi ('Illustrations by Cheng Xiyi on sitting *daoyin* for the twelve months'), by Gao Lian.

Tuna (Breathing) and *Taixi* (Fetal Breathing)

Youzhen Xiansheng Funei Yuanqijie ('Rhyming formula by the man of infantile genuineness for absorbing internal *yuanqi*'), by Youzhen Xiansheng (Tang Dynasty period, AD618–906).

Taixijing ('Classic on fetal breathing'), by Youzhen Xiansheng (Tang Dynasty period, AD618–906).

Yunji Qiqian ('Seven notes of the house of the books of the cloud', 1028), by Zhang Junfang.

Nei Dan (Internal Alchemy)

Zhouyi Cantongqi ('Pledge for the union of the three in relation to the *Yijing*'), by Wei Boyang (1st century AD, referred to in the Tang Dynasty period, 618–906); together with *Wuzhen Pian* this is the most ancient and influential text on internal alchemy.

Jinbi Guwen Longhujing ('Classic of the dragon and the tiger'), by Zhang Boyuan (?–1082).

Wuzhen Pian ('Awareness and genuineness'), by Zhang Boyuan (?–1082).

Lingbao Bifa (Secret procedures of the magic jewel'), 11th century, attributed to Zhongli Quan.

Xuanyao Pian, Wugen Shu, Xuanji Zhijiang, by Zhang Sanfeng (Yuan Dynasty period, 1279–1368).

Bueryuan Junfayu, by Jun Buer (Jin Dynasty period, 215–420).

Guizhong Zhinan, by Chen Zhongsu (Yuan Dynasty period, 1279–1368).

Xingming Guizhi, by unknown author (Ming Dynasty period, 1368–1644).

Xiuling Yaozhi, ('Essential principles for cultivating age', 1442) by Ling Jian.

Shoushi Baoyuan ('Reaching longevity by preserving the source', 1615), by Gong Tingxian.

Tianxian Zhenli Zhilun ('Treatise on the correct principles of the heavenly saints') and *Xianfo Hezong Yulu* ('General notes on the Daoist and Buddhist saints'), by Wu Shouyang (Ming Dynasty period, 1368–1644).

Jinxian Zhenglu ('Treatise on the trials of the golden saints'), by Li Huayang (Qing Dynasty period, 1644–1911).

Shenshi Bafa, by Liu Yiming (Qing Dynasty period, 1644–1911).

Emotions and the Movement of *Qi*

2

Chinese medical tradition identifies only a limited number of emotions as fundamental. However, the simplicity of this perspective does not imply a reductive simplification of the psychic/psychological universe compared with the refined analysis of sentiments that is often considered the prerogative of Western culture. The Chinese model consists, rather, of recognising the essential by attributing the various emotional manifestations to their roots. The five emotions are therefore equivalent to a sort of concentrate of emotional movements, in which the infinite range of sentiments and dynamic relations are distilled and condensed into the 'nuclei' of the primary emotions.

The essential point is that anger, euphoria, thought, sadness and fear correspond to internal movements and constitute primary movements of *qi*. The various sentiments, such as love, hate, envy, affection, nostalgia, jealousy, liking, compassion, attachment, aggressiveness, shame, fault, dependence, regret, generosity, avarice, worry, inadequacy, etc., concern relations with the exterior world, but the root from which they develop identifies with internal movements of *qi*.

TERMINOLOGY

In both classical and modern Chinese medical language, emotional, affective and in a broader sense psychic aspects are referred to by the term 'emotions'. One speaks of *qingzhi jibing* (情 志 疾 病), illness of/from emotions, in which *qingzhi* is an abbreviation of *qiqing wuzhi* (七情五志) – a term originating from the classics, which speak both of *qingzhi* and of *wuzhi*, often translated as the 'seven passions' and the 'five emotions' respectively. The reader is referred to the end of the chapter for an in depth discussion of the separate emotions, but we note here that *qi* means 'seven', the character *qing* is very similar to *jing* 'essence', *wu* signifies 'five', and *zhi* is the same term used to define the psychic aspect 'willpower' of the kidney.[1]

---

[1] *Jing* (精), 'essence' has the same phonetic part as *qing* (情), but the radical 'rice' in place of 'heart' (Karlgren p. 1085). See the notes on terminology in the Introduction; for a discussion on *zhi* 志 see Chapter 3.

Although there are some variations on the theme, the same principles are already seen in texts from the 'pre-Han period', which precede the compilation of the classic medical texts such as the *Neijing*.

Liji, the Confucian classic on rituals, which presumably dates to before the 4th century AD, discusses *qing*, emotions, which are defined as innate, within which one recognises the grand poles of desire and aversion.[2]

The concept of the five elements (*wuxing*) had already appeared in the *Zuozhuan*, but without reference to the emotions, which are called the six *zhi* and presume the existence of an attraction–aversion pair from which euphoria and joy, anger and sorrow originate.[3] These same emotions appear in the *Xunzi*, but there are called the six *qing*.[4]

The concept of attraction–aversion appears throughout history and is found again in the 'Treatise on causes and symptoms of diseases' – in which we find the definition of the internal causes of disease as emotions and which specifies how 'the internal causes that can produce illness pertain only to the interweaving of the seven emotions, to the conflict between love-*ai* and aversion-*wu*'.[5]

The *Neijing* always defines them as *zhi* and links them to the five *zang* organs. The five emotions euphoria-*xi* 喜, anger-*nu* 怒, thought-*si* 思, sadness-*bei* 悲 and fear-*kong* 恐 were afterwards maintained as fundamentals of Chinese medical tradition.[6]

The denomination of seven emotions, *qiqing*, adds anguish-*you* 忧 and fright-*jing* 惊. However, in the medical tradition this goes back only to the 'Treatise on causes and symptoms of diseases' of 1174.

---

[2] 'What is meant by passions-*qing* in man? Euphoria-*xi*, anger-*nu*, sorrow-*ai*, apprehension-*ju*, love-*ai*, aversion-*wu*, desire-*yu*: man is capable of these without learning them. Drinks, food, man, woman, the great desires are stored in them; death, poverty, suffering are the great aversions, therefore desire and aversion are the two great extremes of the heart'. In: Liji ('Memories of the rituals'), Chapter 7. For a discussion on terminology regarding emotions, see the introduction.

[3] 'In man there are attractions-*hao* (好) and aversions-*wu* (恶), euphoria, anger, sorrow, joy, which originate from the six *qi* [which in this text are *yin* and *yang*, wind and rain, darkness and light]. And these are the six *zhi*. [...] joy originates from attraction, anger from aversion [...] Attraction for things produces joy-*le*, aversion to things produces anguish-*you*'. In: *Zouzhuan*, 'Zhaogong Ershiwu nian' chapter. The *Zouzhuan*, a philosophical encyclopaedia compiled around 240BC, is part of *Lüshi Chunqiu* ('Annals of the Spring and Autumn by Master Lu'). Over 45 descriptions of illnesses appear in it, among which the most ancient is a diagnosis of a Jin prince in 580BC, and the discussion found there by Doctor He on the fundamental principles of medicine dated around 540BC is highly interesting.

[4] *Xunzi*, Chapter 22. The text takes its name from Xunzi, one of the principal exponents of early Confucianism who lived in the 3rd century BC and to whom we owe numerous quotes from the Master which do not appear in the 'Dialogs'. The *Baihu Tongyi* ('General Principles of the White Tiger') also defines the same emotions *liujing*, with the simple substitution of the term love-*ai* in place of *hao*.

[5] Chen Wuzi, *Sanyin Jiyi Bingzheng Fanglun* ('Tractate on the Three Categories of Causes of Disease', 1174).

[6] Certain passages however, present variations, for example, in Chapter 5 and in a passage of Chapter 67 we find *you* in place of *bei*; Chapter 23 attributes *wei* (畏) to the spleen ('apprehension, trepidation, respect') and *you* to the liver; Chapter 39 also adds fright-*jing*.

EMOTIONS AND CLASSICAL THOUGHT

The history of classic philosophical thought, which attributes a profound role to interior experience and the immediacy of feelings in the search for wisdom, is deeply traversed by reflections on emotions. As we have seen, according to Chinese thought any agitation of the heart prevents one from being able to act in accordance with the *dao*.

More prosaically, if nothing else, we can all agree that in general our state of wellbeing or discomfort is bound up with changing emotional states. We know that movement is intrinsic to *qi* – the *qi* of the universe, just as in the *qi* of humans. We know too that the *qi* of humans is also feelings and emotions. Furthermore, we also know that the heart of man – our interior world – is related to heaven, with that which occurs outside of us: 'the *yi* of the heart of man responds to the eight winds, the *qi* of man responds to heaven'.[7]

The term *qing* in the classical age meant that which is essential in something; in particular, the *qing* of man is that which he himself is, those essential qualities humans possess by which we can be called 'human' and which distinguish us from other creatures. The *qingyu*, the essential desires, are those without which we would not be human.[8]

The concepts of measure and control over the emotions are tied to the ability of distinguishing the essential desires. In the pre-Han text 'Annals of the Spring and Autumn' it is stated that desires come from heaven, that eyes, ears and mouth desire the five colours, the five notes and the five flavours, and that these are essential desires which are the same for nobles and the poor, for the knowledgeable and for the ignorant, owing to which 'the sage cultivates measures for controlling desires and therefore does not go beyond the essential when acting'.[9]

In Confucius we read 'When joy and rage, sorrow and happiness have not yet appeared, this is called the centre, when they have appeared but with measure, this is called harmony'.[10]

---

[7] *Suwen*, Chapter 54. 'Responds' is the translation of the character *ying* 应, a term often paired with *gan* (感) 'awaken, stimulate, influence', utilised in Daoist philosophical texts when referring to that immediate and spontaneous response which precedes thought, assimilated to a resonance or an echo. In this regard, also see the introduction to classical thought in Chapter 1.

[8] During the Classical Period, from 500 to 200BC, the period of major splendour in Chinese philosophy which saw the flowering of the Doctrine of the Hundred Schools (*baijia zhixue*), 'the concept of *qing* approaches the Aristotelian 'essence', but is none the less linked to denomination rather than being'. In: A. C. Graham, 1999, p. 130.

[9] *Lüshi Chunqiu*, 'Qingyu' chapter. As specified in the Introduction, we use a translation that strictly adheres to the original text leaving the task and pleasure of choosing a more adequate syntactical structure to the reader.

[10] *Zhongyong*, ('The correct centre'). This passage is recorded by the neo-Confucian Zhu Xi (1130–1200) in his commentary *Zhuzi Yulei* ('The sayings of Master Zhu by category'): 'Euphoria, anger, sorrow and joy are emotions-*qing* (情), when they have not yet been produced then it is nature-*xing*, they have no partiality and are therefore called the centre-*zhong* (中); when they have been produced with measure-*zhong* (中) and regulation-*jie* (节) this is called correctness-*zheng* (正) of emotions, meaning there is no overpowering of one by the other and it is therefore called harmony-*he* (和)'.

We have also seen how the Daoist sages consider it necessary to still desires so that the *dao* can take residence.

According to Graham, *qing* begins to be used in 'the Book of Rituals' and in *Xunzi* to indicate the elements of genuineness which are masked in man by rituals and morality, which assume the significance of 'passions' in the sense of 'hidden naturalness which is at the root and threatens to erupt through the civilised exterior'.[11] Desires, emotions, and passions all belong to the depths of our being and potentially hold great danger with respect to both the rules of society and the tranquillity of the heart.

The awareness that 'the seven emotions are the normal nature of man' and that 'the seven emotions which move with measure and regulation do not of themselves cause illness',[12] which we find in medical texts of later periods, is already clearly present in pre-Han literature. Emotions can become damaging – for example, 'if sorrow and joy are out of step, there will necessarily be negative consequences'. However, no emotions are useful or damaging in an absolute sense: 'there are no attractions or aversions that are good or damaging (in and of themselves); benefit and injury are in their adjustment'.[13]

The idea that emotions are elements of disturbance which can alter the state of balance of *qi*, injure the heart and the *shen*, becoming in the end true causes of illness, is certainly a concept that precedes the appearance of the first medical texts known to us, even though the description of the pathological processes aroused by the various sentiments does not always correspond exactly with the systemisation that took shape over time. In texts that precede the *Neijing*, we read, for example, that: 'With worry and apprehension the heart is fatigued and illnesses are produced', or that: 'Great euphoria, great anger, great anguish, great fear, great sorrow – if these five manage to take over the *shen* there will be injury', or furthermore that: 'Great anger breaks the *yin*, great euphoria strikes down the *yang*, great worry collapses the interior and great fright generates terror.'[14]

EMOTIONS AS CAUSES OF ILLNESS

The *Neijing* is the first text that analyses emotions as a cause of illness in a detailed way, examining the factors which can produce emotional alterations

---

[11] A.C. Graham, 1999, p. 336. See further on for a number of passages translated from Chapter 7 of the *Liji* and Chapter 22 of the *Xunzi*.

[12] Chen Wuzi, *Sanyin Jiyi Bingzheng Fanglun* ('Tractate on the three categories of causes of disease'). The term *zhongjie* is the same as that we have seen utilised by Confucius in the *Zhongyong*.

[13] *Zuozhuan*, Zhuanggong Ershinian chapter and *Mozi*, Jingxia chapter. The Moist commentary text *Mobian Fahui* underlines: 'we are speaking here of the fact that attraction and repulsion must be adequate because everyone has a heart with attractions and aversions, but only if they are adequate they are beneficial, if they lose their adequacy-*yi* (宜) then they are damaging; saying that attraction is beneficial and aversion is negative does not correspond to this principle'.

[14] Respectively in: *Zuozhuan*, Zhaogong Yuannian chapter; *Lüshi Chunqiu*; *Huainanzi*, Chuanyanxun chapter.

including socioeconomic factors, the quality and characteristic of aetiological processes, relations among the emotions and the individual differences in responses.[15] As with all stimuli, individuals of an emotional type also act in different ways according to the pre-existing energetic situation, therefore provoking different alterations in the state of *qi*.

Illness can occur if there is an internal deficiency or where the emotional stimuli are excessive in relation to the specific situation of the individual: 'Where *xie* strike, *qi* is empty; if *zhenqi* in the interior is stored, then the *xie* cannot attack.'[16] Concise while simultaneously richly informative, the *Neijing* recognises in this statement that: (1) illness is the product of interaction; (2) the response is individual; (3) the internal state of balance is decisive.

Illness can derive from an interaction with external pathogens of a more concrete nature, or from stimuli of a different type also defined as 'internal components' in our contemporary culture, which were already called 'internal causes' in classic Chinese nosography. The *Neijing* takes into consideration that we are profoundly influenced by feelings and fatigue; it also recognises the existence of individual differences – both innate and deriving from interaction with the environment – and therefore invites us to observe the patient attentively in order to understand the situation – in other words, to make a diagnosis. 'Huang Di asks: 'Is it true that [the *qi* in the] channels of man changes according to his habits in life, his activities, and his constitution?' Qi Bo responds, 'Fright, fear, anger, fatigue and rest can all influence changes. In strong people *qi* circulates and therefore illnesses are resolved [...] In weak people *qi* becomes stuck and the result is illness. Therefore the attentive observation of the constitutional tendencies of the patient, his strength or weakness, his bones, muscles, and skin, in order to understand his condition is a part of the ability to diagnose properly'.[17]

This passage is also extremely interesting because it connects the power of *qi* with its ability to maintain movement and interprets illness as a result of the stagnation of *qi*. A more detailed discussion of the pathologies due to constraint and stagnation will be approached later, but it is worthwhile to note here how a two thousand year old saying is still widespread in our times: 'Flowing water does not spoil and a door's hinges are not eaten by worms.'[18] Furthermore, the most ancient medical texts already illustrated exercises for maintaining health and the primary action of needling is moving *qi*.

---

[15] Please also see the discussion regarding the doctor-patient relationship and methods of investigation and diagnosis in reference to passages in the Neijing (Chapter 15).

[16] *Suwen*, Chapter 62. We remind the reader that in the *Neijing* all causes of illness are called *xie*, a term which later assumed the restricted meaning 'perverse energies' or 'external pathogens'. The term *xie* (邪) 'bad, irregular, deviant' counterpoises the term *zheng* (正) 'upstanding, correct, right', from which the modern translation of *zhengqi* as 'anti-pathogenic *qi*' derives. (Karlgren p. 791, Weiger p. 112i, Karlgren p. 1198).

[17] *Suwen*, Chapter 21.

[18] This saying appears in the *Lüshi Chunqiu*, Chapter 12 and is taken up by Sun Simiao in the 'Yangxing' section of the *Qianjin yaofang*. For a discussion on *yu*-constraint, please see Chapter 4.

To enjoy good health it is important to 'nourish life', to remain in a proper relationship with the macrocosm (the four seasons), to maintain flexibility in respect both to factors originating from the surroundings that do not depend on us (heat and cold) and also to internal emotional movements (happiness and anger), to be calm in everyday life, to have a balanced sexual life, and to continuously integrate the opposing and complementary aspects of life: 'The sage nourishes life, conforms to the four seasons and adapts to heat and cold, harmonises anger and happiness, remains serenely in one place, balances *yin* and *yang*, and regulates hard and soft. In this way, illness and perverse energies do not encroach and one lives a long life.'[19]

The enormous potential of internal attitudes, which can exhaust all resources, seriously injure nutritive and defensive *qi*, destroy the *shen*, and render acupuncture useless and healing impossible, is recognised: 'Desires without limits and worries without end consume *jing*, cause nutritive *qi* to congeal and defensive *qi* to be expelled; it is then that the *shen* departs and the disease is not curable.'[20]

Modern Chinese classifications of the causes of illness go back to the Song Dynasty and are divided into 'external causes', 'neither internal or external causes' and 'internal causes', which consist of the seven emotions, *qiqing*.[21] This nosography therefore proposes a complete coincidence between passions and the internal causes of disease, but the *Neijing* had already recognised emotions as a fundamental factor of pathologies: 'If happiness and anger are not regulated then they will injure the organs, when the organs are injured, the illness originates in the *yin*.'[22]

The text relates the origins of disease to *yang* (climatic causes) or to *yin* (diet, life style, emotions and sexual activity): 'the causes of disease can originate in the *yin* or the *yang*. Wind, cold, and summer heat originate in the *yang*. Diet, life style, euphoria and anger, *yin* and *yang* have origin in the *yin*.'[23]

None the less, the *Neijing* not only distinguishes between internal and external origins, but also recognises that the consequences of each are substantially different, attributing the possibility of directly attacking internal organs to internal factors, whereas injury deriving from external factors mainly regards

---

[19] *Lingshu*, Chapter 8. The term 'nourish life' *yangsheng* (养 生) refers to the internal practices discussed in Chapter 1; 'happiness and anger' is a typical metonymy which stands for all emotions; 'to balance *yin* and *yang*' can refer to sexual activity; 'hard and soft' are opposite and complimentary terms which allude to the trigrams of the *Yijing* (*I King*), in which the continuous and divided lines are defined as 'hard and soft'.

[20] *Suwen*, Chapter 14.

[21] Chen Wuze, *Sanyin Jiyi Bingzheng Fanglun* ('Tract on the three categories of causes of disease'). The 'external causes' are the *liuqi* (六 气), the six climatic *qi* (wind, cold, summer heat, dampness, dryness, fire), which become *liuyin* (六 淫), 'excessive, overflowing'; the 'neither internal or external causes' include excesses of mental, physical, and sexual activity, improper diet, trauma, parasites, poisons and improper treatment.

[22] *Lingshu*, Chapter 66.

[23] *Suwen*, Chapter 62. According to many commentators, 'yin–yang' refers to sexual activity.

the body and initiates from the external layers: 'Wind and cold injure the form; worry, fear and anger injure the *qi*.'[24]

EMOTIONS, MOVEMENT OF *QI* AND ORGANS

Chinese medicine views emotions as physiological events, a response of the *shen* to stimuli from the outside world. Emotions are movements of *qi*, each movement being characteristic, and the qualities of response of *qi* vary according to the emotion involved. In the case of an excessive emotional force there will be an alteration of the physiological movements of *qi* and therefore illness.

The two chapters in the *Neijing* in which the consequences of pathological emotions are described in detail state in similar terms that when anxiety and worry manage to injure the *shen* one has a continuous fear of everything, and loses all resources.

In particular, sadness consumes *qi* and life, euphoria disperses the *shen*, thought and anguish obstruct the flow of *qi*, anger leads to bewilderment and a loss of control, fear confuses and agitates the *shen*, descends *qi* and does not contain it.

The *Suwen* offers a very concise description: 'I know that all diseases originate from *qi*. Anger, then *qi* rises. Euphoria, *qi* is released. Sadness, *qi* dissolves. Fear, *qi* descends. Cold, *qi* contracts. Heat, *qi* overflows. Fright, *qi* becomes disordered. Fatigue, *qi* is exhausted. Thought, *qi* is knotted'.[25]

The images presented by the *Lingshu* are just as effective:

> So it is, sadness and sorrow, worry and anguish injure the *shen*, injured *shen* is followed by fear and apprehension, which drain and overflow without stop; sadness and sorrow move the centre, therefore exhaustion and consumption, loss of life; euphoria and joy, the *shen* is frightened and disperses, it is not stored; thought and anguish, then *qi* halts and is obstructed, it does not circulate; strong anger, then confusion and shock, there is no control; fear and apprehension, then the *shen* oscillates and is frightened, it is not contained.[26]

---

[24] *Lingshu*, Chapter 6. 'Form' here is the translation of the term *xing* (形), in other words, that which one sees and has a specific form, the body. In the character there are three lines that represent shade (in other words, a solid body), while the other part of the ancient form of the character was a well, which however, according to Henshall stands for the structure, the model (*jing* 精 represented a field divided into nine lots the central one of which – with the well – was public) (Karlgren p. 1084, Henshall p. 104).

[25] *Suwen*, Chapter 39. See also the 'Clinical notes' at the end of this chapter. 'Is released' is the translation of *huan* (缓), the same term used for the pulse, which can have a different valence depending on whether it means 'moderate' or 'slowed down'; 'disordered' is the translation of *luan* (乱), a recurring term which defines disorder, the chaos in the movement of *qi* when it does not follow its usual paths; 'knotting' is the translation of *jie* (结), another common term which describes the conditions of *qi* which are later called constraint-*yu* (郁) and stagnation-*zhi* (滞).

[26] *Lingshu*, Chapter 8. As specified in the 'Introduction' we chose a translation that is very close to the text, leaving to the reader the pleasure and task of selecting the most appropriate syntactic structure.

These alterations in the movement of *qi* constitute the root from which the various clinical patterns with their somatic manifestations develop. The history of Chinese medicine, leading up to the differential diagnosis as it is formulated in TCM, offers an extremely refined analysis of the imbalances of *qi* and blood, the accumulation of pathogens, and the relation with the functions of the organs, but it is fundamental to remember that in any case the primary origin of disease goes back to the consumption of *qi*, its exhaustion, its knotting and its disorder.

Just as *yin* and *yang* do not have an autonomous existence and are not independently determined, but exist only as polarities in a complementary pair, so too psyche and soma are not conceived of as distinct entities, but are defined by their juxtaposition, constituting an indivisible and dynamic unit. In Chinese medicine, psyche and soma do not only interact sporadically, but coexist, each rendering the other's life possible, thanks to which as doctors, we find we do not need to choose between the material–physical–biological dimension and the spiritual–emotional–affective one.

The concept of *qi* causes our viewpoint to shift: that which is physical and that which is metaphysical are simply two expressions of the same thing. Emotions can give rise to somatic disorders as well as psychic illnesses; organic illnesses can, in turn, give rise to emotional alterations and psychic pathologies.

On the other hand, the 'organs' of traditional Chinese medicine also possess a sort of intermediate status between the substance of the body and the more subtle characteristics of *qi*; as 'energetic structures' these functional systems, which are obviously very different from their Western counterparts, still have a certain substantiality with specific manifestations and actions.

As such, emotional movements, which originate in the organs and at the same time act on the functional and organic systems, cannot be considered as in any way separate from the body. This implies that psychic disorders should be treated starting from the energetic system of channels and organs, utilising the usual diagnostic process, the same principles of treatment and the same therapeutic tools.

The following passage well illustrates these diverse aspects: firstly, it affirms a relationship between man and heaven, it notes that the organs produce the emotions through transformation and that emotions are *qi*, and lastly it states that emotions and external pathogens strike at different levels. 'Heaven has four seasons and five elements to generate, grow, gather, bury and produce cold, heat, dryness, dampness and wind. Man has five organs which produce five *qi* for transformation: euphoria, anger, sadness, thought and fear. Euphoria and anger injure the *qi*, cold and heat injure the body.'[27]

---

[27] *Suwen*, Chapter 5. If we refer to the triadic model with the three layers Heaven–Man–Earth, the emotions are positioned at the intermediate level 'Man', between the *shen* in its various expressions corresponding to the 'Heaven' and the organs with the structures and functions depending from them and corresponding to the 'Earth'.

Emotional disorders can give origin to somatic illnesses:

> If euphoria and anger are not regulated, if lifestyle does not have a proper rhythm, if one is fatigued, all this can injure the *qi*; if the *qi* is stagnant, fire is exuberant and invades the spleen–earth. The spleen governs the four limbs; if the heat is oppressive, there is no strength for movement, one is lazy in speech, when moving there is a shortness of breath, there is heat on the surface, spontaneous sweating, restlessness of the heart and no peace.[28]

A modern text on psychiatry and TCM specifies:

> Under external stimulation, emotions encounter change and they move internally; therefore alterations also occur on the level of the organs, channels, *qi*, blood, and liquids. Consequently, the regularity or lack of regularity in the functions of the organs and the vigour or weakness of *qi*, blood and liquids can be reflected in the change of emotions, while an excess or deficiency of emotions can directly influence the functions of the organs and the transporting and transformation of *qi*, blood and liquids. For example, the heart governs the *shen*, in the group of five emotions it corresponds to euphoria; an excess of euphoria influences the interior, injuring the heart, if the heart is injured *shen* becomes dull and loses its functions. According to the classics, it was the heart that took responsibility for the ten thousand things, and this function of the heart depends on the *shen*; if the latter is sick, upright *qi* accumulates and does not flow. This inevitably results in illness characterised by a loosening of the heart's *qi*. The liver governs the *hun*, its emotion corresponds to anger; a strong and unstoppable anger displaces the *hun* and injures the liver, if the *hun* is displaced the liver is injured, it loses control of its function– of regulating free flowing circulation – and the *qi* tends to rise perversely upward; if the *qi* rises and does not descend, constraint and knotting of liver *qi* occur.[29]

A number of points can be schematised as follows:

- Man's *qi* corresponds to heaven's *qi*, with a continuous interaction between internal movements and external stimuli.
- Emotions are movements of *qi*.
- The movement of *qi* can be altered: *qi* can rise inversely, disperse, knot, be depleted, become disordered.
- Emotions are expressions of the organs, just as are the colour of the face, the state of the tissues, and the climactic factor, and correspond to all the other aspects considered in the five elements model.
- Emotional disorders can crop up following alterations in the *qi* of the organs.
- Emotions generally act on the *shen* and its five forms, *wushen*.

---

[28] Li Dongyuan, *Lanshi mizang* ('The secrets of the orchid chamber', 1276), chapter 'Yinshi laojuan' ('Tiredness and exhaustion, food and drink').
[29] Li Qingfu and Liu Duzhou, *Zhongyi jingshen bingxue* ('Psychiatry in Chinese medicine'), 1984, p. 103.

- The five *shen* (*shen, hun, po, yi* and *zhi*), which reside in the five *zang* organs, influence emotions and vice versa.
- Excessive emotional movements injure the organs, in other words, they alter the normal physiology of their energetic structures.
- Emotional disorders can generate somatic illnesses.
- The control-*ke* cycle has a fundamental role in emotional dynamics.

THE 'BENSHEN' CHAPTER OF THE *LINSHU*

These elements are expressed in the chapter of the *Lingshu* whose title refers to *shen* and its root/rooting-*ben*. The passage follows the description of the genesis of *shen*; we cite a translation that sacrifices English syntax in order to remain true to the original text and offers the possibility of following its original flow. A reflection on the passages referring to the spleen follows, which can, by analogy, be applied to the other organs.

Heart: anxiety, worry, thoughts and apprehensions, the *shen* is injured, injured *shen* then fear and terror, lost control, the muscles are consumed. The hair becomes fragile, the appearance is of premature death, one dies in the winter.

Spleen: oppression and anguish that do not dissolve, the *yi* is injured, injured *yi* then restlessness and disorder, the four limbs do not lift up. The hair becomes fragile, the appearance is of premature death, one dies in the spring.

Liver: sadness and sorrow convulse the centre, the *hun* is injured, injured *hun* then mania-*kuang* and oblivion, no *jing*,[30] no *jing* then abnormal behaviour, the genitals retract and the muscles contract, the ribs do not lift up. The hair becomes fragile, the appearance is of premature death, one dies in the autumn.

Lung: euphoria and joy without limits, the *po* is injured, injured *po* then mania-*kuang*, in the grip of mania the mind does not see others, the skin dries out. The hair becomes fragile, the appearance is of premature death, one dies in the summer.

Kidney: intense and incessant anger, the *zhi* is injured, injured *zhi* then one forgets what has been said, the flanks and spinal column are painful and do not bend forward and backward. The hair becomes fragile, the appearance is of premature death, one dies at the end of summer.

Fear and apprehension without end injure the *jing*, injured *jing* then pain in the bones, atrophy-*wei* and reversal-*jue*. There is often spontaneous descending of the *jing*.

The five zang organs store *jing*, they must not be injured, if injured they no longer protect, *yin* becomes empty, empty *yin* there is no more *qi*, no more *qi* then one dies.

---

[30] In this context the interpretation of *jing* is controversial; it can refer to a loss of *jing*-essence, *jing*-sperm or *jing*-mental clarity.

Therefore, one who uses needles observes the state of the patient in order to learn if *jing* and *shen*, *hun* and *po* have been maintained or lost. If the five (*zang*) are injured the needles can not heal.

The liver stores the blood, blood is the residence of *hun*, if the liver is empty there is fear, if it is full there is anger.

The spleen stores nutritive *qi*, nutritive *qi* is the residence of *yi*, if spleen *qi* is empty the four limbs do not function, the five organs are not in harmony, if it is full the abdomen is swollen and menstruation and urination are difficult.

The heart conserves the vessels, vessels are the residence of the *shen*, if heart *qi* is empty there is sadness, if it is full there is uncontrollable laughter.

The lung stores *qi*, *qi* is the residence of *po*, if lung *qi* is empty the nose is obstructed, the passage of air is difficult and the breath is short, if it is full one has laboured and hoarse breathing, fullness in the chest and needs to lift the head to breath.

The kidney stores *jing*, *jing* is the residence of *zhi*, if kidney *qi* is empty there is reversal-*jue*, if it is full there is swelling and the five zang organs are not calm.

The form of the illness of the five organs must be examined to learn the fullness and emptiness of their *qi* and regulate it in a wise way.[31]

If, for example, we examine the spleen, an organ which in our society and culture has a front line role, we find a situation where psychic pain, depression, and the weight of sorrow do not manage to 'find a way out', in other words to resolve themselves or, in the words of the Chinese text, to dissolve. This oppression acts on the *yi*, and the capability of thinking. Psychic and physical consequences derive from this, with agitation and disorder of the spirit and fatigue of the body, which in turn no longer responds properly, and 'the four limbs do not lift up'.

Utilising the typical feature of a single part to represent the whole, it is said that 'the hair becomes fragile' to indicate a body which is suffering, which shows signs of extreme consumption with 'signs of premature death', and the phrase is repeated identically for all five *zang* organs.

One dies in spring, the season that belongs to the element that in the control-*ke* cycle dominates the spleen, which is too weak to sustain balance. For each element it is said that death occurs in the season that dominates it, to indicate the fundamental importance of the control-*ke* cycle in emotional pathologies.

After the description of the events which regard the individual organs, the text continues by reminding us how continuous fear injures the *jing*, the deepest level, and how injury to the organs signifies compromising the ability to store *yin*. If there is no more *yin*, then there is no more *qi* and one dies.

---

[31] *Lingshu*, Chapter 8. A complex work of translation and interpretation of this chapter was carried out through the years by C. Larre and E. Rochat de la Vallée (see for example *Les Mouvements du Coeur*, 1992).

The analysis of the various organs is then resumed, to remind us that the spleen stores nutritive *qi*, the residence of *yi*, and if spleen *qi* is lacking then the body does not function, relinquishing the regulatory system of the organs, while if it is full the stagnation manifests itself mainly at the abdominal level. For other organs (heart and liver) the consequences of their emptiness or fullness are seen primarily in the psychological domain – for example, they may produce fear or anger, sadness or uncontrollable laughter. The fundamental principles according to which an 'organic' (in the Chinese sense) alteration can cause both somatic and psychological disorders are derived from this analysis.

PATHOGENIC PROCESSES

Emotions alter the movement of *qi*. In general, emotive alterations first compromise the 'functional' level of *qi*, after which they produce organic damage:

> In the *Lingshu*, 'Benshen' chapter the pathological changes that occur when organs' associated emotions are damaged are described in great detail. Normally, the emotions injure the organs' *qi* first, producing functional changes in the organs themselves along with emotional changes. If the illness progresses, the emotions will then injure the *jing* of the organ, in other words the body, so that organ-related symptoms emerge – for example when it is said: 'the hair becomes fragile, the appearance is of premature death'.[32]

The change in the movement of *qi* can be a cause of pathology, with the involvement of blood, compromising of the organ's function, and syndromes of stagnation or emptiness.

A modern Chinese text introduces the subject by stating:

> The movements of *qi* are the physiological basis of emotions. When the intensity of the emotional stimulus exceeds the organ system's capacity for regulation and in particular the ability of the liver to drain and release *qi*, the circulation and movements of *qi* cannot occur in a normal manner and they fall into disarray and the state of balance and harmony among the organs is shattered. In this way, emotional illnesses are generated and, for example, stasis of blood and *qi* stagnation are produced.[33]

---

[32] Zhu Wenfeng, *Zhongyi xinlixue yuanzhi* ('Principles of Psychology in Chinese medicine'), 1987, p. 101.

[33] Li Qingfu and Liu Duzhou, 1984, p. 104. 'To drain and release' is the translation of *shuxie*, discussed in the Chapter 4 on constriction-*yu*; 'movements of the *qi*' is the translation of *qiji*, that is the movements of coming in and going out, downwards and upwards, 'emotional illnesses' is the translation of *qingzhi jibing*, as specified in the Introduction.

The pathogenic process is complex and, as always, numerous factors intervene, of which the foremost is the patient's energetic balance – or, in other words, the sum of pre-heaven and post-heaven *qi*. In general, emotions have greater effect in a 'terrain' that is not the ideal one of dynamic equilibrium between *yin* and *yang*, free flowing *qi*, and harmony among the five organs. Great sadness will have different impacts and pathological developments in a person with a good reserve of *jing*, in a person with deficiency of lung *qi*, and in a person with spleen deficiency and an accumulation of phlegm.

The first changes following an emotional stimulus occur at the level of *qi*, causing alterations in its basic physiological flow. These are short term changes that can be compared to the automatic responses of the vegetative nervous system: 'The organism's physiological reactions which appear following changes in the movement of *qi* such as, for example, the free flowing of blood in the vessels due to joy, redness in the face and ears due to anger, heavy breathing and sobbing due to sadness, stagnation and non-transformation of foods due to worry, and sweating and trembling due to fear, are all reversible changes. At this stage, it is sufficient to remove the emotional stimulus and the movements of *qi* will return to normal.'[34]

It is, rather, in the next stage that these changes are consolidated, accompanied by compromise at various levels. At first the changes become chronic, so worsening the alterations in the flow of *qi*: for example, a 'perversely' rising *qi* can be produced, in which stomach *qi* rises instead of descending, spleen *qi* drops downward and does not maintain its supporting function, lung *qi* does not descend and diffuse, liver *qi* does not manage to produce a free flow, heart *qi* does not harmonise and kidney *qi* does not control opening and closing.

In any case, when *qi* movements are altered they become laboured and therefore consume *qi*, with specific consequences on the various organs.

A deficiency of *qi* can, in turn, cause deficient circulation, which predisposes to stagnation/stasis and the formation of various accumulations – for example *qi* stagnation, blood stasis, accumulation of dampness and phlegm, transformation into fire and emission of internal wind.

Stasis and accumulations then attack the more substantial aspects and excess syndromes transform into deficiency syndromes, with consumption of *yin*, blood, and *jing*.

The same modern text describes the 'phases of becoming chronic' thus: 'One can then have: (a) concurrent presence of full and empty, and injury to both *yin* and *yang*, pre-heaven and post-heaven; (b) the production of phlegm or stagnation which further aggravates the pathological conditions; (c) further strengthening of the emotional alterations. The flow of *qi* and blood will have even more difficulty returning to normal. The treatment will be very

---

[34] Li Qingfu and Liu Duzhou, 1984, p. 104. 'Worry' is the translation of the contemporary term *yousi*, 'preoccupation, anxiousness'.

complex: you will need to take action using the psychic method to eliminate the causes of illness and using prescriptions to regulate and eliminate phlegm, stagnation, etc'.[35]

RELATIONS AMONG EMOTIONS AND THE FIVE ELEMENTS-*WUXING*

The *Neijing* recognises five emotions, which have specific relationships with the five elements and the five *zang* organs. As with other correspondences in this analogical model, such as dryness which belongs to metal and at the same time easily injures the lung, so too emotional manifestations of *qi* are both expressions of the corresponding element – whichever has the most resonance – and at the same time specific areas of danger.

The *wuxing* system is regulated by physiological relationships of generation and control and can be subject to pathological changes due to deficiency or excess of an element and the related consequences on the other elements.[36]

EMOTION	CORRESPONDENCE	CYCLE OF CONTROL-KE
xi(喜) euphoria	corresponds to heart – fire	dominates sadness – metal
si (思) thought	corresponds to spleen – earth	dominates fear – water
bei (悲) sadness	corresponds to lung – metal	dominates anger – wood
kong (恐) fear	corresponds to kidney – water	dominates euphoria – fire
nu (怒) anger	corresponds to liver – wood	dominates thought – earth

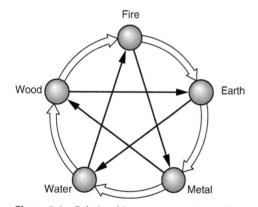

Figure 2.1 Relationship among emotions and organs in the *wuxing* system

[35] Li Qingfu and Liu Duzhou, 1984, p. 104. 'Psychic method' is the translation of *jingshen liaofa*, which is a generic term.
[36] *Wuxing* 五行: we have kept the translation 'five elements' which is now commonly used even though the term 'phase', 'processes', 'motions' or 'movements' would give a better idea of the concept of movement encompassed by the character *xing*. Moreover, unlike the Four Elements of the Greek and Medieval philosophies, they are not conceived as elements constituting things, instead they imply a continuous movement through links of generation-*sheng* and control-*ke*.

The cycle of domination or control-*ke* assumes particular relevance when considering the interaction among corresponding elements: every emotion dominates, controls and limits the emotion that follows the next one in the sequence (the 'grandchild'), and so it is necessary to take this into account in evaluation and treatment.[37]

> Illnesses that appear suddenly do not necessarily have to be treated according to the cycle of generation-*sheng*, since they may not follow this order, especially in suddenly appearing emotional disorders. Thought, fear, sadness, euphoria, and anger often do not follow the cycle of generation and for this reason can cause more serious disorders. Therefore an excess of euphoria provokes emptiness [in the heart] and kidney *qi* exercises too much control. Anger, liver *qi* exercises too much control [on the spleen]. Sadness, lung *qi* exercises too much control [on the liver]. Fear, spleen *qi* exercises too much control [on the kidney]. Thought, heart *qi* exercises too much control [on the lung]. These are illnesses that are provoked by emotions, which do not follow the cycle of generation-*sheng*, but rather the cycle of control-*ke*. Therefore the basic illnesses are five, but there are 25 variations.[38]

As will be noted, the overwhelming of an element can depend on an actual excess of an element, which therefore subdues its controlled element, or on a deficiency, which causes the weak element to be invaded.

Wang Bing, the great commentator of the *Suwen* of the Tang Dynasty, discussing the phrase 'anger dominates thought', specifies: 'When there is anger there is no thought, in the impetus of rage one forgets one's misfortunes, and this is the victory (of anger over thought).'[39]

Famous clinicians used this relationship in the course of various procedures in their treatments. This type of therapy was particularly developed by Zhang Zihe:

> Sadness can treat anger: one must move the patient with sad, painful and bitter words; euphoria can treat sadness: one must entertain the patient with jokes, wisecracks, and practical jokes; fear can treat euphoria: one must frighten the patient with threatening words about death or bad luck; anger can treat thought: one must provoke the patient with insolent words; thought can treat fear: one must divert the patient's attention towards another subject, so that he forgets the cause of his fear. [...] I have tried the method of imitating the moves of the witchdoctor and the courtesan to treat knotting due to sadness.[40]

---

[37] In Italy it is sometimes referred to as 'grandfather–nephew'. The cycle *ke* acts on the element following the generated -*shen* 生 one (that is the one following immediately). The character *ke* 克 means: 1. 'power, being able to'; 2. 'dominating, controlling, submitting'; 3. 'containing, limiting'; 4. 'digesting'; 5. 'setting a limit in time' (Wieger p. 75k, Karlgren p. 415).

[38] Wang Bing, *Zhu huangdi suwen* ('Commentary to the *Huangdi suwen*'). The sentence can be found in Chapter 67 of the *Suwen*, 'Wuyunxing dalun' ('Great treatise on the five movements').

[39] Wang Bing, *Zhu huangdi suwen* ('Commentary to the *Huang Di suwen*'). The sentence can be found in Chapter 67 of the *Suwen*, 'Wuyunxing dalun' ('Great treatise on the five movements').

[40] Zhang Zihe, *Rumen shiqin* ('Confucian responsibilities towards family and parents'), chapter 'Jiuqi ganji gengxiang weizhiyan' ('Treatment of illnesses of the nine *qi*'). 'Imitating the moves of the witchdoctor and the courtesan' means 'to amuse, distract, induce laughter'. On this issue see also Chapter 14 on the treatment with emotions in the classics.

CLINICAL NOTES

In Chinese clinics, little time is spent on the baring of the patient's soul and the pangs suffered, yet it is always surprising how the doctors manage to determine the weight of eventual psychic components in a short time. When we listen to their conversations and the questions and answers, we find ourselves in what is an alien universe for us, but then the patient is cured and we can only accept the results.

Such a prudent attitude towards emotional labours is often difficult for us to comprehend, so much so that one can have the impression that modern Chinese doctors simplify the psychic universe to a level which is crude and banal, and it is easy for us to suspect that the five or seven codified emotions are a superficial reduction with respect to the refinement of our analysis of feelings.

The fact that the Chinese do not show their emotions also seems strange to us, even more so given that hiding emotions implies being untrustworthy in our iconography.

Certainly, Chinese culture is profoundly different from our own, which particularly since the 1800s and in contemporary thought has placed personal aspirations and the feelings that link us to others at the centre of attention. This process finds full expression in the development of psychoanalysis and our general way of perceiving and referring to ourselves nowadays. However, that which seems obvious to us – specifically the expression of feelings, or the introspective search for the person's internal truths and his psychological aspects, cannot in reality be identified as absolute human traits.

Chinese tradition, for example, attributes a different role and importance to emotions: in Confucian ethics the individual – and therefore his personal affairs including those of an emotional nature – is of secondary importance to his role as part of a collective; in Daoist thought, in order to adhere to the *dao* one must calm the *shen* to avoid its being disturbed by external and internal events; in Buddhist tradition, the first step towards understanding consists of distancing oneself from the various attachments of the soul.

In any case, we cannot forget that even in Western civilisation the question of the identity of the individual only goes back to the first centuries of the Christian era. In Ancient Greek society, taking care of oneself did not mean turning oneself into an object of consciousness, but rather constituting oneself as a subject of action with respect to world events, asking oneself what one's obligations were with respect to the family or as a citizen in the *polis*.[41]

---

[41] On this issue see also the article by Frederic Gros on the last Faucault, 'what do we want to do with ourselves?', Il Manifesto, 21.6.2001.

Diagnosis

In Chinese thought, theoretical reflections on feelings and passions followed specific paths: as we said in the beginning of this chapter, the five emotions can be compared to primary nuclei, equivalent to a sort of concentration of internal emotional movements.

However, just as the treatment of prevalently emotional syndromes is carried out on the basis of the general picture which includes signs and symptoms of a somatic type, so too the diagnosis will be based on the four methods, whose integration is particularly valuable in those patterns where emotions play an important role.

The words the patient uses regarding a specific emotional problem are, in fact, only some of the methods we have available for perceiving where and how *qi* flow has altered. The verbal explanation can be limited or even lead us astray; in this case the somatic symptoms and the objective elements based on observing and touching can be of great help.

When interpreted according to traditional systems of correspondences, we can also put mental states, movements of the soul or other conditions that do not coincide with the five classical emotions (for example, shame, guilt feelings, frustrations, feelings of abandonment, etc.) into context. In this regard, the reading of the pulse and the palpation of the points (especially *shu* and *mu*, the *yuan* of the three *yin* channels and the *he* of the three *yang* channels of the foot, and, naturally, the symptomatic points), the examination of the tongue, and the accurate observation of the patient's being (the *shen* of the eyes, the complexion, signs on the face, the state of various tissues, attitude, movements, etc.) are fundamental.

However, even if a definite diagnostic hypothesis is indicated by all these signs and symptoms, it is still essential to listen closely to what the patient is saying, without taking anything for granted and without making premature inferences.

Since emotions are movements of *qi*, physical experiences correspond to them. If – as often happens – a patient tends to tell an abstract story, it is necessary to find a means of arriving at an understanding of what his real physical sensations are.[42]

Perception of Emotions

This is not the proper place to enter into a debate over whether or not there is greater somatisation of psychological disorders in China compared with

---

[42] See also Chapter 16 on the events related to acupuncture and case study 6.1.

more developed countries, or the decreased capacity for interaction that this hypothesis often implies. We should remember, however, that a somatising tendency is also decidedly relevant in studies on Western populations. Feelings of malaise are extremely frequently referred to as somatic symptoms in the absence of objectively demonstrated organic pathologies – so much so that, according to certain studies, psychiatric disorders are referred to as somatic by patients in over 90% of cases.[43]

Emotions can injure *qi*, blood and organs, but above all they are movements of *qi* and pathologies derive from a disorder in the physiological movements of *qi*. *Qi* is constrained, knotted, rises inversely, stagnates, sinks, and hesitates in abnormal excesses and deficiencies and so forth, and this produces physical and emotional sensations.

Knowing that people often lack both the habit of direct perception of emotions and their verbal expression, it can be useful for us to direct our attention to a number of elements that help in recognising the five emotions in themselves and in the clinical setting. The following sections review the observations and language encountered in daily clinical practice so that we may better understand how best to deal with both the complexity of patients' emotions and the reactions that these produce in us.

It is a good rule to recognise emotions as authentic and genuine movements of *qi* (for example, rather than 'producing *qi* which rises perversely', anger is in itself '*qi* that rises upward'); we need to appreciate fully that rather than cause and effect, it is a matter of concurrence.

Knowing that words are often used to explain and rationalise, it is important to discern and acknowledge every emotion as a specific internal sensation inside ourselves, revealing and identifying every movement of *qi* as a direct experience (and the various forms of practice with *qi* help with these aspects). This refining of our own sensibility simplifies the job the patient has to perform in order to discover his emotions beyond the words with which he usually describes them.

In basic manuals, the relationship between emotions, organs and movements of *qi* is explained; however this information is often restricted to the general context and difficult to apply to clinical practice.

Anger-*nu* (怒)

Pertains to wood–liver.

Nu means 'anger, rage, ire'; like many of the terms which refer to the mental/emotional area, it contains the radical 'heart', while the phonetic

---

[43] Goldberg, D., *Epidemiology of Mental Disorders in Primary Care Settings*, 1995. A first explanation of this mechanism is in the fact that dysphoric emotions are socially stigmatised, while somatic symptoms are more easily accepted.

part utilises the semantically quite suggestive character *nu*, meaning 'slave'.[44]

Being angry is feeling 'the rage mounting', which corresponds precisely with the classic description 'anger, then *qi* rises'; 'with anger, *qi* rises in an unstoppable way, heat rises attacking the heart, breathing is short as though one is about to die, there is no air to breathe'.[45]

However we certainly cannot ask a patient if he gets angry often; quite apart from the fact that direct questions often produce wrong answers, the term 'getting angry' generally evokes scenes of furious rage in which the person quite honestly does not recognise himself.

This movement of *qi* rising is important to take into consideration; it is a sudden internal movement, immediate and uncontrollable, a type of 'internal excitement' following the most varied events. It is like an internal cry (the crying–shouting of the liver), it is an irritable response to even little things that happen or do not happen, that others do or do not do, or that we ourselves do or do not do – events that are often of little importance, but are in effect destabilising. It can also manifest as simple intolerance without bad moods or ruminations, but rather an ever-present readiness to snap, and we can detect that everything about the person remains tense, like the *xuan*-wiry pulse, typical of the liver.

This movement may not have an immediate direct expression in words or deeds, due to its natural tendency to subside – if it is not too powerful – or due to a constraint which keeps it on hold, considering it inopportune, with enormous and unhappy effects on the psychological balance.

Furthermore, we note that the relationship between anger and aggressiveness was already recognised in the *Nejing* in its affirmation that when liver *qi* is empty there is fear.

Euphoria-*xi* (喜)

Pertains to fire–heart.

The difference between *xi* and *le* is that, whereas the first represents a type of happiness closer to a euphoric state, the second is a more harmonious form of joy; euphoria or 'excess of joy' is expressed in the patient mostly as a state of excitation, possibly slight, but continuous – a form of being constantly 'out of bounds'. Such people are generally hyperactive, they communicate a

---

[44] The character *nu* 怒 'slave' is composed of 'woman' and 'hand' (Wieger p. 67c, Karlgren p. 674).
[45] Chao Yuanfang commenting the sentence 'rage, thus the *qi* rises' *nu ze qi shang* 怒 则 气 上 in the *Suwen*, Chapter 39. In: *Zhubing yuanhoulun* ('Treatise on the origin and symptoms of illnesses', 610). In the general medical tradition there is also a more specific reference to *yunu* 郁 怒 'contained rage', *baonu* 暴 怒 'exploding rage' and *fennu* 愤怒 'resentment-indignation' (for example in *Lingshu*, Chapter 6).

sense of nervousness, they fill their lives with commitments and amusements, and often the more they are agitated the more they have to do.

Fire, with its agitating flames, can also manifest itself through grandiose maniacal behaviour.[46]

A specific indicator is a slight laugh at the end of a sentence even when communicating painful events (laughing pertains to the heart).

It is said: 'euphoria, *qi* slows down';[47] we also certainly recognise this movement of *qi* that is dispersed, which unravels like a fraying fabric. The *qi* is no longer united, it loses its centre, and everything escapes. As the harmony of the heart and its integrating action is diminished, the whole breaks apart.

The patient suffers from an internal agitation, complaining of not being able to concentrate, sleeps poorly, has no sense of where he actually is or cannot recognise his part in what is happening around him. In extreme cases, the various personality parts fragment explosively; these are delirious states of psychosis, where the patient loses all grasp of reality.

Thought-*si* (思)

Pertains to earth–spleen.

The character *si*, whose lower part is made up of the radical 'heart' and whose upper part represented the head or brain in ancient times, means (1) 'think, consider, deliberate'; (2) 'think about, having nostalgia'; (3) 'thought'.[48]

We recall here that in the classic Chinese conception, in contrast to the Greek–Jewish tradition, thought is considered to mediate an immediate response to the conditions in which the answer rings like an echo, follows like a shadow and accurately expresses adaptation to the *dao*.[49] In our culture, thought is considered pathological when it becomes cold intellectualisation that excludes feeling, a process of rationalisation that allows no room for emotions or sentiments. In clinical practice, the most common manifestation is

---

[46] In psychiatry a maniacal behaviour is defined as a 'psychological condition characterised by great euphoria, disinhibition, unlimited confidence in oneself, dispersive racing of initiatives and ideas that fly out of every biographical context, and to which the subject relates in an absolutely uncritical way'. In: Galimberti, *Dizionario di Psicologia*, 1992. For a definition of manic or hypomanic episode see the notes on diagnostic framing in conventional psychiatry notes, in Appendix B.

[47] X *i ze qi huan* 喜则 气 缓, *Suwen*, Chapter 39. On this issue see also the discussion on the clinic of *shen*, *hun* and *po*, in Chapter 3.

[48] The upper part now matches with the character *tian* 田 'field' (Karlgren p. 813).

[49] In the Homeric conception of thought (*fronein*) it has a wider meaning, embracing the sphere of sensations and emotions. See also Onians, 'The origins of European thought', 1998, for a description of how knowledge and intelligence were thought to be placed in certain organs, and for the relationship between perception, physical emotion, thought and propensity to action: 'Where cognition and thought are so connected with sensation and propensity to action, the relationship between moral qualities, virtues, and knowledge is deeper than when cognition is more "pure".' p. 40.

obsessive rumination, in which endless thought circles do not transform or result in action.

Thought belongs to the spleen, whose *qi* performs the functions of transformation and transportation: in a similar way as with a heavy meal, heavy thoughts overburden this movement and become ruminations.

Thought as a form of reflection, a moment in which one stops and elaborates sensations, perceptions, and fantasies, is a correct movement of transformation of earth; if this function becomes excessive, though, if it develops into preoccupation – or in other words it preoccupies all the space – it then produces knotting of *qi*.[50]

If we try to imagine ourselves as being knotted, in other words bound up, we can immediately understand what happens to *qi* in these cases and it is not a pleasant sensation. *Qi* that 'blocks and closes up' corresponds to a monotone voice, along with somatic symptoms such as oppression, bloating and heaviness, while the feeling that the patient transmits to us is one that reminds us of sinking in a swamp.

During conversation with patients, one must take into account that many describe themselves as 'anxious', but what they intend by this term is a tendency to ruminate, to return in their thoughts to things that have already happened. They are worried by recurring thoughts and on waking their thought processes are already at work, to the point where they may suffer from actual obsessions in which the mind has no choice but to retrace the same path infinitely.

Obsessive thought is a good example of the *ke* cycle's mechanism of control: the fear of water can be moderated by the reflection of the earth, but if the system becomes inflexible it cannot hold together indefinitely and the attempt to control the world in order to defend oneself from its dangers becomes an obsessive–compulsive pathology.

Sadness-*bei* (悲)

Pertains to metal–lung.

We translate *bei* or *bei ai* as 'sadness, pain, suffering, anguish, melancholy'.[51] While there should apparently be no major problem in recognising

---

[50] Zhang Jiebin comments on the sentence of the *Suwen* Chapter 39, 'thought, knotting *qi*', *si ze qi jie* 思 则 气 结: 'Anguish and excessive though, thus the *qi* knots itself, if the *qi* is knotted transformation can not take place'. In: Zhang Jiebin, *Jingyue quanshu* ('The complete works of Jingyue', 1640), Chapter 'Yige' ('Blocking of the diaphragm').

[51] The character *bei* 悲 is composed by the phonetic part *fei* 非, negative particle, and the radical 'heart' (Wieger 170a, Karlgren 27). An example of a reading of this character is: '*bei*, the heart refuses: the person opposes to himself (back to back) in his heart, falling into contradiction, negation, and negativity. The weariness caused by this fight destroys the breaths in the heart and lung region.' In: Larre and Rochat de la Vallée, 1994.

these emotions, in practice the contrary is often the case because when faced by great pain, whether recent or in the past, the patient is evasive, since the wound is so deep that in order to maintain the little life that remains he withdraws, as though every contact and communication risks allowing a little *qi* to escape.

'Sadness, *qi* dissolves.'[52] We know how pain consumes life. *Qi* is exhausted, and this is exactly the sensation we feel, of having nothing left.

Obviously, in the majority of cases the pain is neither so pervasive or destructive, rather there is a diffuse anguish, sadness that is the suffering of living, the existential ennui mentioned in romantic and psychiatric literature. These feelings are decidedly difficult to identify, as we are poorly prepared to perceive them and even the words used to express them are obsolete.

The patient often refers to being 'depressed', a very widespread term to which a wide range of meanings are attributed, all of which therefore need to be investigated. Due to the fact that modern society tends to focus on 'action', a pathological condition can be identified by the non-action of depression.

A whining–wailing tone of voice (whining and wailing pertain to the lung) can also be of help in identifying sadness.

Fear-*kong* (恐)

Pertains to water–kidney.

Pertaining to the kidney, fear is therefore a part of the deepest *yin*, the root of life. It is also the root of all the other emotions: the anger of aggressiveness, the sadness of abandonment and loss, the thinking that attempts to control everything, the euphoria that hides the panic of desperation are all connected to it, and fear embraces all of them.[53]

We note here that in the definition of the seven emotions the term *jing* appears, meaning 'fright, alarm'.[54] Zhang Jiebin had already pondered this point:

> We ask ourselves why, while both fright and fear belong to water, the damage wreaked on man by fear-*kong* is so much more serious than that provoked by fright-*jing*. The latter comes from something which is temporary and being temporary permits a return (to the original situation), fear however, accumulates in a progressive manner and being progressive cannot be resolved, when

---

[52] *bei ze qi xiao* 悲 则 气 消, *Suwen*, Chapter 39. We recall how in our society it is difficult to find a space and way to live the mourning after painful events and how the suffering consequently fails to be contained by the gathering movement of the lung.

[53] The character *kong* 恐 is composed of the radical 'heart' and by the phonetic part *gong*, an ancient term for 'hugging', where the pictogram was composed by 'work' and by a person stretching his arms (Karlgren p. 469).

[54] The simplified form of *jing* 精 'fright' contains the radical 'heart'; the complete one contained the radical 'horse' (Karlgren p. 396).

it becomes serious the heart weakens and *shen* is injured, *jing* withdraws; the
yin therefore atrophies, is extinguished and withdraws as time passes.[55]

Whereas fright is the response to a sudden and usually real threat, fear and apprehension are rather related to a continuous expectation of something dangerous, and in many cases refer to a persistent, pervasive and often undefined sensation.

Fear-*kong* frequently appears together with apprehension-*ju*, whose ancient form contained the radical 'heart' and the doubled radical 'eye' above that for 'bird' – interpreted by Karlgren as a frightened, timid, nervous appearance like that of the eyes of a bird. Wieger, however, relates it to the vigilant state of birds, which must remain alert for their survival. It in any case contains the idea of a continuous state of alarm.[56]

Whereas fright strikes with force, ruffling and rendering the *qi* chaotic, fear causes *qi* to sink.[57]

More than fear of something specific, this emotion is often apprehension that something might occur, fear of what the future may bring us; we usually refer to this as anxiety. We are speaking of that state of continuous restiveness which the patient may refer to, for example, as 'constantly feeling my heart in my throat, even if I know no one is chasing me' – a state which the *Neijing* describes under the symptoms of the kidney channel as 'kidney *qi* deficiency, easily frightened, the heart beats as though someone is grabbing at you'.[58] This manifests as the symptom 'easily startled by sudden sounds' that is included in the descriptions of these syndromes, also those patterns of commotion and deep fear which invade some people as soon as someone dear to them is late, or the actual disorder of panic attacks.[59]

NOTES ON THE GALL BLADDER AND DETERMINATION

Even today, in the common usage of China a courageous or fearful person is said to have a big or small gall bladder. This connection goes all the way back

---

[55] Zhang Jiebin, *Jingyue quanshu*, chapter 'Zhenzhong jingkong' ('Palpitations from fear and fright'). Zhang Zihe in the chapter on the reciprocal control of emotions states: 'Fright-*jing* is *yang* and comes in from the outside, fear-*kong* is *yin*, it comes out from the inside'. In: Zhang Zihe, *Rumen shiqin*, chapter 'Jiuqi ganji gengxiang weizhiyan'.
[56] Wieger p. 158g, Karlgren p. 490.
[57] In *Suwen*, Chapter 39 reads: 'fright, thus the *qi* is messed up' and 'fear, thus the *qi* descends': *jing ze qi luan* 惊 则 气 乱 (*luan* means 'mess, licence, chaos, confusion', Wieger p. 90b, Karlgren p. 582) and *kong ze qi xia* 恐 则 气 下 (*xia* means 'under, down below, downwards'). The relationship with the heart is also highlighted by many texts since '*kong* moves the heart and the kidney reacts-*ying*'. In: Yu Chang, *Yimen falu*.
[58] *Lingshu*, Chapter 10.
[59] See also Chapter 9 on classical syndromes for a discussion of the *bentun* illness, where: 'The *bentun* illness starts from the lower abdomen, rises and attacks the throat, when it burst out one feels like he is dying, it comes back and then stops, it all comes from fright and fear'. In: Zhang Zhongjing, 'Jingui yaolue' ('Prescriptions in the golden chamber'), Chapter 8.

to the *Neijing* and the assessment of the consequences of a weakness of gall bladder *qi* appears throughout the history of medical thought.

The gall bladder is spring and *Shao Yang*, its *qi* rises and allows the other *qi(s)* to flow upward.[60]

It is, furthermore, a curious or extraordinary viscera, *qiheng zhifu*, in that it fills and empties like all the other viscera, but at the same time it acts like a *zang*-organ since it preserves fluid-essence, *jingzhi* (惊志).[61]

The first aspect, 'viscera of the centre's *jing*', which is already present in the *Neijing*, is incorporated into the *neidan* internal alchemy practices; these consider bile as pure *jing*, associating it with fire and attributing to it a precise function in the process of birth and development of the spiritual 'fetus' in the *dantian*.

The correspondence with emotions belongs, first, to the organs-*zang* aspect, but the viscera-*fu* gall bladder aspect has nevertheless a particular role in the expression of the human soul. A substantial difference between the two is, however, evident: that aspect which corresponds to the gall bladder is not an internal emotion or movement of *qi*, like fear and anger, so much as a way of relating to the outside world.

The *Neijing* states: 'the gall bladder presides over justness and correctness and from these determination and decision are derived'.[62] Judgement enables choice and therefore action; 'deciding' signifies 'arriving at a final judgement ending all pre-existent doubts and uncertainties, choosing'.[63] Deciding therefore corresponds with the moment of choice; it coincides with the initial moment of action when one passes from the all-possible to something concrete that is being actualised. The human, being finite, must choose with respect to the potentially infinite. It is therefore natural that this moment of passage called decision belongs to the gall bladder, which is *Shao Yang*, the beginning of *yang*, of movement, of externalisation.

---

[60] 'The gall bladder is the *qi* of the rise, of the spring, of the *shaoyang*. If the *qi* of the spring rises the ten thousand things are in peace. If the gall bladder *qi* rises all other organs follow it.' In: Li Dongyuan, *Piweilun*, chapter 'Piwei xushi zhuanbian' ('Transformation of emptiness and fullness in spleen and stomach'). And when he speaks about its role in sustaining the function of the spleen in transforming food he says: 'The defensive *qi*, the *qi* of the cereals, and the original *qi* are all one, that of gall bladder [...] Food and drink come into men through the stomach, the nourishing *qi* rises and this happens thanks to the gall bladder *qi*.' In: Li Dongyuan, *Lanshi micang*, chapter 'Yinshi laojuanmen' ('Tiredness and exhaustion, food and drink').
[61] 'The gall bladder is the viscera-*fu* of the *jing* of the centre.' In: *Lingshu*, Chapter 2.
[62] *Suwen*, Chapter 8. In this chapter all the *zangfu* are connected with a function, using for each one the same syntactic construction of which one can give apparently multiple translations. Here the term 'presides' is the translation of *guan* 脾, which means both the functioning and the role; 'justness' is the translation of *zhong* 中, the 'centre' in the classical sense of correctness, which also means 'to hit the target'; 'correctness' is the translation of *zheng* 正, the term is also used to define the correct *qi*; 'determination' is the translation of *jue* 决, whose character contains the idea of the water getting round the stones in the river, and 'decision' is the translation of *duan* 断, a character which also means 'to interrupt' and has in its ancient form many silk threads and a chopping axe (*zhong* Karlgren p. 1269, *zheng* Karlgren p. 1198, *jue* Karlgren p. 440, *duan* Karlgren p. 331).
[63] Zingarelli, *Vocabolario della Lingua Italiana*, 1994. 'To decide' derives from the latin *caedere* 'to cut' and *de* 'away'.

The *Neijing* explains it this way: 'All *qi*(s) are important, but the gall bladder makes the final decision because it supports all the *qi*(s) that begin to arise.'[64]

Determination has its origin in discernment of that which is just and correct; as well as being the effect of deciding, the term 'decision' also signifies 'resolution' in English. In this sense, determination does not signify obstinacy or stubbornness, but rather derives directly from the person's understanding of and adjustment to the *dao*, the way. When there is no disconnection from the unfolding of the *dao* there is also no problem of choice, and action then has the characteristics of immediacy, spontaneity and inevitability.

In everyday life, 'having a good gall bladder' means being able to make a choice and carry it out: being able to see the situation with lucidity, to make decisions without excess difficulty, and at the same time to possess sufficient determination to transform these into action. It is in this sense that we speak of judgement, decision, determination and courage.

Insufficient gall bladder *qi* causes fearfulness, *danqie*, 'a cowardly gall bladder'. The meaning that comes closest to *qie* in English is 'fearfulness, apprehension'.[65] It can also be a case of timidity, in the sense of insecurity – in other words, that feeling of discomfort and inadequacy that comes from the lack of an immediate connection with the situation.

An emptiness of gall bladder *qi* therefore manifests as fearfulness, uncertainty, indecision, lack of initiative and courage; it can also be accompanied by an emptiness of heart *qi*, producing a state of apprehension, anxiety and a continuous state of alarm.

The *Yanglingquan* point, GB-34 was suggested by Sun Simiao in those patterns where there is 'apprehension and fear as though someone is grabbing at you' and successive texts also referred to this susceptibility to being frightened, speaking of 'easy fear, apprehension, as if someone is grabbing at you, this comes from an emptiness of heart *qi* and gall bladder *qi*'.[66]

The concept that 'when one encounters an external danger and is frightened, those who are strong of heart and gall bladder are not injured, but those who are weak of heart and gall bladder will be easily frightened by just coming into contact with it' is returned to in the following contemporary case

---

[64] *Suwen*, Chapter 63. We also recall that the gall bladder corresponds to *jia*, the first of ten celestial trunks and to *zi*, the first of the 12 earthly branches. The character *jia* 甲 represents the part which protects the seed (Karlgren p. 344); *zi* 子, whose pictogram represented a child, means 'child, seed, young' (Wieger p. 94a, Karlgren p. 1089).

[65] The character *qie* 怯 is the opposite of brave, it means: 1. 'fearful, coward, shy, craven'; 2. 'gross, clumsy'; it is formed by the phonetic part *qie* and by the radical 'heart' (Karlgren p. 491). The relationship between the gall bladder and braveness is highlighted by Zhang Zihe in the chapter on the reciprocal control of emotions: '*Shao Yang* of the gall bladder belongs to the liver-wood, the gall bladder is *gan* 脾 "braveness, to dare".' In: *Rumen shiqin*, chapter 'Jiuqi ganji gengxiang weizhiyan' ('Development of the treatment of the illnesses of the nine *qi* through the reciprocal alternance').

[66] Sun Simiao, *Qianjin yaofang* ('Remedies worth a thousand golden pieces for urgencies', 625); Gong Tingxian, *Shoushi baoyuan* ('Reaching longevity preserving the source', 1615). Regarding the 'Emptiness of the gall bladder and heart *qi*' see also the clinical discussion in Chapter 11.

studies, which outline its features with respect to stress-related pathologies.[67] If gall bladder *qi* is strong enough it can withstand agitation, tension, and the fear that derives from violent change and one is able to overcome the emotive changes that follow due to the pressure of external solicitations.[68]

Case Study 2.1

Hiccups

One of my patients arrives with her 50-year-old brother, whom she had spoken to me about a few days earlier. The man has been hiccuping continuously for the last 8 days with a worsening after meals.

The hiccuping is not violent, but it is without pause, present during the night and with a burning sensation in the back at the level of T7. The only time the hiccuping was interrupted, for about one hour, was after an inhalation of ether. Investigation of the case shows the presence of a peptic ulcer and a hiatus hernia, but no pathologies involving the phrenic nerve.

I really have no time for proper data collection so I listen to his brief story; he informs me about nausea (absent, however there had been two episodes of vomiting), thirst (strong), and bowel movements (a tendency to constipation); I ask if he can relate the beginning of the hiccuping to something that may have occurred. 'A fit of anger', he responds.

Observing his physique, he seems strong, although his state of weariness is evident. The tongue is red with a greasy yellow coating, the pulse is full on the right and strong on the left.

Diagnosis
Anger that causes *qi* to rise.

Therapeutic Principles
Regulate perversely rising *qi*.

Treatment
First treatment:

---

[67] Li Zhongzi, *Yizong bidu* ('Essential readings of the medical tradition', 1637). Similarly: 'The heart is threatened so the gall bladder becomes cowardly.' In: Cheng Guopeng, *Yixue xinwu* ('Medicine revelations, 1732). The relation with this heart *qi* and with the fright also pass through the closeness of sovereign fire and minister fire: 'When the fright-*jing* 惊 hits, from the heart it immediately reaches the gall bladder and the gall bladder reaches the liver, it follows that the sovereign fire *junhuo* 君火 ruled by the heart and the wood-wind of the liver and gall bladder minister fire *xianghuo* 相火 suddenly rise. This because the fright received from the outside moves the wood, fire, wind on the inside.' In: Ye Tianshi, *Lingzhen zhinan yian* ('Guide cases in clinic', 1766).
[68] For a discussion on the current interest in this concept and its clinical application see also the work by Qiao Wenlei in Chapter 18.

- LIV-3 *Taichong*, LIV-2 *Xingjian*

During the treatment, the hiccuping calms down. The next morning the patient mentions that it disappeared for three hours after the treatment, but started again in the evening and during the night, albeit in a lighter form, and in the morning it became rare.

Second Treatment:

- LIV-3 *Taichong*, LIV-2 *Xingjian*, BL-17 *Geshu*

Since it is Friday and at the moment I have no space to fix an appointment for the next week, I tell him to call me on Monday to see what can be arranged.

I do not hear from him, but at the end of the week I see his sister, who tells me that he no longer has the hiccups.

Comments

The primary points for hiccups are generally different, but in this case the precision of his answers guided me in the direction of liver *qi*, which appeared to have reversed its normal flow.

From the few indications gathered and the brief interaction that we had, it seemed probable that lifestyle, psychological and emotional balance and *qi* all suffered from constraint-*yu* and stagnation-*zhi*. An event that had generated strong anger had knocked the system off-balance, further knotting-*jie* the *qi* and unleashing a violent counterflow-*ni*, which also manifested physically as contraction of the diaphragm, causing hiccuping.

The internal path of the liver channel enters the abdominal cavity, circumvents the stomach, connects to the gall bladder and liver, and ascends past the diaphragm into the hypochondria: by choosing two points on the same channel, the effect on the *qi* is strengthened.

In the first treatment the stimulation of the two points was quite substantial, with the intention of regulating *qi*, liberating its constraints and guiding it downwards.

In the second treatment I used a gentler stimulation, attempting to consolidate the proper movement of *qi* and furthermore to free the diaphragm by acting upon its *shu* point, which was also indicated by the location of the burning symptom.

Follow-up

At an interval of 3 weeks, the symptom has not reappeared.

Case Study 2.2

When Mood Improves by Moving *Qi*

This patient, a 53-year-old chemist, is sent to me for a problem of trigger finger that began 8 to 9 months previously without any apparent cause or correlations.

Functional impediment and pain are present when moving the interphalangeal joint of the index finger of the right hand.

During the examination, intestinal disorders such as borborygmi, swelling, and flatulence are revealed, although the pain has become more sporadic since the patient has reduced his consumption of bread, dairy products and sugar; bowel movements are regular. He also presents non-itching rashes that appear only in the area of the cheekbones and which recede after taking antibiotics (amoxicillin). Appetite and sleep are good.

The tongue is lightly tooth marked with a thin yellow coating at the base and two skinned zones in the liver and gall bladder area. The pulse is full and rapid.

Diagnosis

Blood stasis and *qi* stagnation in the right lung channel.

Qi stagnation with heat and dampness in the viscera and in the stomach channel.

Therapeutic Principles

Circulate blood and *qi* in the lung *jingluo*; activate and regulate stomach *qi* and release dampness-heat.

Treatment

First to third treatment at an interval of 2–3 days:
- LI-4 *Hegu*, LU-11 *Shaoshang*, LU-10 *Yuji*, LU-7 *Lieque* (all one sided)

To activate *qi* and blood in the directly involved channel and its paired channel.

The flexing–extension of the finger has already returned to normal by the second treatment and no longer jerks, and in the third session all that remains is a light pain during forced extension.

Fourth to Tenth Treatment, With Weekly Frequency
- LI-4 *Hegu*, LU-11 *Shaoshang*, LU-10 *Yuji*, LU-7 *Lieque*
- ST-2 *Sibai*, SI-25 *Tianshu*, ST-36 *Zusanli* and ST-44 *Neiting* (or ST-37 *Shangjuxu* together with ST-39 *Xiajuxu*), SP-4 *Gongsun*, P-6 *Neiguan*, Ren-6 Qihai.

The ST-44 *Neiting ying* point activates the *qi* in the channel and is supported by ST-36 *Zusanli* and ST-25 *Tianshu*, while it is guided towards its cutaneous zone by the local point ST-2 *Sibai*.

ST-36 *Zusanli*, ST-37 *Shangjuxu* and ST-39 *Xiajuxu* are the lower *he* points of the main *fu*-bowels involved and they release heat-dampness, an action shared by ST-25 *Tianshu*, which together with Ren-6 *Qihai* regulates *qi* and resolves stagnation.

The two *luo* help activate the flow of *qi*, with a specific effect on the *Chong Mai* – the extraordinary vessel most implicated in these digestive disorders – and the involvement of the *shen*.

From the fifth session onwards, he no longer has any dermatological manifestations, the movement of the finger is normal, and flatulence and abdominal swelling are markedly diminished. The intestinal disorders still appear with certain foods (he loves onions and baked peppers), but he pays more attention in general to what he eats.

Normally, I attempt to summarise the situation at a certain point during the therapy; generally this is in response to a specific request on the part of the patient, or when the treatment cycle is finished and I foresee only one concluding session, or, in chronic illness, before interrupting the treatment, for instance over a holiday. This point of review also includes the psychological aspects, which may not have previously been mentioned specifically and which I purposely do not solicit directly.

During the ninth session, 2 months after the first treatment, I ask: 'What do you think of your general mood?'

Response: 'I didn't intend to say anything, but it seems to me that it has improved greatly, and I feel better. I always slept well, but now I sleep better, maybe due to the fact that I am less weighted down, having eliminated various foods.'

Comments

During the first three sessions, the treatment is restricted to the specific problem in the involved channel. Only later, when considering the results obtained, is a more general intervention considered.

During the subsequent seven sessions in which the points for the lung channel are retained, the stimulation used is, however, of lower intensity since the strength of the manipulation is less important than the intent, as the initially pressing call for *qi* has now become more of a memory of a problem which may still persist.

The releasing of *qi* stagnation and clearing of heat-dampness are performed through action on the stomach channel, whose disorders manifest themselves both on the level of the viscera and through cutaneous signs.

This case does not have particularly important psychological aspects; however, it is presented here specifically because it is one of those truly innumerable examples in which a treatment that takes its cue only from somatic symptoms actually has effects at various levels (in this regard, please see the notes on the psychological effects of acupuncture in Chapter 16).

As often happens, this patient already knew what would be considered more proper behaviour, for example regarding eating habits; what he acquired was the possibility to put them into action.

Another interesting element is that, although he initially defined himself as a person who is not impatient, anxious or who mulls over things, he now considers his mood to be generally improved.

Follow-up

After 6 months, I see the patient again for a pain in the elbow: his mood has remained good, he has had no further disorders in the face or abdomen and he continues to eat properly.

His tongue is still slightly tooth marked and continues to have a thin yellow coating at the root, but the two areas of skinning have disappeared and the pulse is full.[69]

---

[69] A swelling due to an accumulation of liquid had appeared on his right elbow 2 weeks earlier; this accumulation had already been drained twice, but it had reformed and now presented as a painless and non reddened mass of 7 cm. We proceed with four treatments in the space of a week (after which New Year's holidays begin) using points on the channel and points adjacent to the mass, which is rapidly reduced due to reabsorption of the liquid. In January the patient confirms that the syndrome has regressed and the joint has returned to normal.

The Psychic Souls:
Shen, Hun, Po, Yi and *Zhi*

3

Translating or defining the terms *shen* (神), *hun* (魂), *po* (魄), *yi* (意) and *zhi* (志) is extremely difficult, not only owing to the absence of corresponding concepts in our culture, but also because these terms are in themselves polysemous, in that their meaning varies according to the context in which they are found.

An initial level of complexity relates to the fact that *shen, hun, po, yi* and *zhi* appear not only in the context of traditional medicine, but also in philosophical thought as well as certain aspects of popular belief systems. In all these cases, the concepts refer to psychic aspects of life, possessing a range of meanings that extend from the field of human physiopathology through to forces that almost have the status of autonomous entities.

SHEN

As will be better seen later in the text, there are many possible examples of this multiversity. Legends and stories of different periods and places are animated by *shen*; the practising Daoists who withdrew to the mountains carried a mirror to reveal *shen*-foxes hiding themselves behind visions; the precocity with which the Emperor Huang Di started speaking was a sign of an extraordinary *shen*; the most ancient medical text tells us that in the absence of *shen* it is useless to attempt to heal a patient; *shen* harmonises emotions, governs consciousness and allows perception; *shen*, being antecedent to definition and shape, transcends *yin* and *yang*.

In all of these very different contexts the same term *shen* is used; however even the translation of an apparently simple phrase such as '*shen* of man' immediately presents dilemmas. For example, since the Chinese language does not define whether a noun is singular or plural, we have to choose whether to say 'spirit' or 'spirits' of man. If even a grammatical choice already implies a particular interpretion, then every other semantic choice further narrows the concept in a specific direction.

Furthermore, there is an intrinsical ambiguity in all the terms used to describe the less tangible aspects of man, since the more significance a word possesses, the wider is its range of meanings – if for no other reason than the fact that it is used in diverse theoretical structures, in different historical periods and in world images that do not necessarily overlap.

Just as the terms '*yin*' and '*yang*' are not normally translated, so we can keep the use of the term '*shen*'; however, we still need to know what it refers to.

Etymologically, the ideogram *shen* is formed by the phonetic part *shen* 'explain' and the root *shi* 'show, indicate', which in the ancient character was composed of two horizontal lines (the heavens) from which three lines come down (that which descends from heaven). Contemporary Chinese dictionaries translate *shen* as: 1. 'divinity, god'; 2. 'spirit, mind'; 3. 'supernatural, magical'; 4. 'expression, look'; 5. 'vigorous, intelligent'; 6. 'vitality, energy'.[1]

French authors for the most part use '*les esprits*', in the plural form; many Anglo-Saxons, including Wiseman, translate *shen* as *spirit*, while others use the term *mind*, defining instead as *spirit* the whole group of the five *shen*. 'Individual configurative power', on the other hand, is the translation chosen by the German sinologist Porkert.[2]

Shen as an Extraordinary or Transcendent Aspect

Shen has no definition nor limits; it precedes *yin* and *yang*.

The *Yijing*[3] states: 'That which is beyond *yin* and *yang* is called *shen*' and similarly the *Suwen* states (Chapter 66): 'The birth of things is called transformation, the limit of things is called mutation, the immeasurable of *yin* and *yang* is called *shen*.'

Shen refers to a different universe from the one that manifests in the imminent world, to which the movement of *yin* and *yang* and the ten thousand things also belong.

In a wider sense *shen* is understood as a transcendent aspect of the universe and man. The term had already been used in this sense in early philosophical texts to describe that which is transcendent in the universe: the divinity to

---

[1] The radical *shi* (示), 'to indicate, omen' recurs continuously in the characters that concern rites and sacredness and in the ancient form in the shape of a simple T used in oracle bones it probably represented an altar with sacrifices (Karlgren p. 868 and 882; Weiger 3d).
[2] Respectively in: Granet, 1934; Faubert, 1974; Eyssalet, 1990; Larre and Rochat de la Vallée, 1992; Wiseman and Ye, 1998; Maciocia, 1989; Porkert, 1974.
[3] *Yijing* ('Classic of Changes'), '*Dazhuan*' ('Great Comment'). Also see in this regard the clinical contribution of Zhang Shijie, Chapter 23.

whom sacrifices are offered, the spirits that populate the earth, and strange and mysterious natural phenomenon.

The Confucian classic on rites defines *shen* as 'all the strange things' that are seen in mountains, forests, streams, valleys, and on the hills where clouds, wind and rain rise.

Xunzi, describing the movement of the heavenly bodies, the cycle of the four seasons, the transformation of *yin* and *yang* and of the ten thousand things, says: 'That whose effects are seen, even while it itself can not be seen, this is what we call *shen*', and further on he speaks of a *shen* that belongs to man once his body is completely formed.[4]

That which in humans, goes beyond the normal, which is extraordinary is also an expression of *shen*; philosophical texts refer to this superior knowledge and define the sage as a *shen*-man; they consider *shen* as the highest level of the virtue/power-*de*, and they describe *shen* as 'knowing that which others do not know'.[5]

The nature of the extraordinary capabilities identified with *shen* varies depending on what different traditions consider most important. For instance, tradition has it that Confucius described the emperor Huang Di as someone whose *shen* was so powerful from birth that he already knew how to speak as an infant. Growing up he became sincere and intelligent, and in maturity was sagacious and wise.[6]

In a more general sense the term is comparable to the Greek term *daimon*. '*Shen* is used more as a conditional verb than a noun, to indicate the power and intellectual capabilities that radiate from a person or thing.'[7]

In the medical texts *shen* also appears as a divine–spiritual aspect of man, for example when comparing the normal way of diagnosis, called *xing* (形) ('form' in the sense of 'tangible'), and the *shen* way – sudden revelation after intense mental concentration while ignoring irrelevant signs in order to remain mentally open and clear, so that intuition may arrive 'like the wind that blows away the clouds'.[8]

Shen is thus both a quality possessed by the doctor and that which the doctor must observe in the patient and upon which he must act. The

---

[4] The *Liji* ('Memories of the rites'), probably older than the 4th century BC, is one of the six Confucian classics and Xunzi who lived in the 3rd century BC, is one of the principal exponents of early Confucianism.
[5] Respectively in *Zhuangzi*, a text which takes its name from the famous Daoist master Zhuangzi, who lived in the 4th century BC; Mengzi or Mencius, who lived at the beginning of the 4th century BC; *Huainanzi*, a Daoist text compiled by court members of the prince of Huainan around 140 BC
[6] This description is also found in the *Liji*. Huang Di, the Yellow Emperor, is the mythical figure to whom the title of the classical text *Huang Di Neijing* refers. Already present in sources of the 4th century BC, it is to him that the teaching of medicine, the invention of the calendar, and wheeled vehicles are attributed, while the discovery of the breeding of the silk worm is attributed to his wife.
[7] A.C. Graham, 1999, page 133.
[8] *Suwen*, Chapter 26. See also discussion in Chapter 15 on the space shared by the patient and the acupuncturist.

Neijing begins by stating that 'a capable doctor is the one who can see the patient's *shen*'.[9]

Shen as Vitality

As such, *shen* is therefore identified with those aspects of the human that are closest to the transcendental. However, it is also simply what allows life; it is the 'basis of life', and there is death when it leaves the body. It is therefore the difference between life and death: 'He who has *shen* lives; he who loses it dies'.[10]

Shen does not simply influence mental conditions, but it also makes 'the eyes bright, the words clear, the complexion beautiful and the breath regular'.[11] The vitality of people can be seen in the *shen* of their eyes; the *shen* of the pulse is an important prognostic sign.[12]

Qi Bo's description of the origin of *shen* is quite interesting in his answer to the emperor's question on *shen* and on the various energies and possible physical and psychic disorders: 'That which heaven gives man is the power/virtue-*de*, that which the earth gives man is *qi*; *de* and *qi* move towards each other, then there is life; the origin of life is called *jing*, when the two *jings* mutually grasp each other this is called *shen*.'[13]

The passage therefore starts by describing two principles of universal order, which produce life as they move towards each other, and continues by attributing the origins of life to *jing*, which is a more human element – matter of a denser quality. The joining of the two *jings* (generally interpreted as the joining of the essence of father and mother) produces *shen*; *shen* relates therefore to a specific point in time and space and gives birth to human existence. This is followed by the description of the process of individualisation discussed later.

Man is an individual and functioning being when all the aspects of *qi* are present and interacting, as Qi Bo explains: 'What is *shen*?' 'A man is formed when *qi* and blood harmonise, nutritive *qi* and defensive *qi* communicate, the five *zang* organs take shape, *shen* settles in the heart, *hun* and *po* are both present'.[14]

---

[9] *Lingshu*, Chapter 1.
[10] *Lingshu*, Chapter 54. The references to shen as 'foundation of life' are also found in texts that are not mainly medical, such as *Shiji*, ('Historical Memories of Sima Qian'), text of the Western Han period (206 BC–24 AD).
[11] *Suwen*, Chapter 13.
[12] If the pulse shows 'shen, stomach and root' it is a good sign, also in cases of severe illnesses (on this subject see also Appendix A on classical pulses). Tongue and skin colour are also referred to as 'having *shen*'.
[13] *Lingshu*, Chapter 8. Similarly in *Lingshu* Chapter 30: 'The two *shen* meet, join together and the form stems from their union; such a substance, which comes before the body, is called *jing*'. For a discussion on the term *de* 德 'power, virtue' see Chapter 1.
[14] *Lingshu*, Chapter 54.

These very concise images show us the fundamental aspects which define man: the balancing of *yin* and *yang* (expressed in physiology as *qi* and blood), the interaction between the more internal and the more external energies (*yingqi* and *weiqi*), the performing of various functions (*zangfu*), the presence of psychic activity (*hun* and *po*) and the settling of *shen* in the heart.

Shen as an Aspect of Physiology

In the sphere of physiology, *shen* is *qi* – in its most refined form – and its root is *jing*.[15] *Qi, jing* and *shen* are called 'the three treasures'; the conservation and nourishment of *jing* are fundamental for a long life, in which the light of *shen* shines forth.[16]

Shen resides in the *zang* organs and it is stored specifically in the heart. It is injured if these organs are injured and in turn influences *qi, jing,* and the organs.[17] It is formed when maternal and paternal *jing* join ('pre-heaven') and draws nourishment from the pure *qi* of air and food ('post-heaven').

Shen has cognitive functions: intelligence, awareness, thought, reasoning, judgment, and consciousness all depend on *shen*. Wisdom and intuitive knowledge originate from its integrating function.

It harmonises and governs the world of feelings, and if the emotions reach the degree where they injure the *shen* this can alter or constrain the flow of *qi*, exhaust or disperse *jing*, damage the organs, and cause disorder and agitation of the psychic aspects *hun* and *po, yi* and *zhi*.

This emotional activity of *shen* was already recognised in the *Jiayijing*, which considers the emotions as a type of exteriorisation of the heart, in whose interior *shen* resides: '*Shen* resides in the heart; the external movement of the nature of the heart is called the emotions'.[18]

Lastly, perception also depends on *shen*: it is through *shen* that the senses unfold their functions; for example: 'the nose relies on the lungs, but its functions depend on the heart'.[19]

---

[15] Li Dongyuan highlights the fact that *jing* and *shen* originate from the *qi* and that the *qi* nourishes them and keeps them connected to the plant – it is both the root and the petiole; 'The *qi* is the ancestor of the *shen*, the *jing* is the son of the *qi*, the *qi* is the root and the petiole of *jing* and *shen*. It is necessary to accumulate *qi* for it to become *jing*, to accumulate *jing* to maintain the *shen* intact, to purify and calm and protect the *shen* with the *dao*.' In: *Piweilun* ('Treatise on spleen and stomach', 1249), chapter 'Shengyan' ('Saving words').

[16] 'If we treasure the *jing*, the *shen* shines, if the *shen* shines it will have a long life.' Cao Xiaozhong, *Shenji zonglu* (Imperial Medicine Encyclopaedia, 1117).

[17] See also the discussion on the relationship between emotions, organs and *shen* in Chapter 5 on emotions.

[18] Huangfu Mi, *Zhenjiu jiayijing* (The systematic classic of Acupuncture and Moxibustion, 282). This is the first work specifically on acupuncture and the quote is taken from the comment to Chapter 31 of the *Suwen*, called 'Yijing bianqi' ('Modifying the *jing* and changing the *qi*').

[19] *Nanjing*, Chapter 14.

The Five *Shen*

In traditional medical thought also, *shen* appears as a polysemous term with interwoven but also distinct meanings.

First, *shen, hun* and *po, yi* and *zhi* are specific psychic aspects or 'souls' of the individual organs: 'the heart stores *shen*, the lungs *po*, the liver *hun*, the spleen *yi*, and the kidney *zhi*'.[20]

It is also said that: '*Hun, shen, po, yi* and *zhi* take *shen* as their ruler, therefore they are called *shen*' and that 'the *shen* of the heart gathers itself and unites *hun* and *po* and combines with yi and *zhi*.'[21] In this sense *shen* is singular – the 'ruler' that resides in the heart, the 'emperor' of the organs – but there is another level in which the five *shen* that reside and are stored in the five *zang* organs, share an equal status.

This latter is the sense in which the five *shen* are inserted into the system of *wuxing*, in analogical correspondence with the five organs, directions, seasons, moments of the day, climates, colours, tastes, odours, sense organs, body tissues, emotions, etc.

Therefore, *shen* can, on the one hand, be seen as that which gathers and integrates, and can be articulated within the system of five psychic aspects, or from another perspective a person's *shen* can be seen as the individual expression of a more universal *shen*, in which *po* and *hun* constitute a pair with *yin* and *yang* polarity – partially autonomous forces that act upon the individual – while *yi* and *zhi* relate to a sort of unfolding of the subject in the world.

HUN AND *PO*

Po (魄) and *hun* (魂) are translated in contemporary Chinese dictionaries respectively as: 1. 'soul'; 2. 'vigour'; and 1. 'soul'; 2. 'spirit, mood'.[22]

Po contains the radical *gui*-ghost, preceded by the phonetic part *bai*-white, which is the colour of the element metal–lung–autumn, related to *po*.

Hun contains the same radical *gui*-ghost, preceded by the phonetic part *yun*, the same as 'cloud' and 'talk' and also the same as 'colza seed, to roll'; therefore it has a strong idea of movement (just as, on the other hand, it has the element connected with *hun*, that is, wind–liver–spring).

---

[20] *Suwen*, Chapter 23.
[21] Respectively in the comment which today is considered to be the closest to the original text of the *Neijing Suwen*, the *Huang Di neijing taisu*, by Yang Shangshan of the Sui period, and in Yu Chang's text of the Ming period *Yimen falu* (Principles and prohibitions of the medical practice).
[22] N. Wiseman *Chinese–English Dictionary*, 1991.

French authors traditionally use the term *entites viscerales*, while Anglo-Saxons generally translate them as *corporeal and ethereal souls*. Porkert defines them as 'specific structural and active forces'.[23]

The concepts of *hun* and *po* appear in the first medical classics through very concise yet extremely meaningful references; they reappear in the course of medical history in a non-systematic, yet suggestive way; they seem to find little space in theoretical discussion and contemporary clinical work.

Like *shen*, both *hun* and *po* are also terms that derive from an established philosophical discourse preceding the first medical texts and they were as forces well-recognised inside the belief system, with their own specific cults and ceremonies.

As forms of *qi* are essentially connected to psychic life they belong to the individual, but at the same time have strongly impersonal aspects.

Earth and Heaven

Po and *hun* are also a pair of opposite polarity which mutually influence each other; sometimes we also find them connected with other pairs such as earth–heaven, *yin–yang*, *jing–qi*, *jing–shen*, shape–*qi* and *ling–shen*.[24]

Yin, whose character represents the shady side of a hill, represents night, stillness, the interior, humidity, density, matter and earth; *po* is called 'the *qi* of earth' whereas *hun* is the '*qi* of heaven'. *Yang*, the sunny side of the hill, represents movement and subtle energy.

The most complete and suggestive description is probably that by Zhu Xi: '*Hun* is *shen*, *po* is *ling*; *hun* is *yang*, *po* is *yin*; *hun* is movement, *po* is stillness. At birth *hun* enters *po* and *po* encloses *hun*; at death *hun* disperses, fluctuating and returning to heaven, *po* falls, sinking and returning to earth. When man is born *hun* and *po* unite, at death they separate. That which moves and acts is *hun*, that which does not move and does not act is *po*. The dark side of the moon is *po*, its light is *hun*; *Hun* is the flame of *po*, *po* is the root of *hun*. Fire is *hun*, the mirror is *po*; the lantern has fire, matter is burned by it. The mirror reflects the images, which are, however, on the inside. The flame of the fire is external light, the water of metal is internal light; one is *hun*, the other is *po*. *Yin* governs concentration and gathering, therefore *po* can record and

---

[23] Wiseman also proposes 'animal soul' as a synonym of *hun*. The bibliographic references are identical to those suggested for the term *shen*.

[24] In its full form the character *ling* 灵 is composed of *wu* 巫 'sorceress' and of the phonetic part *ling*, in its turn composed of 'rain' and of three drops. It has similar translation to *shen*: 1. 'spirit', 2. 'intelligent', 3. 'effective', 4. ' mysterious', 5. 'elf', but it also differs from it because of its closer bond with materiality. It can refer to talents, capacities or specific abilities, but it is also the spirit of things (for example, *hualing* 'spirit of the plants') and the way they manifest themselves.

remember on the inside, *yang* governs movement and action, therefore *hun* can give rise to action'.[25]

So *po* is the dark side of the moon, and *hun* the bright side. Just as *yin* nourishes *yang* and *yang* moves *yin*, so *po* and *hun* are respectively the root and flame of each other. It is also interesting to note the stress given in this text to the internal function: the mirror reflects images that in reality are on the inside.

Po and *hun* appear as partially autonomous forces that join in the single individual and separate at death. They are that which is still and that which moves, respectively in relationship with the denser body and the subtler *qi*.

There is a *yin* and a *yang* aspect in everything: *yang* is a subtle aspect which in *qi* is called *shen* and in the body is called *ling*, therefore even the most dense matter has its own spirit-*ling*, through which it can, for example, 'record and remember internally'.

Po is also that through which the body relates to the outside world, that which allows it to perceive, to move and to express itself: 'at the moment of birth the perception of the eyes and the ears, the movement of the hands and the feet, the sound of crying and breathing, all this belongs to *ling* and *po*. The *shen* which is based on *qi* is instead the thought and consciousness acquired progressively.[26] This type of intelligence, of consciousness and memory of the body is present throughout one's entire life and it moulds its quality. If *po* is vigorous then the eyes are sharp and clear and one is able to remember; in the aged who have dull eyes, dull ears and poor memory, this is due to weakened *po*'.[27]

Po and *Jing*

The description of the genesis of *shen* in the 'Benshen' chapter continues confirming the fundamental ties between *po* and *jing*, which is the most ancestral aspect of *qi*: 'That which exits and enters with *jing* is *po*'.[28]

Po therefore refers back to *jing*, the vital pre-heaven essence – a denser aspect than *qi*, a profound quintessence that is inherited through parents and ancestors and defines our constitutional set.

Jing and *po*, *qi* and *hun* can grow through correct lifestyle, but they are also subject to exhaustion: 'The two are not separated at the root, therefore if *jing*

---

[25] The quote is ascribed to Zhu Xi taken from Zhang Jiebin in the *Leijing* ('The classic of categories', 1624), book III, Chapter 14. Zhu Xi (1130–1200) belonged to the School of Principle-*li*, which resumed the Confucian theories with a deep influence by Buddhism.
[26] Kong Yida (574–648), *Wujing zhengyi* ('The correct meaning of the five classics'). Zhuangzi is said to have declared: 'That of the *xing*-shape which rests upon *ling* is called *po*, that of the *qi* which rests upon *shen* is called *hun*.'
[27] Zhu Xi, quoted by Zhang Jiebin, *Leijing* ('The classic of categories', 1624), book III, Chapter 14.
[28] *Lingshu*, Chapter 8.

accumulates, *po* also accumulates, if *qi* accumulates then *hun* accumulates, and this is man; when *jing* is exhausted and *po* collapses, then *qi* scatters, *hun* floats and one no longer is aware of anything'.[29]

Po – which relates to *jing* and to form – has a particular relevance during intrauterine life and, even though *hun* is also present from the third lunar month onward, performs the main functions. It is said that it enters the embryo on the third day (an analogy with the crescent moon that appears on the third day) and the seven *pos* are believed to be established by the *ling* of *yin* in the fourth month of gestation. The maternal *po* supports that of the embryo and fetus until the eighth month, when the latter becomes autonomous and is allowed 'to wander'.

Po resides in the lungs. In the cycle of the five elements it corresponds to the rise of *yin* within *yang*, to the west, to sundown – that is, the process of densification of *qi*. In this phase *qi* tends to assume a shape, with a framing and structuring movement. In the system of analogies and resonances the tissue that corresponds to lung–metal is the skin, a system of exchange with the exterior and at the same time a limit of the body.

Po is certainly an 'earth' force, tied to concrete forms and to the body. This constituting of dense forms that is a precondition of individual life is, however, also that which tends to separate and distance the individual from the original all: *po* contains the germs of death, but bones and flesh are potentially already death.

These aspects are particularly present in Daoist texts that aim to overcome the frailness of mortal form through internal alchemical practices: '*po* is *yin*, the deep and turbid part of *yin*, it relies on the heart of what has a form-*xing*; *po* turns towards death, everything that loves the colour and movement of *qi* is *po*, *po* after death benefits from blood'.[30]

The same chapter, however, notes the importance of this more material aspect that allows a consciousness and a continuity in time: 'Men create their bodies with intent-*yi*, the body is not limited to the seven feet that make up the body, in the centre of the body is *po*, *po* attaches to the conscience-*shi* and therefore acts, the conscience rests on the body and is therefore born; *po* is *yin*, it is the substance of the conscience; the conscience is not interrupted, it creates and continues to create in the centuries and centuries; the changes of the form of *po* and the transformations of matter do not stop'.[31]

---

[29] Xhu Xi, quoted in Zhang Jiebin, *Leijing*, book III, Chapter 14. We recall: '*Jing* is the root of life' (*Suwen*, Chapter 4); 'At the beginning of a man's life the *jing* is formed first, after the *jing* the brain and marrow form' (*Lingshu*, Chapter 10); 'the kidney receives the *jing* of the five organs and of the six viscera and preserves it' (*Suwen*, Chapter 1).

[30] *Taiyi jinhua*, Chapter 2. It has been passed on orally for centuries (it was printed for the first time in the 19th century) and translated and commented by Wilhelm and Jung in 1929 (*The Secret of the Golden Flower*). The term 'colours' refers to all the pleasures of the senses, while 'benefiting from the blood' refers to ritual offerings.

[31] *Taiyi jinhua*, Chapter 2. In the Zhou system the 'foot' corresponds to 10 *cun* 'thumbs' (that is 19.9 cm).

Other texts allot a higher value to *hun* than to *po*: 'In the light and transparent, *po* conforms to hun, which ascends; in the heavy and turbid, *hun* conforms to *po*, which descends. The sages restrain *po* through *hun*, common men use *po* to absorb *hun*'.[32]

Hun is the *yang* aspect, the fire; it accompanies *shen*, it moves and acts whereas *po* remains still. It can be construed as the 'spirit' of acting rather than actual movement in a concrete sense, so much so that it is said: '*yang* governs movement and action; therefore *hun* can give rise to action'.[33] *Hun* allows us to move freely in the world of thought, imagination and sensations.

If we see *po* as the body, or more accurately as the 'spirit of the body', as consciousness through the body, then *hun* is situated at the opposite pole, it is the extreme of thought: that which one comes to know through imagination, the movement of dreams: 'In dreams there is activity, but the body does not act in accordance with it, this is the movement and the stillness of *hun* and *po*; the movement is *hun* and the stillness is *po*'.[34]

'*Hun* lives in the eyes during the day, in the night it resides in the liver; when it lives in the eyes it sees, when it resides in the liver it dreams. Dreams are the wandering of *hun* through the nine heavens and the nine earths'.[35]

Although similar to *shen*, *hun* differs from it because it is less integrated: the attributes of *shen* are brightness, clarity, consciousness and intelligence; while fluctuating, dreaming, hallucinatory and visionary states belong to *hun*.

Hun follows *shen*; therefore if *shen* is not still, integrated and well rooted then *hun* wanders. 'If we say that *shen* and *hun* are both *yang*, what does it mean that *hun* comes and goes following *shen*? The virtue-*de* of *shen* belongs to the category of brightness, clarity and consciousness. If we speak instead of *hun*, the states of dreaming and sleeping, floating and absentmindedness and mutating hallucinations belong to it. *Shen* is stored in the heart, therefore if the heart is calm *shen* is pure; *hun* follows *shen*, therefore if *shen* loses consciousness then *hun* wanders'.[36]

---

[32] *Xingming guizhi* ('Precious compendium of nature and fate'), chapter 'Hunposhuo' ('Discourse on *hun* and *po*'). We do not know the exact date of the text; the first manuscript version is by Yin Zhenren, a master of the Ming period.
[33] Zhang Jiebin, *Leijing*, Book III, Chapter 14.
[34] *Ibidem*.
[35] *Taiyi jinhua*, Chapter 2. Likewise: 'When *hun* is in the eyes it allows us to see, when it is in the liver it makes us dream.' In: *Xingming guizhi*, chapter 'Hunposhuo' ('Discourse on *hun* and *po*').
[36] Zhang Jiebin, *Leijing*, Book III, Chapter 14.

Gui-Ghost

The character *gui* (鬼) is translated in contemporary dictionaries as: 1. 'ghost, spirit, secret'; 2. 'terrible, evil, damned, clever'[37]

The ancient character represents a vaporous human form: a ghost. It represents man after death, the spirits or ghosts. After the introduction of Buddhism it also represented demons called *preta*.

In the medical classics the term *shengui* refers to deep psychic alterations, hallucinations and delirium.[38]

In state and family cults, sacrifices are offered to *gui* and *shen*, which are the spirits of dead humans, just as they are offered to the mountains and rivers. In the classics we find *gui* as 'spirits of the earth', in opposition to *shen*, the 'spirits of the heavens'.[39]

At the moment of death, while the decomposition of the tissues takes place, the *po* withdraws ever more deeply, into the areas which are more *yin*, all the way to the bones, but it continues to maintain a certain existence; it remains in the corpse, mainly in the bones, and it dissolves into the earth together with it. The corpses of fantasy stories are animated by *po*. 'The five flavours, turbid and humid, form the shape, the bones, the flesh, the blood, the vessels, the six emotions-*qing*; these *gui* are called *po*, *po* are feminine; they enter and exit through the mouth; they communicate with the earth.'[40]

Granet recalls that *gui* can exit from the inferior world through the cracks produced by the sun. In other words, they exit from the depths of the earth following a trauma, a tremor of the terrain, and in such cases it is necessary to pacify them and have them return to the earth by performing sacrifices that nourish them.

'One speaks of *gui* when an unexpected, disturbing, illicit manifestation occurs. The sages do not believe that the rocks speak, that the dragons fight

---

[37] Wieger p. 40c, Karlgren p. 460. Different authors of the French School insist on the euphony between *gui* 'ghost, spirit' and *gui* 'to return', but the two terms are written in a completely different way and they also have a different tone (under *gui* one can enumerate 88 different characters, among which are other equally charming terms that share also the third tone, such as: path, scheme, to preserve, a ceremonial vase, the tenth Heavenly Branch and a type of shade).

[38] On this issue see also Chapter 8 on madness-*diankuan*.

[39] For example in the Book of the Rituals we read: '*Qi* is the fullness of *shen*, *po* is the fullness of *gui*.' In: *Liji*, Chapter 24. 'Their knowledge could compare that which was due to the higher and to the lower ones; their wisdom could lighten them up from far away and make them visible; their sight could recognise them in all their magnificence; their hearing could distinguish their voices. The luminous *shen* would then descend upon them, on the men and on the women called shamans.' In: *Guoyu*, 18.559, quoted in Graham, 1999, p. 132.

[40] *He Shangong*. It is the most ancient text commenting the *Daodejing* and it owes its name to He Shangong, a Daoist master who possibly lived in the fourth century AD. Flavours have *yin* qualities, they belong to food, earth and they shape the body and organs, they are more dense and damp than smells and air. Here emotions are also linked to a more *yin* aspect of the essence of the five organs: 'The genes of the five natures are called *hun*, they are masculine (in gender); the demons of the six passions are called *po*, they are feminine (in gender).' Authors such as Eyssalet interpret the tradition with a strong connotation as in this case where he translates the terms *gui* as 'génie', masculine and *po* as 'démon', feminine (Eyssalet, 1990, p. 468).

and battle or that the dead return to kill their enemies. This last case is the most frequent; the sages calm the public's emotions by authorising a sacrifice: every being that eats is placated.'[41] The perturbing power of the *gui* derives from this origin which is tied to the depths of the earth together with the darkness of that which has no name.

The rituals offer to the *gui* the blood that comes from raw flesh, while the *shen* are nourished by the smoke, the smells of the burning herbs, the *qi*, by that which is most subtle, released from cooked foods.

In Chinese culture the act of giving a name defines the act of belonging to the world of humans: it is said that the *shen* enters an infant at the moment it is given a name, and the names of defunct nobles are inscribed on the tablets of the ancestors so that their *shen* can receive offers according to the rituals.

Rites also define what belongs to humanity; they are rules that mark and regulate time – forms that, like words, give an order to the world. However, while for the *shen* there are ceremonies of fixed seasonal offerings with rituals in which the emperor participates, these spirits-*gui* do not receive regular tributes; they belong mainly to the confused world of popular beliefs.[42]

Clinical Hypotheses

In China when one is 'scared to death', they say that the '*hun* flies and *po* scatters'. *Hun* and *po* are therefore terms that are still part of the common language: used in relation to powerful events, their disorder is dangerous.

A description of the clinical situation is more difficult. First of all, as usual, the traditional Chinese description and the biomedical description do not coincide or overlap with respect to the way that symptoms and signs are grouped and interpreted. Therefore every concept, definition or syndrome can only be referred back to the relative theoretical model. In the same way that alterations of *po* and *hun* do not correspond to established Western psychiatric models, neither can they be assimilated into specific psychological structures.

Unfortunately, as acupuncturists, we often do not have a clear idea of the possible alterations of *hun* and *po* and their relative clinical consequences. We may not know that much about *qi*, blood, channels and organs, but by now they are like old friends with whom we are familiar: we have an image of them inside of us and a frame of reference for treatment. *Hun* and *po* remain,

---

[41] M. Granet, 1971, p. 299.
[42] According to Eyssalet this polarity expresses the constant tension and conflict between the body, the darkness, the centripetal aspect and the expansion forces, the refining of our energy and spirit, the sense of totality of the *shen*. Gui are dangerous because of their egocentric character, their fixed quality and their predisposition towards fragmentation. While the cults regarding *hun* relate to ancestors, the sacrifices for *po* relate especially to relationships among human beings. The '*gui* are the main source of our relational problems and of our problems in general.' (Eyssalet, 1990, p. 468).

however, definitely more vague and elusive concepts that leave many of us indifferent and many others somewhat frustrated.

Contemporary medical texts rarely treat the pathologies of *hun* and *po* specifically; rather, they are restricted to general discussions of man in the broadest sense, and areas where different levels of observation and practice intersect: physiology in the strictest sense, internal 'alchemical' practices of 'nourishing life', heterogeneous philosophical thoughts, and ritual ceremonies related to the cult of ancestor worship and popular beliefs. The hypotheses that follow derive therefore from classical descriptions of *hun* and *po*, from the integration of these images with the other aspects of traditional physiopathology and only lastly from the indications that come from clinical experience. These hypotheses therefore require further verification, but nevertheless we can use them as a starting point for looking at theoretical and clinical work in Chinese medicine.

As we have seen, the Chinese viewpoint recognises various *shen* in the human being, which in some ways lead back to different orders of consciousness: two of these are *po* and *hun*, of which we have described 'localisation', origin, references, functions and manifestations.

Just as in the case of the *yin–yang* pair, pathology may initially affect only *hun* or *po* individually, but the ultimate result is an alteration of the dynamic balance between the two; finally the excess of one of the pair causes it to prevail, to the point that it becomes unable to express itself through interacting with the other. The isolation of either one of the two prevents movement and produces illness, whereas the natural state is that in which *yin* and *yang* enter one into the other, so there is a flowing integration and transformation of the various components (another frame of reference would define this condition as that state in which information circulates freely and permits a continuous readjustment of the system in response to internal and external changes).

Po, which relates to the dense, to matter, in everyday language represents strength, vigour and the condition of general health.

The classics also relate the strength of the body (form) to the vigour of *po*, which accompanies *jing*, the dense essence from which the body derives. '*Jing* is a turbid and heavy matter with its own consistency; form-*xing* is made of it. *Po* is a function-*yang* that allows movement and action, the perception of pain and itching. *Jing* is born from *qi*, therefore if *qi* accumulates *jing* flourishes; *po* accompanies *jing*, therefore if the form is strong *po* is vigorous.' [43]

One can therefore see a weakening of *po* in those serious pathologies of a degenerative type, with strong genetic components in which we recognise a weakness of *jing*.

Jing is what precedes the forming of the body: 'The two *shen* meet, unite and originate the form. This substance that precedes the body is called *jing*'.[44]

---

[43] Zhang Jiebin, *Leijing* ('The classic of categories', 1624), Book III, Chapter 9.
[44] *Lingshu*, Chapter 30.

Using a different frame of reference we can draw an anology between *jing* and the genetic code, and between *po* and its phenotypical expression.

Po regards the body but does not identify itself with the body: the description of *po* which 'can register and record internally' refers to a type of consciousness which belongs to the body, which is its intelligence, its memory and its language.

Its pathologies are those in which the organism produces a dysfunctional response, for example autoimmune diseases, hypersensitivity and tumours, are pathogenic behaviours of the organism towards itself; in these conditions the body is confused, and lacks memory and recognition.[45]

In other cases dependence prevails, as if development had stopped at a symbiotic stage – that is, like a *po* that did not separate from its mother *po* and did not reach autonomy. Of course, this element of dependence can be a bare hint or feature quite strongly; it can appear in love relations or manifest itself as compulsions, such as eating disorders or drug addiction.

When *po* predominates, it can end up functioning in an internally closed circuit, losing the complementary polarity of *hun* and the integration of *shen*: this loss of movement and imagination naturally belonging to *hun* leads to clinical conditions in which elements of fixation, repetition and rigidity prevail.

These situations can seem very varied, but are linked by the sensation that only *po* exists, without the *hun* pole; we can detect disquieting repetitions in the clinical history, possibly not so much the symptoms themselves, but rather in the way they are told. The patient communicates a sensation of heaviness, when he speaks only of his symptom without being able to connect it with anything else, without being able to 'move' it in his mind. We can note an abnormal weariness in the conversation, which has an inflexibility that does not allow him to consider other possibilities or alternative routes.

Having lost the connection, interaction, and exchange with *hun*, *po* remains depleted of the movement-*hun* of thought; being incapable of integrating itself in the conscience-*shen*, it then shows only in more undifferentiated sites. In the most serious cases, *po* thinking remains as primitive, concrete thinking, with no access to the symbolic realm.

Since it is also *po* which establishes our relationship with the outside world – that which allows us to perceive, move, and express ourselves, 'the perception of eyes and ears, the movements of the hands and the feet, the sound of crying and breathing' – when a person perceives, elaborates and expresses himself only through the body, this is a sign that *po* is overwhelming and the complementary activity of imagination is relatively lacking. This situation is seen in somatic disorders, in which the person is unable to bring the suffering into

---

[45] A similar interpretation can also be found in contemporary medical texts, in which *po* is said to include also 'every compensatory function regarding the regulation of biological activities', for example in the article by Zao Youchen, in: *Liaoning zhongyi* ('Spirit therapy with traditional medicine'), 1979.

the mental realm. Therefore, it can only be expressed through the body, which then manifests the symptoms, but without the capacity of expounding on them: the passage of *po* in the *shen* is lacking.

The isolation of *po*, however, can impede the expression of *hun* and *shen* not only with regards verbal expression, but also in their actions, leading to situations where the individual acts without thinking. This dynamic can assume many different forms: it can manifest in a tendency to restlessness, that is an internal agitation which pushes one to 'do' continuously in order to relieve the anguish, to the expression of feelings using only gestures and actions rather than thought and words, the inability to explain oneself can lead to risky behaviour (violence, abuse and mistreatment towards oneself and others) and it can be seen in repetitive 'acting out' during psychotherapy sessions.[46]

If *hun* – 'the movement of dreams' and 'pertaining to the fluctuating states' – is inadequate, then all that remains is the solidity of *po*, with the various types of lack of imagination described above.

A weakness of *hun* can also cause insufficient flow of emotions: if the movement that enables the emotions to circulate is deficient, they cannot harmonise and mutually balance, and a single emotion can easily dominate, becoming inflexible and stuck.

The example of the spleen – an organ which has functions of transforming and transporting and is related in the *wuxing* system to thinking and worrying – can be helpful. Thinking means also worrying and taking charge but if the spleen does not function then digestion – of food as well as thoughts – suffers, leading to a tendency to brood, to the point of turning into a clinical obsessive–compulsive disorder.

Hun is *yang*; in various texts it is from time to time called external light, fire, the flame of *po* (which is its root), *qi* of heaven that 'governs movement and action' and is also defined as 'that which gives rise to action': these are characteristics related to the essence of movement, they express that which is furthest from matter – that is, pure mental activity.

Whereas *po* can be traced to the conscience of the body, *hun* 'belongs to dreams and sleep, trance, mutating hallucinations, fluctuating states'; it corresponds to what we know through the imagination, 'in dreams there is activity, but the body does not correspond'.

---

[46] Also called *acting out*, they indicate 'the attempt of the patient following an analytic treatment to avoid confronting himself with his unconscious conflicts, searching for solutions at the level of reality' (Galimberti, 'Psychology dictionary', *Dizionario di Psicologia*, 1992, p. 19). They show themselves both in behaviours outside the treatment and in actions such as being late for or missing sessions. In a psychoanalytic sense this type of action denies the secondary process which is characterised by stable representations that allow the deferring of the satisfaction based on the reality principle.' We have highlighted how *shen* derives from the union of the virtue-*de* of the heaven–father with the *qi* of the earth–mother. But in this case, where the law of order is denied (the fatherly is also 'the third, the outside' that breaks the dual symbiosis with the mother and opens towards the sociality) and the time deferring the desire is excluded, the imbalance of *hun* and *po* corresponds to an absence of the heaven, to an absence of the clarity of the word-law (*de*) as opposed to the darkness of the earth (the material, nourishing *qi*). It corresponds to an annihilation of time (the heaven of the round back of the turtle).

If, therefore, the equilibrium of the pair *hun/po* is lost, *hun* becomes isolated, the 'spirit of movement' which does everything by itself; its link with the denser and more material mental aspect is broken and *hun* feeds back only to itself, resulting in mental activity without any relation to actual reality.

Severed from the boundaries imposed by matter, the imagination of *hun* remains isolated, to the point of creating its own perceptions by hallucinating.[47] We can therefore see extreme pathologies of *hun* in psychotic conditions, with their hallucinatory forms. However, since *hun* follows *shen*, 'the progressively acquired consciousness', and if *shen* is lost, *hun* fluctuates and goes wandering without return, leading to a detachment from reality and logical thought – that is, to true delirium.[48]

Imbalances of *hun* are also found in less extreme but more frequent cases: we find clear traces of it where patients lose contact with internal and external reality, their responses no longer fit the situation, mood and feelings swing dangerously, and the body suffers.

In fact, *hun* is tenuous, it ascends, it tends to disperse, it 'fluctuates' when life is exhausted, and its excess can affect the body: 'Just as the flame burns matter, *hun* can consume *jing*'.[49]

This image suggests a dynamic in which an excess of thought consumes matter, losing contact with the real and concrete. This excess with regards to imaginative thought can substitute reality with illusion and block its recognition as such. It can also be identified with a sort of spirituality that denies the needs of the body, as happens in anorexic patterns. It can furthermore manifest as a rationalisation that denies the perception of emotions.

However, the potentials of *hun* and *po*, and the existence of particular states of consciousness are not merely pathologies. In the internal practices linked to mystical ecstasy, the attainment of enlightenment presupposes a state of 'empty heart' – a state through which the 'critical point between life and death' can be reached. This process is described as a separation of *yin* and *yang* (an event that normally implies death), a transformation that happens in dreams – in other words in an altered state of consciousness. In dreams one can be transformed, but in waking life one cannot: this is the separation of the unity of *yin* and *yang*; this separation comes from emptiness, whereas unity comes from fullness. This is a sign of *hun* and *po* and in reality it embodies the subtle distinction between life and death. 'If one manages to completely empty his heart,

---

[47] 'All of a sudden it as if the body is splitting into two people, but only the one self can see the other'. In: Chen Shiduo, *Shishi milu*, ('Secret notes of the stone chamber'), chapter 'Lihun' ('The leaving *Hun*').
[48] See also the systematisation of the contemporary psychiatrist Zhang Mingjiu, Chapter 21. He focuses on the relationship between *shen* and the disorders of the conscience, speech and thought (for example deliria), and between *hun*, perception disorders (classified on the basis of the alteration of time, space, own body, hallucinosis, hallucinations) and affective area disorders (indifference, paradox reactions, emotional instability, anxiousness, aggressiveness, euphoria, etc.).
[49] *Taiyi jinhua* ('The secret of the golden flower'), Chapter 2.

then it will be clear and still, and in dreams one will reach the critical point between life and death and his consciousness will reach great depths'.[50]

YI AND ZHI

In medicine, *yi* (意) and *zhi* (志) usually belong to the system of resonances and interactions of the five elements (phases) and are related respectively to the spleen and the kidney, in which each is respectively stored.[51]

However *yi* and *zhi* refer not only to the field of medicine: like *shen, hun* and *po*, the terms also represent mental states and activities belonging both to philosophical systems and to everyday language. Since these different frames of reference do not precisely overlap the terms have a number of meanings making them somewhat difficult to translate.

The Process Developed in the 'Benshen' Chapter

To see the sense of the various meanings of *yi* and *zhi*, we can start from the 'Benshen' chapter of the *Lingshu*, the first parts of which we already examined when speaking of emotions and movements of *qi*: in this context, the five *shen* are included in a process of creation, formation and structuring of thought.

Although translations and interpretations do not always dovetail perfectly, they generally agree in so far as all recognise a progression from the less specific forms like *hun* and *po* to a thought sequence that starts with the persistence of a memory, continues with the forming of an idea and its elaboration, then finally through forward planning decides on the correct course of action: 'That which comes and goes with *shen* is called *hun*, that which enters and exits with *jing* is called *po*, that which occupies itself with things is called heart, that which the heart remembers is called *yi*, the persistence of *yi* is called *zhi*, conserving and transforming through *zhi* is called thought-*si* (思), making long term projects through thought is called deliberation-*lü* (慮), dealing with things through deliberation is called wisdom-*zhi* (志).[52]

---

[50] Zhang Jiebin, *Leijing*, book III, Chapter 9.

[51] *Suwen*, Chapter 23. The term 'to store' is the translation of *cang* 藏, the same character as 'organ' *zang* 臟. But the latter usually has the radical 'flesh' in front of it (Karlgren p. 1084). In the *Nanjing* it is said that: 'The spleen stores the *yi* and the *zhi*' (Chapter 34).

[52] *Lingshu*, Chapter 8. 'To occupy oneself with, to take care of' is the translation of *ren* 任, The same character of the *Ren* channel, which is composed of a stick with two weights at its ends for transportation on shoulder and of the radical 'man'. It means 'to sustain, to take something on oneself, to occupy oneself with, to allow, to serve in a specific role' (Wieger p. 82c; Karlgren p. 934). According to Zhu Wenfeng (1987, p. 22), the role of the heart in 'taking care of things' *renwu* 任惡 expressed here corresponds to the moment when things 'are perceived' *ganzhi* 知. Larre and Rochat de la Vallée (1994, p. 69) translate: 'That which takes care of living beings is called heart'.

These passages described in the *Neijing* refer to the operations which neuropsychology calls retention of memory traces, organisation in concepts, consolidation in categorical systems, cognitive elaboration, development of hypothetical thought and operational execution.

We also find this line of interpretation in contemporary Chinese texts, for which *yi* corresponds in a more specific way to the mind's ability to grasp external reality, to register it and to transfer it into memory: 'Therefore *yi* encompasses the entire process of the forming of thought which includes the sequence of directing attention, remembering, deliberating, conjecturing, and analysing'.[53]

Yi belongs therefore to that moment when the heart – that is, the consciousness, the spirit, the emotions, the mind – enters into contact with external reality. It corresponds to the possibility of grasping images in a broad sense and keeping them over time. Yang Shangshan, the great commentator of the *Neijing*, restates the above definition: 'That which the heart that occupies itself with things remembers is called *yi*'.[54]

Inside the process of forming thought, *yi* refers in particular to that initial phase in which there is the passage from no-shape to individuation: 'We call *yi* that crucial moment of the *shen* of heart which moves but has no form'.[55]

Zhang Jiebin clearly sees *yi* as the first phase of thought, when an idea appears but is not yet stabilised: 'When a thought is first born the heart has a direction, but it is not yet stabilised, this is called *yi*'.[56]

A contemporary comment specifies: 'The image of memory left when the heart occupies itself with things that come from the outside is called *yi*'.[57]

Yi as an 'Idea' and as 'Intent'

In modern Chinese *yi* signifies: 1. 'idea, significance'; 2. 'desire, intention'; 3. 'trace, nuance, suggestion'; 4. 'attention'; 5. thinking, expecting'.

The character is composed of *yin* (音) 'sound' and the radical 'heart': this structure suggested interpretations that either stress the significance of 'that

---

[53] He Yuming, *Zhongguo chuantong jingshen binglixue* ('Mental illness pathology in Chinese medicine'), 1995, p. 34.

[54] *Yang* Shangshan, *Huangdi neijing taisu*. Larre and Rochat de la Vallée (1994, p. 75), who translate *yi* as 'intention' say: 'When the heart applies we will speak of intention' and comment: 'To apply oneself implies an active sense of approaching thought, of remembering, of recalling: from this stems the idea of a certain application of the spirit, who considers what is happening, what appears and what represents itself to him.'

[55] Wu Jian, *Yizong jinjian* ('The golden mirror of medicine'). 'Crucial moment' is the translation of *ji* 机, which means 'turn, mechanism' (Karlgren p. 328).

[56] Zhang Jiebin, *Leijing* ('Classic of categories'), Book III, Chapter 9. In this phase 'thought' is the translation of the term *nian* 念 and 'stabilised' the character *ding* 定 'to fix, calm, stable' often used with reference to the heart or mind.

[57] Guo Aichun (ed.), *Huang Di neijing lingshu jiaozhu yuyi* ('Commented and translated critical edition of the *Huang Di neijing lingshu*'), p. 81.

which resonates in the heart' or which favour the sense of 'sound-voice that comes from the heart'.[58]

In this term, therefore, two aspects are included: one belonging to the concept of idea (or significance, being derived from something significant) and the other regarding a subjective area such as intention put into action, the purpose inside action.

This is not a contradiction in Chinese thought; it shows that there is no clearcut separation between mind, its aspects regarding the impulses of the soul, and methods of application in concrete action. In this sense the ancient philosophical texts consider *yi* as cognitive intelligence that moves in with the *dao*. Graham translates *yi* as 'idea, image', but also as 'intent, intention' since the term 'includes both the image and the idea of a thing as much as the intent to act that is inseparable from it (with the single exception of abstractions such as the idea of the circle in late Moist geometry).[59]

Given the complexities of the philosophical implications of this concept, it is easy to understand why the term *yi* in medicine assumes different values and several meanings that are at times apparently distinct from each other.

Starting from the definition in the *Neijing* of 'that which the heart remembers is called *yi*' we find different meanings, pertaining to both an analytical–rational and an emotional–subjective area. *Yi*, in fact, can be translated as 'idea', 'thought', 'opinion', 'meaning', but it also means 'intention, 'proposal', 'attention', 'aspiration', 'desire' and 'feeling'.

In the *Neijing* itself the term *yi* appears not only in the sense of an image that structures itself in an idea, as described in the 'Benshen' chapter, but also in the various nuances just seen.

It assumes, for example, the value of 'meaning' in the question about the various types of needles: 'I heard of the nine chapters about the nine needles [...], I would like to understand completely its meaning-*yi*'.[60]

It becomes an expression of opinion when it is said: 'I have heard that in man there are *qi*, essence, liquids, blood, vessels; I believe-*yi* that it is all one *qi*'.[61]

The subjective component of desire and intent appears in the phrase: 'the *yi* of man's heart responds to the eight winds'.[62]

Yi is also found to refer to a feeling of an emotional order: 'When one has a belly ache it is called *jue*-turning over, the *yi* is not happy, the body is heavy, and there is restlessness.[63]

---

[58] From its structure the character *yi* 意 is translated as 'the sound of the heart' (Karlgren p. 203) or as 'the voice of the heart' in the sense of 'the intention put in the pronounced words, the ability to repeat images which present themselves to the conscience' (Larre and Rochat de la Vallée, 1994, p. 183). In Wiseman and Ye, 1998, *yi* does not appear except in *Yishe* BL-49, translated as 'reflection abode'.

[59] A. C. Graham, 1999, p. 179.

[60] *Suwen*, Chapter 27.

[61] *Lingshu*, Chapter 30.

[62] *Suwen*, Chapter 54. In modern Chinese *yixiang* 意 向 means 'intention, expectations, aspiration'.

[63] *Suwen*, Chapter 69. Here 'happy' is the translation of the character *le* 乐.

Lastly, *yi* has a meaning specific to medical thought and practice: it is the intent that one must have when performing therapy. For this to be effective, the *Neijing* with its typical conciseness states: 'Hold the needle without leaving it, stabilise *yi*'.[64]

During the Ming Period a specific debate developed about the role of intention-*yi* in the practice of medicine: on one side the importance of an empathetic–intuitive attitude in the act of curing was underlined, while on the other side the necessity of knowledge based on a solid and substantial structure was stressed. The discussion also unfolds by playing with the homophony between the two different characters of *yi* (医) meaning 'medicine' and *yi* (意) meaning 'idea, intention', but also 'meaning' and 'clue, trace'.[65]

Scheid and Bensky throughout discussion on *yi* find these various connotations, from the more intellectual to those more tied to intention, suggesting a significance of intelligence in the most complete sense:

> As we know from the texts and from experience, the spirit (*shen*) simultaneously manifests itself in the integrity of our actions and in the clarity of our understanding. Both in a medical context and in a philosophical one, we can therefore speak of *yi* (意) as a type of intelligence, an intelligence that comes from knowing and that manifests itself in doing, which nonetheless is an intelligence that surpasses intellectual knowledge.[66]

In this sense, remembering the aspect of self-cultivation which is also implicit in the process necessary to become a good doctor, they propose to translate *yi* as *signification*, meaning the act of signifying, where:

> … signifying implicates both that something is important because it has a special significance (a significance which in any case is specific and not absolute), that this significance can be communicated (even if often with a loss of significance) and that it is this special significance which is manifested in action'. In this way signification becomes 'effective action based on a clear vision in accordance with that which is necessary and possible.[67]

---

[64] *Suwen*, Chapter 62. In *qigong* practices we use the modern term *yinian* 意 念 referring to the act of thinking in the sense of concentrating.

[65] On this issue see the discussion in Chapter 15 on the space shared by patient and acupuncturist and in particular the debate between Yu Chang and Zhang Jiebin. The meaning of *yi* as a sense/intention of something that is consequently also a sign of itself can be found in the *Yixian* ('The antecedents of medicine': 'Medicine is *yi* 医 assume the initial *yi* 意 of the illness and cure it.'

[66] V. Scheid, D. Bensky, Medicine as signification, *The European Journal of Oriental Medicine*, vol. 2, n. 6, 1998, p. 35.

[67] *Ibidem*, p. 35 and p. 37. See also the following number of the same journal for the debate that stemmed from it. Also on the dialectic between signification and method, on medicine as art and science and on the concept of 'Chinese medicine'.

Zhi as 'Will'

The meanings of *zhi* are also varied. In the classics, *zhi* (志) can assume the meaning of: 1. 'will'; 2. 'emotion'; 3. 'mind'; 4. 'memory, sign' (preceded by the radical 'word').

The character *zhi* is composed of the radical 'heart' and the phonetic part *shi*, which was originally *zhi* (志). In the original radical *zhi* (志) a 'foot' was included, thereby suggesting semantically the idea of 'direction' of the heart.[68]

The capacity for directional movement is underlined by Larre and Rochat de la Vallee as an intention of the heart that persists in time and develops 'like the plant that begins to raise itself from the ground' and also by Wiseman and Ye who connect *zhi* (志) in its meaning of 'emotion' to the concept of 'direction of the heart'.[69]

In the 'Benshen' chapter *zhi* follows *yi*: 'The persistence of *yi* is called *zhi*'. A contemporary critical edition explains: 'Knowledge formed through the accumulation of thought is called *zhi*'.[70]

We see how the movements of accumulating, storing and conserving are tied to concepts of duration in time, of stabilising and concentrating – in other words to the functions of the kidney and *jing*. The discussion on *zhi* that runs throughout the history of Chinese philosophical and medical thought refers back to these processes, using the same terms as for *jing*, which, like *zhi*, is stored in the kidney.

The *Yijing* already attributes to *zhi* the qualities of being concentrated, straight and true: '*Zhi* in stillness is concentrated; in movement it is straight'.[71] Medical texts from different periods relate *zhi* to *yi* saying: 'When remembered *yi* remains concentrated, it is called *zhi*'.[72] 'When *yi* is already stabilised and it rises straight it is called *zhi*'.[73] '*Zhi* is concentrated *yi* that does not move'.[74]

---

[68] *Zhi* 志 served as an object pronoun, as a connecting particle and as the verb 'to go'. Now *zhi* 志 is translated as: 1. 'will'; 2. 'annals, documents' (Wieger p. 79b; Karlgren p. 1210, 1216).

[69] 'The movement of the heart is oriented towards an aim: the plant represents the process of the development of life; the heart has the power and tension of the phallus: the plant is characterised by the strength of the stem. [...] The expression which unites will and intention orients the very base of all animation, starting from a mentality which is well built and inspired.' Larre and Rochat de la Vallée, 1994, p. 185. The idea of direction is also in Wiseman when he highlights that *zhi*, being preserved in the kidney, must be interpreted as will or 'memory', 'in which a person finds his orientation in time'. (Wiseman and Ye, 1998, p. 396.)

[70] Guo Aichun (ed.), 1989, p. 81.

[71] *Yijing* ('The classic of changes'), ' *Xici*' ('Added sentences', part 1).

[72] *Yang* Shangshan, *Huangdi neijing taisu* (610 approximately). 'Concentrated' is the translation of *zhuang* 专. Often we also find 'concentrated in the one, unified' *zhuangyi* 专一.

[73] Zhang Jiebin (1563–1640), *Leijing* ('Classic of categories', 1624), Book III, Chapter 9. 'Stabilised' is the translation of *ding* 定, 'to fix, to stabilise, calm, stable', a term which also recurs in classic texts on 'the nourishment of life' *yangsheng* and in contemporary *qigong*. 'To rise straight' is the translation of *zhi li* 直立.

[74] Tang Zonghai (1846–1897), *Zhongxiyi huitong yijing jingyi* ('Essential meaning of the classics in the connection between Chinese and Western medicine', 1892).

Intrinsic to the kidney, *zhi* and *jing* are aspects of gathering, concentration, endurance and stability: we can then understand how firmness, determination, desire, decision and their related action derive from these characteristics, and how the term *zhi* can assume all of these meanings.

The stabilisation of ideas is confirmed by the act of choosing: 'When one thinks of something, decides, and acts, this is called *zhi*'.[75] The ability to pursue a goal and to carry out one's intentions overlaps with the present definition of will, which is 'the faculty of willing, the ability to decide and initiate a certain action'.[76] Decision, determination and tenacity are linked to *zhi*: 'The determination of a sage to the *dao* is such that if he has not finished a chapter he goes no further'.[77]

We recall that willing is a movement which springs forth from adjustment to the *dao*, from an immediate clarity in which spontaneity combines with knowledge of the inevitable. In this sense, we translate *zhi* as 'will, willing', but also as 'intention', 'purpose', or 'intent'.

Graham, who translates it as 'intent', chooses this term because it comes closer to our concept of will, but he underlines: '*Zhi* (志) is far from being a Kantian will detached from spontaneous inclinations and is rather an impulse which was awakened by the spring and stabilised by the autumn'.[78]

Zhi as 'Emotion' and as 'Mind'

Willing is also something that is more individual: it is subjective desires and aspirations, as we read in the *Neijing*: 'Everyone desires that their will/feelings-*zhi* be fulfilled'.[79] This switching from a will that coincides with the actualisation of the *dao* to more personal aspects can clarify the reason why the same term *zhi* also assumes the meaning of 'emotions'.

As we have already seen in the discussion regarding terminology and in the chapter on emotions, *wuzhi* – 'the five emotions', is the general term that defines the emotions, intended as internal movements of the soul, sentiments, and passions which can easily cause illness.

In the first classics, *zhi* is used to define the specific emotions in relation to the five *zang* organs, but also as a more general term for feelings and emo-

---

[75] Zhang Jiebing, *Leijing* ('Classic of categories', 1624), Book III, Chapter 9. Larre and Rochat de la Vallée (1994, p. 77) translate the passage from the 'Benshen' chapter: 'When the intention (*yi*) is permanent we will speak of will (*zhi*).'

[76] Vocabolario della Lingua Italiana Zingarelli. *Yizhi* 意 志 in modern Chinese it means 'will'.

[77] Mengzi, chapter '*Jinxinshang*'. In Confucius's 'Dialogues' we find: 'When I was fifteen I was determined-*zhi* in studies', in *Lunyu*, chapter 'Weizhen'.

[78] A. C. Graham, 1999, p. 485. In a different context *zhi* is translated as 'memory', the equivalent of storing (p. 346).

[79] *Lingshu*, Chapter 29. In this phase 'all' is the translation of 'the people with a hundred names'. For some references to classical thought and terminology relating to emotions see the first two chapters.

tions: 'The east generates the wind [...] as for emotions-*zhi*, it is anger'.[80] 'If the pathogens stay in the body without being released, one has feelings-*zhi* of aversion or attraction; *qi* and blood get into a state of disorder'.[81]

Zhi also means mental activity in a broad sense.[82]

Often when referring to mental activities, one speaks alternatively of *zhi* or *shen* or heart, with overlapping meanings. In contemporary texts the current term for 'mind' is *shenzhi*, but the same term is also found in the classics. In medicine, it is often said: 'calm the *shen* and stabilise the mind' (*anshen dingzhi* 安神定志).

The specific meaning of 'mind' is clear, for example, in the passages that describe madness-*diankuang* as 'loss of *zhi*', or in phrases like: 'If nutritive *qi* and defensive *qi* are both empty, there is numbness and loss of function, the muscles are insensitive, and body and *zhi* do not exist for each other'.[83] In this sense, *zhi* (志) also means 'intelligence, intellect', which is not to be confused with *zhi* (知) 'knowing, knowledge, talents, cognitive faculties' or with *zhi* (智), which means 'wisdom, knowing' and has the radical 'sun'.[84]

Notes

A reading of the five *shen* as specific aspects of the relationship between man and the universe acknowledges *shen* as an individual expression of a more universal *shen* and as part of it; *po* and *hun* as a *yin–yang* pair, partially autonomous forces which also characterise body and mind; *yi* and *zhi* as the realisation of man in the world.

Yi and *zhi* are those qualities that enable us to avoid dispersing ourselves mentally and physically, to adapt ourselves to the external conditions of reality, to avoid falling prey to the emotions and to avoid becoming ill. '*Zhi* and *yi* are that which protect *jing* and *shen*, gather *hun* and *po*, adjust hot and cold, harmonise euphoria and anger [...]. If *zhi* and *yi* are in harmony, then *jing* and *shen* are concentrated and straight, *hun* and *po* do not disperse, rancour and anger do not arise and the five organs are not overcome by pathogens'.[85]

In terms of the self's integration with external reality, *yi* and *zhi* are an aspect of integration with reality; they correspond to that which is specifically human.

---

[80] *Suwen*, Chapter 5.
[81] *Lingshu*, Chapter 58.
[82] Wiseman translates it in the first place as *mind*: '*Zhi*: Synonym: mind-spirit. 1. 'will, determination'; 2. 'ability to think, feel, answer'; 3. 'love, emotion', 4. 'memory, will'. In: Wiseman and Ye, 1998, p. 395.
[83] *Suwen*, Chapter 34. This also relates to difficult aspects as when in Chapter 2 the *Suwen* says that it is necessary to put *zhi* in harmony with the four seasons: it must give during spring, be free of rage in summer, calm in autumn and secret in winter.
[84] Karlgren p. 1218. In Mozi's 'Principles' we also find a third graphic form, containing the radical 'heart' (Graham, 1999, p. 334).
[85] *Lingshu*, Chapter 47.

SECTION II

CLASSICAL ASPECTS OF PATHOGENS, SYMPTOMS AND SYNDROMES

CHAPTER 4 CONSTRAINT-*YU*

CHAPTER 5 EMOTIONS AND HEAT

There are elements that play a fundamental part in the processes leading to illness and in their consequent clinical patterns. These elements appear to be substantially identical in pathological conditions with dominance of psychic symptoms and in illnesses that are definitely somatic.

In both cases there can be mechanisms of invasion or accumulation by pathogenic factors, disorders in the movements of the *qi*, stagnation of *qi* or blood stasis, exhaustion of the *yang* or consumption of the *yin*, alterations at the level of the channels or of organs and viscera. But when the psychic aspect prevails there are certain aetiopathogenetic processes that we find in traditional Chinese thought and are still essential in contemporary clinic.

In passing from the theoretical guidelines of the first section to the part devoted to clinical applications I felt the necessity to recall concepts such as 'constraint' or 'heat'. These are precise but also very complex concepts that are often regarded with a certain confusion or superficiality.

In any case they are worth understanding, since they have a great explicative power with respect to many pathological conditions and to their related implications regarding the therapeutic path. Moreover they can be used in a wider medical sphere.

CHAPTER 6 AGITATION AND RESTLESSNESS-*FANZAO*

CHAPTER 7 INSOMNIA

For the same reasons we found it useful to focus on the concept of *fanzao*-'agitation and restlessness', a symptom which, together with insomnia and palpitations, tends to characterise 'emotional illnesses'.

The 'being troubled', whether in its more inner/mental manifestation of restlessness or in its more behavioural/movement form of agitation, has been long debated during the history of medicine. This symptom reveals itself as a fascinating core nucleus of attraction in thought on the dynamics of *yin* and *yang*.

We have also chosen to include a chapter on insomnia since it seemed important to offer colleagues something which has been written by great clinical doctors. The following part of the text rearranges some diagnostic material categorised by type of insomnia. It may be useful as a corollary to the definition of patterns following TCM guidelines.

In contrast, palpitations, the other specific symptoms seen with emotional involvement, are only briefly examined since they are quite clear and straightforward.

CHAPTER 8 MANIC-DEPRESSION–*DIANKUANG*

CHAPTER 9 CLASSICAL SYNDROMES – *ZANGZAO, BENTUNQI, BAIHEBING* AND *MEIHEQI*

The severe *diankuang* pathology and the syndromes *zangzao, bentunqi, baihebing,* and *meiheqi* are patterns appearing in the early medical texts and they are part of contemporary definitions and clinical presentation.

As it is often the case for material prior to TCM systematisation, the Western study of Chinese medicine tends to leave these patterns to one side, so that they appear more obscure and are less used. We nevertheless recall that these syndromes are an issue taken into consideration by classical texts and that many contemporary Chinese clinical doctors continue to use them in their practice linked to psychic illness.

The contributions from Jin Shubai, Zhang Mingjiu and Zhang Shijie, the personal annotations and the examined cases propose an interpretation that combines these syndromes with points of view belonging to our modern thought. This is done with the intention of keeping them alive by bringing them closer to the real contemporary practice of medicine.

Constraint-*Yu*

4

Medical texts and modern clinical practice have established the closeness of the relationship between the emotions and liver *qi* stagnation. Since one of the liver's main functions is to help *qi* circulate in a smooth, fluid manner, if the emotions become blocked and no longer flow smoothly the first results are stagnation of *qi* and constraint of the liver (*ganyu qizhi* 肝郁 气 滞). In Qing Dynasty texts we find the statement: 'Illnesses of the seven emotions all reside in the liver, because the liver governs the function of spreading and draining *qi* and has an important role in regulating its movement; if this activity is impaired, alterations at the emotional level appear easily.'[1]

A modern clinical text states:

> The initial phase of the constraint syndrome (*yuzheng* 郁 证) is always trace-able to emotions that attack and cause knotting at the *qi* level. The symptoms are depression, 'low' moods, a sense of oppression in the chest and pain in the ribs, frequent sighing, lack of appetite, etc. The main thing is to release the liver and regulate *qi*. As is stated in the *Yifanglun*: 'In all *yu* illnesses the *qi* must be the first to fall ill; if instead *qi* is free and flowing, how can there be *yu*?'[2]

Given, however, the correspondence between the anatomical level (*qi*, blood, channels, organs) and the psychological one, the concepts of *qi* constraint and emotional constraint tend to dovetail, such that emotional constraints can cause stagnation of *qi* flow while, vice versa, *qi* stagnation can effect changes in emotional states.[3]

---

[1] Wei Zhixiu, *Xu mingyi leian* ('Continuation of clinical cases of famous doctors', 1770). Another Qing Dynasty author, Zhou Xuehai, writes: ' The nature of the Liver loves to go upward and loathes going downwards; it loves spreading and detests contraction; easy transformation of the organs' and chan-nels' *qi* and the absence of illness depends on the spreading and draining action of Liver and Gall bladder *qi*.'

[2] Wang Zhanxi, *Neike zhenjiu peixue xinbian* ('Revision of the pairing of points in internal medicine in moxa-acupuncture', 1993). (*Yifanglun* is a text by Fei Boxiong from 1865).

[3] Julian Scott's discussion of the fact that small children have strong emotions, but that they live them in an immediate fashion is interesting. Only around the age of 5 do they start to have the sen-sation and awareness of emotions and attempt to control them; the relative possibility of developing Liver *qi* stagnation accompanies this development.

THE TERM *YU*

The term *yu* is often translated in English as 'depression', or 'depressed' (when considered as an attribute), superimposed on which is the modern clinical term *yiyu* (抑郁), which translates as 'mental depression'.

Discussions of *yu* syndrome in modern texts often refer to Wang Lu's explanation that: 'the origin of the majority of illness is *yu*. *Yu* means stagnation (*zhi* 滞) and consequential non-passage (*butong* 不通).[4]

Within the character *yu* (郁) (not to be confused with *yu* 瘀 referring to blood stasis) are depicted two trees, which suggests the idea of density.[5]

In English, 'constraint' is probably the term that comes closest to the all-encompassing meaning of *yu*, which denotes a difficulty in the movement and passage of *qi*.

We note here that whereas in modern usage the term *yu* is commonly used mainly with respect to liver *qi*, in earlier medical literature – as we shall see later in the text – there is found also both the concept of autonomous *yu* and a definition of *yu* in relation to individual emotions or specific pathogens – so that, for example, one finds references to the *yu* of anger or the *yu* of fire.

The concept of *yuzheng* – a '*yu* syndrome' of a specific and autonomous nature – was first formally elaborated in a medical context during the Yuan Dynasty (1260–1368). The relationship between the two terms – as is always the case in Chinese syntax – can be understood both in the causal sense (illness resulting from constraint) and as a specific label (illness called constraint).

The term encompasses a whole variety of clinical cases produced by *yu*, all linked by the same aetiological characteristics; all of them are traceable back to repressed emotions and knotting-*jie* (结), and stagnation-*zhi* (滞) of *qi* flow, after which blood stasis, phlegm accumulation and constrained fire easily follow.

SPREADING AND DRAINING – THE *SHUXIE* FUNCTION OF THE LIVER

No direct link between liver *qi* and its action on the flow of *qi* is mentioned in the *Neijing*, although – as we have already seen regarding emotions – good *qi* circulation is a prerequisite to good health. For example, the answer to

---

[4] Wang Lu (1332–1391), *Yijing suihuiji* ('Collection of memories of the classics of medicine'), chapter 'Wuyulun' ('Tractate on the five constraints'). The concept of *yuzheng* is introduced, for example in: Li Qingfu and Liu Duzhou, *Zhongyi jingshen bingxue* ('Psychiatry in Chinese medicine'), 1989, p. 103; in: Jin Shubai, *Zhenjin juliao jingshenbing* ('Acupuncture in the Treatment of mental Illness'), 1987, p. 62.
[5] The term *yu* is no longer used on its own in modern Chinese, where we find instead *youyu* (忧郁) 'sad, depressed, sadness'. In its non-simplified form *yu* shows a vase between two trees, which a roof separates from the sacrificial wine and the feathers in the lower part of the ideogram (Weiger p. 130c, Karlgren p. 555).

the question posed about the fact that *qi* varies from person to person states: 'Fright, fear, anger, fatigue and rest can all influence change. In strong people *qi* circulates and therefore illnesses resolve themselves. (...) In weak people *qi* becomes stuck and the result is illness.'[6]

The concept of *shuxie* (疏 泄) 'spreading and draining' is closely linked to that of *yuzheng* '*yu* syndrome' and its use in this sense goes back to the same period. From then on this connection between the emotions, liver *qi* circulation and constraint remains a fundamental element in medical thought, as in the following expression: '*Yu* is caused by the lack of draining-*shu* of the emotions, which results in progressive knotting of *qi*; *yu* protracted in time causes innumerable pathological changes.'[7]

In fact, in the *Neijing*, all it says is that the body of the earth is *shuxie* in the sense that the earth needs to be well drained and released in order to foster birth and growth, without implying the specific meaning that it has today, or a direct link to the liver.[8]

In Qing Dynasty (1644–1911) texts, however, the role of the liver becomes central: 'The nature of the liver loves to flow upwards and loathes descending; it loves spreading and loathes contraction, because the ease of transformation of the channel's and *zangfu*'s *qi* and the absence of illness all depend on the action of liver and gall bladder *qi* to drain and release.'[9]

'Among the five organs of man, the liver is the one which moves easily, but calms down with difficulty. When the other organs fall ill, only that one is sick, and the only way the illness can extend to other organs is when it continues over a long period and the mutual control–generation cycle is altered. As soon as the liver falls ill, however, the illness immediately spreads to the other organs.'[10]

The two characters *shu* and *xie* are usually connected with the free circulation of liver *qi* and are translated as course/dredge and discharge, spreading and draining, and also as free flowing of *qi*.[11]

'Drain and release' can also be used as an effective translation since the words *shu* and *xie* have meanings that at least partially overlap and both refer to a draining action that permits water, and by comparison *qi*, to flow freely.[12]

---

[6] *Suwen*, Chapter 21.

[7] Xu Chunpu, *Guyin yitong dacheng* ('Great compendium of ancient and modern medicine').

[8] *Suwen*, Chapter 70. Zhu Danxi, when referring to the fact that both Liver and Kidney *yin* possess the minister fire *Xianghuo* 相火, speaks specifically of the *shuxie* function of the Liver: 'It is the Kidney that governs closing and storing (*bicang* 闭藏); it is the Liver that guides *shuxie*'. In: Gezhi yulun, 1347, chapter '*Yang* youyu, *yin* buzu ('*Yang* in excess, deficient *yin*').

[9] Zhou Xuehai, *Duyi suiji* ('Notes from medicine readings').

[10] Li Guanxian, *Zhiyi bibian* ('Necessity of distinguishing the knowledge of medicine').

[11] For a discussion on the two distinct functions of *shu* and *xie* and their interaction and relationship to the endocrine functions, please see Garvey and Qus' article, *The Liver Shuxie Function*, 2001.

[12] The character *shu* (疏) is composed of the phonetic part *shu* together with *liu*, the thin hair of new born infants, and is now translated as 'sparse, thin, scarce, draining, spreading' (Karlgren p. 904). The character *xie* (泄) contains the radical 'water' and the phonetic part *shi* and is translated as 'unload, release, liberate, let free, spread'. In Italian the term 'liberate' can refer to knots and constraints and to emotions, but, just as in Chinese, it also applies in the specific sense of obstructed channels.

EMOTIONS AND *YU*

Even if the most ancient texts such as the *Neijing* do not speak of *yuzheng*, they do define the relationship between the liver and anger: the emotional expression which comes from finding ourselves faced with something with which we feel no correspondence and which we do not like. Anger is usually generated when an obstruction appears to thwart our will or our desire – whether it is an active impulse towards something or a 'passive' need for confirmation or love – and this corresponds to the situation where *qi* instead of bending flexibly like wood and finding another path around the obstacle instead ascends impetuously to crash against it.

In '*yu* syndrome' there is therefore constraint of desires, constraint of the typically explosive movement of rage and constraint of the free flow of *qi*.

The concept of *yu* and its relationship with emotions is, however, also found in the most ancient classical texts. According to Guanzi, we already find that 'anguish-*you* and constraint-*yu* produce illness, if the illness becomes difficult then one dies.'[13]

The *Neijing* takes *yu* into consideration both in relation to the macrocosm and with respect to the internal world. There is a *yu* of each of the five elements (wood, fire, earth, metal, water) in response to the invasion of the corresponding seasonal *qi*, just as there exists a precise relationship between emotions and movements of *qi*, according to which 'when there is anguish-*you* and worry-*chou*, *qi* is blocked and obstructed and does not flow.'[14]

The concept of stagnation/blockage/constraint was often defined as knotting-*jie* (节): 'When there is thought-*si*, then the heart withdraws, the *shen* pauses, correct *qi* withdraws and does not circulate, and in this way *qi* becomes knotted.'[15]

Knotting and constraint are also among the causes of those syndromes described by Zhang Zhongjing (AD200) in which the pathologies of the movement of *qi* are manifested through symptoms which do not correspond to well defined somatic illnesses.[16]

During the Sui Dynasty (AD581–612) similar cases were called *qijiebing* (气 结 病) (illness of knotted *qi* or due to knotted *qi*) or *qibing* and referred to emotions that knot heart *qi*. In that period, rather than to the liver, the main

---

[13] *Guanzi* (4th–2nd century AD), Chapter 16.
[14] *Lingshu*, Chapter 8. Constraint of the five elements (*muyu* 木 郁, *huoyu* 火郁, *tuyu* 土郁, *jinyu* 金 郁, *shuiyu* 水 郁) is discussed in detail in the Suwen, Chapter 71, where we read for example, 'When Earth's *yu* is manifested one suffers from abdominal swelling, intestinal rumbling, and repeated bowel movements; in serious cases there is pain in the heart and fullness in the chest, nausea, vomiting and violent diarrhoea with vomiting.'
[15] Suwen, Chapter 39. Zhang Jiebin makes these comments on this passage: 'Anguish and worry in excess, then *qi* is knotted, if *qi* is knotted, transformation cannot take place', in: *jingyue quanshu* ('The complete works of Jingyue'), Chapter 'Yige' ('Constraint of the diaphragm').
[16] Please see the discussion on classic syndromes (*bentunqi*, *meiheqi*, etc.) in this regard in Chapter 9.

reference was to the heart – the ruler that controls all the *zangfu*, and the organ of awareness and feeling whose state of *qi* reflects on the entire system. Going back to the *Neijing*, it states: 'Illnesses of knotted *qi* are produced by worry and concerns. The heart withdraws, *shen* pauses, correct *qi* withdraws and does not circulate and therefore knots up internally.'[17]

In any case, it was Zhu Danxi (1281–1358) who attributed a major role in the aetiological process to *yu*, recognising the origin of all pathological changes in the constraint of *qi*.

According to Zhu Danxi: 'When *qi* and blood flow freely, the ten thousand illnesses do not arise; when there is constraint-*yu*, all illnesses may arise, therefore illnesses of the human body originate mostly from *yu*', specifying further that 'if there is suffocated *yu* all illnesses derive from it, therefore all the illnesses of the human body originate mainly from *yu*.'[18]

Zhu Danxi therefore clearly identifies the concept of constraint-*yu* as a cause of illness and further articulates the concept in describing the six specific *yu*s of *qi* constraint, dampness, heat, phlegm, blood and food. When *qi* is constrained it produces dampness; prolonged constraint of dampness causes internal heat, which over time consumes the liquids causing the formation of phlegm. Phlegm obstructs the vessels and circulation and if blood stagnates and does not circulate freely, foods are not transformed.[19]

This is how the six manifestations of *yu* are described in detail:

> When there is *qi* constraint there is pain in the chest and hypochondria and the pulse is deep and choppy. In constraint of dampness there is pain in the whole body, or pain in the joints that manifests with cold, the pulse is deep and fine. In constraint of phlegm there is shortness of breath during movements, the pulse in the *cun* position is deep and slippery. In constraint of heat there is confused vision together with restlessness, red urine, a deep and rapid pulse. In constraint of blood the limbs have no strength, one cannot eat, the stools are red, and the pulse is deep. In constraint of food there is acid reflux, full abdomen, one can not eat, the carotid pulse (*renying* 人迎) is soft-*huan* (缓) while the radial pulse is extremely wiry.[20]

---

[17] Chao Yuanfang, *Zhubing Yuanhoulun* ('Tractate on the Origin and Symptoms of illnesses', 610).

[18] *Danxi Xinfa*, chapter 'Liuyu' ('The six constraints'). *Danxi Xinfa* ('The teachings of Danxi', 1481) is a collection edited by the students of Zhu Danxi. Zheng Shouqian affirms: '*Yu* is not the name of a specific illness, but it is that from which all illnesses originate.' Regarding the relationship among emotions, fire and constraints, see also Chapter 5 on emotions and heat.

[19] The six *yu* described in the relative chapters are *qiyu* (气 郁), *shiyu* (湿郁), *reyu* (热 郁), *tanyu* (痰郁), *xueyu* (血郁) and *shiyu* (湿郁). We note here that Zhu Danxi also placed an emphasis on the constraint of stomach and spleen. Any excess of the six external pathogens, the seven emotions, or fatigue acts on the correlated organ, altering the ascending and descending movements, and in the end damage the spleen and stomach, due to which the *qi* of the middle burner particularly suffers from *yu*.

[20] Attributed to Zhu Danxi, *Jingui guoxuan* ('The mysteries of the *Jingui*'), chapter 'Liuyu' ('The six constraints').

EXTERNAL AND INTERNAL FACTORS

In the musings of the 'heat' school of thought, emotional factors as opposed to external pathogens acquire an ever-increasing relevance. For example, in the above-mentioned chapter 7 of the *Suwen*, which speaks of the five elements and their variations according to seasonal and cosmic mutations, it is asked: 'The majority of illnesses initiate from constraint, which can be due to dominance (by other organs' *qi*) or develop autonomously from an individual organ's *qi*. Could this all be caused by mutations in the five elements?'[21]

An aetiological role for external factors, including foods, is nevertheless also recognised:

> Regarding the six *yu* (…) they are either caused by repression of the seven emotions or the penetration by cold or heat, due to which there are syndromes of suffocated fire, or they are caused by the penetration of rain and dampness or the accumulation of alcohol and greasy foods, due to which there are syndromes of *yu* from accumulations of liquids and dampness.'[22] 'When there is knotted *yu*, accumulation, and absence of flowing, then that which needs to ascend does not ascend, that which needs to descend does not descend, that which needs to be transformed is not transformed, in some cases there is *yu* at the level of *qi*, in other cases there is *yu* at the level of blood, and this is the start of illness (…). Both the six pathogens-*xie* and the seven emotions-*qing* are capable of causing *yu*.[23]

The deficient nature of the root and the excess of the manifestations is also underlined. In weak constitutions, or in patients with chronic pathology, the circulation of *qi* and blood are deficient; when this deficiency overlaps with another in the draining of emotions then internal constraint of *qi* is easily produced: 'In people with deficient constitutions, when things do not go as they desire, they can have dizziness and foggy vision, lack of vitality, flaccidity-*wei* of the tendons and urgent-*ji qi*, just like in other deficiency syndromes.'[24]

The position of Zhang Jiebin in particular is expounded, which recognises that constraint syndromes can originate from the actions of the heart's emotions, but also that constraint may possibly develop secondarily to a problem of an 'organic' order. In other words, *yu* can be the cause which produces pathologies in the organs or, instead, the result of alterations of the *qi* of the five *zang* organs – for example: 'Constraint due to emotions is always linked to the heart, and in this case the illness is due to constraint', but also, 'In all illnesses, constraint of the five organs' *qi* is present and this is constraint due to

---

[21] Wang Lu (1332–1391), *Yijing suihuiji* ('A collection of remembrances from the medical classics'), chapter 'Wuyu' ('The five constraints').
[22] Yu Tuan, *Yixue zhengchuan* ('The true traditions of medicine', 1515).
[23] He Mengyao, *Yibian* ('Fundaments of medicine', 1751).
[24] Sun Yikui, *Chishui xuanzhu* ('The mystic pearl of the purple water', 1573).

illness (of the organ)'. He explains that, for instance, in illnesses of the lung an accumulation-*chu* of phlegm is produced, in illnesses of the heart constraint-*yu* of fire is created, in illnesses of the spleen stagnation-*zhi* of food, in illnesses of the liver knotting-*jie* of *qi*, in illnesses of the kidney still water. In illnesses due to constraint, Zhang Jiebin considers emotions to be the primary cause and describes the symptoms: 'In constraint due to anger, *qi* is full and the abdomen is swollen; constraint due to worry links in the upper regions to lung and stomach and is the origin of coughing and lack of breath, haemorrhages, difficulty in swallowing, nausea and vomiting; in the lower regions it influences the liver and kidneys causing cloudy spotting, uterine bleeding, urinary disorders-*lin*, fatigue and mental fogginess.[25]

The distinction between internal and external origins is very explicit in a more recent passage:

> Entering the body, the six pathogens can all stagnate and cause illness. Cold pathogens remain constrained-*yu* in the defensive layer, on the nutritive level, in the channels and in the organs. The summer heat pathogens and dampness knot in the *sanjiao*, the epidermal pathogens position themselves at the *muyuan* level. (…) In general, when pathogens are not expelled or dispersed, we speak of constraint, in this case generated by the six *qi* of external origin. In this chapter we speak of constraint of the seven emotions, which is much more frequent. Worry damages the spleen, anger damages the liver, and the reason is always in the heart. Because if the emotions remain unsatisfied, there is constraint and illnesses occur. (…) If there is constraint, then *qi* stagnates, if *qi* stagnates for a long time, it turns into heat. If there is heat then the liquids are consumed and do not circulate and the ascending and descending movements of *qi* are not regulated. In the first phase, the *qi* level is damaged, afterwards by force the blood level also. If this becomes protracted it brings chronic consumptive illnesses. (…) *Yu* of the emotions derives from suppressed sentiments and from frustrated and non-expressed proposals-*yi*, which impede the mechanism of the ascending and descending of *qi* and that of opening and closing.[26]

YU SYNDROME, PHLEGM AND BLOOD STASIS

Constraint, or in other words, *qi* that stops, is knotted and accumulates, can easily produce heat and generate phlegm, which in turn obstructs the movement of *qi*.

---

[25] Zhang Jiebin, *Jingyue Quanshu* ('The complete works of Jingyue', 1640), 'Yuzheng' ('*Yu* syndrome') chapter.
[26] Ye Tianshi, *Lingzhen Zhinan Yian* ('Guiding cases in the clinic', 1766). *Muyuan* 幕原, located between the pleura and the diaphragm, is the space between external and internal in which epidemic febrile illnesses tend to nest.

Produced by pathology, and in turn a cause of pathology, phlegm is a turbid and heavy substance that possesses the intrinsic ability to penetrate anywhere, just as *qi* does physiologically. However, phlegm forms because *qi* does not circulate easily, therefore its removal depends on managing to get *qi* flowing properly.

Zhu Danxi, who developed the concept of phlegm obscuring the portals of the heart, said in fact: 'Phlegm, this substance, ascends and descends following *qi*; there is no place at which it does not arrive.(...) Those who are good at treating phlegm do not treat phlegm, but *qi*; if *qi* flows then all the body's liquids flow easily following the *qi*'.[27]

Wang Qinren focuses on blood stasis, around which he develops all of his clinical reflections. From his perspective, many manifestations of irritability are attributed to blood stasis, for example when the early stage of an illness is accompanied by an impatience for even small things: 'Even small things are not allowed to pass, this is blood stasis, a normally calm person that becomes irritable after the commencement of the illness', so that 'that which is commonly called illness of liver *qi*, in which one gets angry for no reason, is actually blood stasis in the thorax'.[28]

Case Study 4.1

A Body That Feels the Weight of Living

The patient, a 42-year-old orthodontic technician, turns to acupuncture for a series of disturbances that he attributes to a problem in the cervical part of the spine. He has already tried both ultrasound treatments and physiotherapy, but with only brief periods of respite. X-rays reveal reduced intervertebral spaces in the section between C4 and C7, together with light calcification.

He complains of tightness in his neck muscles, numbness in his left hand, irritation and lack of strength in the four limbs, tingling at the top of the head, a sensation of instability that worsens when he walks in unfamiliar surroundings, and sporadic episodes of headaches in the left temporal–parietal zone together with nausea.

---

[27] *Danxi Xinfa*, 'Tan' ('Phlegm') chapter. The origin of phlegm is varied, but emotions and constraints are the first cause: 'Due to anguish and constraint, to thick flavours, to the absence of sweat or to tonifying prescriptions, *qi* ascends, the blood boils, the pure is transformed into the turbid, old, dense and liquid, solid and gluey phlegm is mixed.' In: Zhu Danxi, *Gezhi Yulun*, 'Semai' ('Rough pulse') chapter.

[28] Wang Qinren, *Yilin Gaicuo* ('Corrections of errors in w, 1830). 'Thorax' is the translation of *xuefu* (血府), literally, 'the palace of blood'. We remind the reader that the term *yu*-constraint (郁) is not used for blood, but rather *yu* (欲), which we translate as 'stasis'.

The patient suffers periodically from colic pains, with repeated bowel movements of either normal or liquid stools with mucus. Tests had revealed a diverticulosis and he was prescribed an antispastic medicine to be used when needed. Generally, however, bowel movements are regular if he keeps his eating habits under control.

He also says that he is very bothered by the frequent palpitations that he has during the day, and that he is anxious and becomes agitated by anything unexpected, owing to which he always tries to organise everything in advance. He has no incapacitating phobias, but describes himself as being 'at the limit'.

All his symptoms worsen when he is agitated; however, he continues to sleep well.

The tip of the tongue is red; the tongue coating is thick and white, tending to yellow at the root. The pulse is deep and wiry and stronger in the right *guan* position.

Diagnosis

Qi stagnation with damp-heat and diffuse phlegm (*jingluo*, head, chest, intestines and the portals of the heart).

Therapeutic Principles

Activate liver *qi*, resolve dampness-heat and phlegm.

Treatment

Nine treatments at an average of once a week, initially closer together and subsequently further apart over a two and a half month period.

Basic treatment:

GB-20 *Fengchi*, LI-4 *Hegu*, LIV-3 *Taichong* and GB-34 *Yanglingquan* to regulate and activate *qi*; the two points on the gall bladder channel act on the constraint which causes the muscular contraction, on the dampness-heat, and on the 'determination' of the gall bladder; the 'four gates' *siguan* activate *qi* and blood and alleviate the pain and sensory alterations caused by the stagnation.

Furthermore, the following points are alternated:

- Du-14 *Dazhui*, P-5 *Jianshi* and ST-40 *Fenglong*
  and
- Du-16 *Fengfu*, TB-5 *Waiguan*, GB-41 *Zulinqi*.

Du-14 *Dazhui* is the meeting point of all the *yang* channels, it regulates their circulation and removes obstructions in the area; the other two points transform phlegm and free the portals of the heart, but P-5 *Jianshi* in particular regulates the three *jiao*, while ST-40 *Fenglong* activates and regulates *qi* in the stomach channel.

The second combination is addressed to the *yangweimai*; the *yangweimai* was chosen because of its connecting function and the location of the symptoms, and also the fact that the *yin* and *yangweimai* can be implicated in mental disturbances when *yin* and *yang* are unbalanced.

Du-16 *Fengfu*, the 'sea of marrow' point, eliminates wind, calms the *shen*, aids circulation of *qi* to the neck and head, and is a meeting point between *yangweimai* and *Du Mai* (the *Yin* and *yangweimai* meet in the upper body through the *Ren* and *Du Mai*).

A cycle of *tuina* treatments on the *jingluo* and the areas most involved is linked to the other treatments.

During the first 2 months the situation is extremely variable, the various symptoms disappear and reappear, they seem to improve only to show up again later.

The patient remains very courteous, but does not seem convinced about the treatments or satisfied with their progress. At times he asks me about the possibility that the various symptoms might not depend on the condition of the vertebrae, but then immediately excludes this hypothesis.

When it is in any case necessary to interrupt for the summer break, I ask him to give me his evaluation of the situation and he says: 'There have not been great results regarding the sensation of instability, but I feel calmer, I haven't had anymore butterflies in the heart or tingling in the legs or that lack of strength, and I am less impatient and angry. Maybe acupuncture is the only thing that has had any effect.' He does not speak of his intestinal disturbances, but later it turns out that he has not needed to use the antispastic medications in this period.

He spontaneously picks up on my hypothesis of continuing the therapy after the summer with two treatments per month.

Comments

I have included the details of this case because it presents a number of elements that recur in clinical practice, even if the results with respect to the specific symptoms are less impressive than those generally obtained in similar cases.

In conditions of stagnation or constraint of *qi*, the reaction seems to vary independently of the correctness in the choice of points: at times there is an unlocking effect with consequent disappearance of symptoms, a realignment of the entire energetic system and a net improvement in the quality of life; at other times it seems that nothing can remove the blockage, and the stagnation also manifests itself as a sort of hostility on the part of the patient, almost as though he obstinately refuses to get better.

From a Chinese energetic viewpoint, the discrepancy in results also depends on the specific case of stagnation: if it accompanies heat or fire it is easier to resolve, whereas when there is dampness this is intrinsically heavy and boggy so resolution is more difficult (in the first type, however, the heat must be pre-existent, not simply a product of the accumulation of dampness).

It is worthwhile remembering here that unsatisfied patients – those sick in a characteristic way that seems to resist any change, which often causes us to perceive them as very hostile and makes us feel inadequate or frankly incapable – are also communicating their suffering to us in their own way. The difficulty we encounter in these treatments also depends on the fact that patients with stagnation of *qi* often exhibit a lack of fluidity in their thought processes, so that they remain glued to a very concrete explanation and reject other interpretations of events or alternative behaviour.

Even where the aetiological process is clear to us and the 'errors' in the patient's lifestyle that are causing his suffering appear self-evident, we know well how in such cases advice and recommendations are not positively received. In effect, each stagnation is a case of excess, and it is difficult for a person who is already in a state of excess to accept anything more.

It is difficult to say whether a better or correct solution exists. Some doctors require that their patients do *qigong* or other practices and will not agree to continue with treatments unless this condition is met; they feel, in fact, that if the patient's pathology also depends on his continuously transferring responsibility to others, then a fundamental role in the therapeutic process consists of ensuring the patient accepts personal responsibility for making lifestyle changes, and it is therefore necessary to be extremely insistent.

Others, however, think that it is not worthwhile being obstinate or forcing the situation, but better to remain empty so that the other person may in turn, empty himself (without forgetting that helping a person 'unload' does not mean turning oneself into a trash bin). If *qi* stagnates, all we can do is to aid the circulation of *qi*, both through using needles and also by remaining flexible ourselves, attempting to seize the moment when an avenue of communication opens in order to try and suggest other possible explanations, always using extreme delicacy.

Follow-up

After an interval of 3 months the patient says he spent a good summer, without palpitations or strange sensations, even though at times a sensation of feeling dazed or unstable still occurs. He generally feels less irritable and impatient, has decided to continue with follow-up therapy and is evaluating whether to start practising *taijiquan*.

Emotions and Heat

5

In a modern text we find the statement: 'Anger, euphoria and worry easily give birth to fire and this fire which is produced by the emotions damages the organs. In particular, it is the fire of the heart and the liver that is involved, because the heart has a pre-eminent role in emotional activities and liver *qi* has the characteristic of being easily subject to constraint, knotting and counter-rising.'[1]

The relationship between fire and emotions is particularly close from the moment that: 'The heart governs the *shen* and is fire, emotions act through the heart and it is therefore easy for fire to cause psychic and physical illnesses. The first thing that happens is an alteration in the movements of *qi* and when this reaches its peak that which is in excess is fire.'[2]

LIU WANSU AND THE THEORY OF HEAT

The formulation of the *wuzhi huare* (五志 化 热) theory that the five emotions transform into/produce heat goes back to Liu Wansu. The development of this theory had a great influence on successive medical thought and it was particularly expounded in the Jin and Yuan periods by Zhang Zihe, Li Dongyuan and Zhu Danxi (whose works appear respectively in 1228, 1249 and 1347). To summarise briefly, these works describe the pathological process in which excess of emotions tends to produce heat and fire; this fire consumes *yin* and the organs and generates illness: 'The emotions-*zhi* of the five *zang* organs are anger, euphoria, worry sadness, and fear; if the five emotions are in excess then there is exhaustion, if there is exhaustion, the corresponding organ is injured, damage to the five *zang* organs is always from heat'.[3]

---

[1] Zhu Wenfeng, *Zhongyi Xinluxue Yuanzhi* ('Principles of psychology in Chinese medicine'), 1987, p. 91.
[2] Wang Miqu, *Zhongguo Gudai Yixue Xinlixue* ('Ancient Chinese medical psychology'), 1988, p. 238.
[3] Liu Wansu, *Suwen Xuanji Yuanbingshi* ('An examination of the circumstances that give origin to illnesses of the mysterious mechanisms of the *Suwen*'), 'Relei' Chapter, ('The category of heat'). Liu Wansu (1120–1200), founder of the refreshing and cooling therapeutic system, returns to the same seven emotions that appear in the *Liji* and the six desires of the Buddhist tradition, which are related to the five organs and thought-*yi* (意).

Liu Wansu's regards the developing pathology essentially as a consequence of the imbalance between *yin* and *yang*, between fire and water: proceeding from the fact that *yang* is movement while *yin* is stillness, we can understand how the movement of desires and emotions in excess agitates the stillness and how their fire consumes the body (form-*xing*) and *shen*:

> What we intend when we say that *yang* is movement while *yin* is stillness is that if form and *shen* are exhausted then there is agitation-*zao* and lack of stillness, whereas with stillness there is pureness and tranquillity. Therefore the superior good is like water, while the inferior stupidity is like fire. The sages of the past said that the six desires and the seven emotions are the disgrace of the *dao*, and that they belong to fire. [...] The superior good stays far away from the six desires and the seven passions, while the inferior stupidity draws nearer to them.[4]

Of interest is the attention given to the fact that when emotions are in excess they invade the dreams and heat rises even further due to the fact that *shen* is dimmed. 'When you can not overcome the seven emotions, then while dreaming during sleep the heat remains blocked inside and grows.'[5]

The heart–kidney, fire–water axis therefore is of fundamental importance in this perspective that links emotional pathologies to heat: fire has the capability of agitating and disarranging *zhi* (志), which – like *jing* – must remain united, concentrated and solid; if the root of life darts about like flames then you can only have confusion and disorder. 'Doubt and confusion, turbid and disorder, *zhi* is not united, it is irregular like flames, there is confusion and doubt, if fire is in excess water is weakened, *zhi* is lost and there is confusion and disorder, *zhi* is the *shen* of water–kidney.'[6]

LI DONGYUAN AND *YIN* FIRE

Reflections on the role of emotional stimuli in the aetiology of fire is further developed by Li Dongyuan, who analyses the consequences of heat at the level of the consumption of *yuanqi*. 'Euphoria and anger, anguish and fear damage

---

[4] Liu Wansu, *Suwen Xuanji Yuanbingshi*, 'Bei' ('Sadness') chapter. See also the discussions on the role of fire in consuming *yin* and producing agitation and restlessness *fanzao* or the classic syndromes *zangzao*, *baihe*, etc. in Chapter 9 and the discussions on madness-*diankuang* in Chapter 8, in which reference is made to the relationship that Liu Wansu finds between anger, fire, consumption of water and loss of *zhi* with folly.

[5] Liu Wansu, *Suwen Xuanji Yuanbingshi*, 'Zhan' ('Delirium') chapter.

[6] Zhang Yuansu, *Yixue Qiyuan* ('The origins of medical science', 1186), 'Huo' ('Confusion') chapter. Zhang Yuansu – to whom the first diagnostic systemising of the five organs with syndromes of deficit and excess go back – was the direct teacher of Li Dongyuan and a supporter of the *yishui* (易 水) 'changing waters' therapeutic system. See also the discussions on folly-*diankung* in Chapter 8, in which reference is made to the relationship among the disorder caused by excess of fire, the weakening of water, perceptive distortions and hallucinations.

and consume *yuanqi*, they nourish heart fire, fire and *yuanqi* can not coexist, if fire overcomes then it invades the position of earth and this is the reason one gets sick.'[7] Further: 'Anger, ire, sadness, worry, fear, and apprehension, all damage *yuanqi*. Vigorous burning of *yin* fire initiating from the heart generates thickening and stagnation and the reason is that the seven emotions are not calm.'[8]

Li Dongyuan introduces the concept of *yin* fire, *yinhuo* (阴火), in a particular manner. This fire, which is an enemy of *yuanqi*, comes from below and derives from a disorder of *qi*. If stomach *qi* is weak and *yuanqi* is insufficient, then spleen and stomach no longer maintain their central position and they descend, permitting *yin* fire to rise from the lower *jiao* to occupy the earth position and invade the upper *jiao*, until it substitutes the ruling fire of the heart, attacks the lungs, enters the brain and 'cooks the marrow': If spleen *qi* and stomach *qi* are empty then they slide down to the kidney and *yin* fire manages to take the earth position. [...] If *yuanqi* is insufficient there is excess of heart fire. If the heart no longer rules, the ministerial fire substitutes for it. The ministerial fire is the fire of the *baoluo* of the lower *jiao* and a thief of *yuanqi*. 'Fire and *yuanqi* cannot coexist so one overcomes and the other succumbs.'[9] Furthermore: 'If *yuanqi* does not flow, then stomach *qi* slides downward, the fires of the *San Jiao* and the heart overcome the lungs at the centre of the chest, while above they enter the brain and cook the marrow.'[10]

The title 'thief of *yuanqi*' which Li Dongyuan gives to *yin* fire will serve to signify this specific relationship of interdependency according to which if *yuanqi* flourishes then *yin* fire is contained, whereas weakness of stomach and spleen *qi* and emptiness of *yuanqi* permit *yin* fire to blaze upwards: 'The strength of both fire and *qi* cannot coexist'; therefore in the *Neijing* it is said: 'Strong fire draws nourishment from *qi*, *qi* draws nourishment from weak fire, weak fire generates *qi*, strong fire disperses *qi*.'[11]

A number of elements are specific to *yin* fire: it is an empty heat that can also manifest as though it were full, it rises from below, it is related to insufficiency of *yuanqi* and it derives from internal causes. It does not, however, pertain to a specific organ, even if there is a close relationship with the kidney and ministerial fire. A modern commentary quotes the words of Li Dongyuan

[7] Li Dongyuan, *Piweilun* ('Tractate on spleen and stomach', 1249) 'Piwei Xushi Zhuanbianlun' ('Transformations of deficit and excess in spleen and stomach') chapter.
[8] Li Dongyuan, *Piweilun*, 'Anyang Xinshen Tiaozhi Piwelun' ('Calm and nourish heart and *shen* in order to regulate spleen and stomach') chapter.
[9] Li Dongyuan, *Piweilun*, 'Yinshi Laojuan Suoshang Shiwei Rezhonglun' ('The damage of nourishment and fatigue starts as heat at the centre') chapter. 'Ruling fire' is the translation of *junhuo* (君火), also called 'imperial fire'; 'ministerial fire' is the translation of *xianghuo* (相火); we remind the reader that when speaking of *baoluo* (包络) we intend the connecting channel-*luo* of uterus and kidney
[10] Li Dongyuan, *Piweilun*, 'Piwei Xuzi Juqiao Butonglun' ('When spleen and stomach are deficient the nine orifices do not flow smoothly') chapter. Regarding disorders in the movement of *qi*, see also Chapter 6 on *fanzao*.
[11] Li Dongyuan, *Lanshi Micang* ('Secrets of the orchid chamber'), Neijian Yanlun ('About Cataracts') Chapter. The passage referred to is in the *Suwen*, Chapter 5.

'Due to activity and fatigue *yin* fire boils over and rises up inside the kidney' and explains that: 'The *yin* fire we are speaking of here includes heart fire, kidney fire, and ministerial fire, and from this we can conclude that *yin* fire does not indicate a pathological fire of any particular organ.' To support this hypothesis the author cites the fact that in the various works of Li Dongyuan the term '*yinhuo*' appears a total of 40 times (kidney 5 times, spleen 3, heart 2, liver, lung and stomach 1, channels 6, emotions 2, empty fire 6, full fire 2, others, but always of internal origins 15 and external origins 0), therefore 'this tells us that we are talking about fire and heat pathogens of an empty type, or emptiness of the root and fullness of the manifestations, produced by internal causes'.[12]

ZHU DANXI AND MINISTERIAL FIRE

The centrality of the fire–water axis is also noted by Zhu Danxi: 'The heart is fire, it resides above; the kidney is water, it resides below; water can rise and fire can descend, one rises and the other descends, and there is no limit. [...] The body of water is still, the body of fire is mobile, movement is easy, but stillness is difficult.'[13]

Zhu Danxi also picks up on Li Dongyuan's expounding of the relationship between emotions and fire, reasoning in particular about desires and passions. He acknowledges their strength and inevitability as elements of human nature but states, however, that from the *yang* movement of desires and emotions fire is easily generated and *yin* consumed, 'so difficult to produce and so easy to exhaust' – conditions in which ministerial fire blazes and *jing* flows.

Returning to the thoughts of the neo-Confucians Mengzi and Xunzi, Zhu Danxi describes the pleasures of the senses as follows: 'The desire of man is without limit. [...] Warmth and softness fill the body, sounds and voices fill the ears, colours and images fill the eyes, smells and fragrances fill the nose, only in a man of steel could the heart not be moved.'[14]

The chapter on ministerial fire records how *yin* and *yang* are generated from stillness and movement, it underlines the relationship between movement and fire, and describes the distinction between sovereign fire and ministerial fire and their characteristics. It is, however, ministerial fire that is called 'heavenly

---

[12] Qiu Peiran, *Zhongyi Mingjia Xueshuo* ('Theories of famous doctors of Chinese medicine'), 1922, p. 158.
[13] Zhu Danxi, *Gezhi Yulun* ('Extra tract based on the investigation of things', 1347), '*Yang* Youyu, *Yin* Buzu' ('*Yang* in excess, *yin* insufficient') chapter.
[14] Ibid

fire', because it is this fire that activates desire and *jing*, in this way permitting life and the continuation of the species.[15]

However, the ease with which fire rises has unforeseeable consequences and leads to the consumption of *yin*. Zhu Danxi returns to Li Dongyuan's discussion on ministerial fire as a 'thief of *yuanqi*' to affirm the need to contain the fire of the five elements through the stillness of the heart and adjustment to the *dao*, so that the functions of transformation of ministerial fire and generation of life can be explained. 'Ministerial fire rises up easily; when in response to the *yang* fires of the five natures it flares up perversely, it moves in a rash-*wang* way. When the fire comes from disorder its movements are unforeseeable and there is no movement where true *yin*, boiling and slowly cooking is not present. If *yin* is empty there is illness, if *yin* is exhausted there is death. [...] Master Zhuo affirms: 'The sages held the happy medium-*zhong* (中), rectitude-*zheng* (正), humanity-*ren* (仁) and justice-*yi* (义), as the norm and supported stillness-*jing* (静).' Master Zhuo says: 'One must make sure that the heart of the d*ao* constantly governs the entire body and that the heart of man always obeys its orders. This is a good way to confront fire; in this way the heart of man is placed at the orders of the heart of the *dao*, is governed by stillness, the movement of the five fires is under control, the ministerial fire can assist and integrate generation and transformation and give origin to life.'[16]

Fire and the generation of phlegm that follows it are in a close relationship with the concept of constraint-*yu* (郁) introduced by Zhu Danxi as a central factor in the aetiology of emotional illnesses: 'Old constraints cause heat to evaporate and heat generates fire over time.'[17]

Heat that derives from constricted *qi* that halts and knots tends to consume liquids and produce phlegm; 'Constraint of the seven emotions, then phlegm is produced and fire moves.'[18]

---

[15] 'The *taiji* generates *yang* when it moves, *yin* when it is still. *Yang* moves and changes, *yin* is still and joins it. water, fire, wood, metal and earth are each generated with an individual nature, except fire, which has two. These are the ruling fire (*junhuo* 君 火) or human fire (*renhuo* 人 火), and the ministerial fire (*xianghuo* 相 火) or Heavenly fire (*tianhuo* 天火). Fire with *yin* on the inside and *yang* on the outside governs movement. Therefore, any movement should be attributed to fire. [...] Once alive, man, in the same way, is in perennial movement. The reason he is in continuous movement is none other than the work of ministerial fire'. In: Zhu Danxi, *Gezhi Yulun*, 'Xianghuolun' ('Ministerial fire') chapter. Please also see the reading that a modern Chinese text gives of *xinghuo* as *yushen* (欲 神), 'desiring spirit put into movement by the seduction of external things regarding the heart, latent impulse conserved inside, hidden deeply in the liver and kidney of the lower *jiao*, similar to Freudian theory'. In: He Yuming, *Zhongguo Chuantong Jingshen Binglixue* ('Pathologies of mental illnesses in Chinese medicine', 1995) p. 58.

[16] In: Zhu Danxi, *Gezhi Yulun*, 'Xianghuolun' ('Ministerial fire') chapter. Master Zhuo is the philosopher Zhou Dunyi (1017–1073), Master Zhu is Zhu Xi (1130–1200). Similarly: 'the Heart is the ruling fire, it is stirred-*gan* (感) by things and moves easily, if the Heart moves, ministerial fire also tends to move, and then *jing* flows spontaneously. [...] Therefore the sages and saints taught men only to defend-*shou* (守) and nourish-*sheng* (生) the Heart and this principle was very profound'. In: Zhu Danxi, *Gezhi Yulun*, 'Yang Youyu, Yin Buzu' ('Yang in excess, *yin* insufficient') chapter.

[17] *Danxi Xinfa*, 'Liuyu' ('The six constraints') chapter. For a discussion on the pathogenesis and consequences of constraint and phlegm see Chapter 4.

[18] *Danxi Xinfa*, 'Tan' ('Phlegm') chapter.

When *qi* is constricted it produces dampness, and prolonged retention of dampness produces heat, which over time consumes liquids causing phlegm to form.

Constraint, and therefore a *qi* which halts and knots, plus the heat from which it derives can easily give birth to phlegm.

Regarding treatment, the indications of Zhu Danxi, according to whom it is necessary to act on fire through an action of 'releasing, opening, expanding', are interesting.[19] There are cases in which it is possible to bring down fire and others in which in order to eliminate it there is nothing else to do but follow its nature – that is, going along with its upward movement: 'Light fire; it is compatible with lowering, strong fire, it is compatible with raising, adapting to its nature. Full fire, should be drained, [...] empty fire, *yin* should be tonified.'[20]

ZHANG JIEBIN, CONSTITUTION AND CONSUMPTION OF *YIN*

During the Ming and Qing dynasties, the concept of constraint-*yu* was definitively established and the emotional aspects assume an ever-growing relevance.

Zhang Jiebin recognises, for example, that excess derives from the knotting effect of too much thinking or the accumulation of anger, producing fire and the perverse rising of *qi*, with possible manifestations of mania:

> In all the *kuang* illnesses the cause in the majority of cases is fire. This comes from overplanning, which causes the loss of *zhi*, or from constraint and knotting of the thoughts, which fold in upon themselves and do not expand, and therefore anger is not released-*xie*. This leads to pathogenic wood and fire, and perverse ascending of liver and gall bladder *qi*, and these pathogens become a case of excess in the east.[21]

Zhang Jiebin is also well aware how emotive and sexual irregularity, the consumption of alcoholic beverages and excessive activity first exhaust *qi* and later consume *yin*.

---

[19] 'Constraint of fire, it is necessary to release-*fa* (发) it' In: *Danxi Xinfa*, 'Huo' ('Fire') chapter. The character *fa* is formed of an arrow *shu* and a bow *gong* and the phonetic part composed of two feet, which according to Weiger suggests the idea of 'separation, divergence, letting go' (Weiger p. 112h, Karlgren p. 17).

[20] *Danxi Xinfa*, 'Huo' ('Fire') chapter.

[21] Zhang Jiebin, *Jingyue Quanshu*, ('Complete works of Jigyue', 1640), 'Diankung Chidai' ('Dementia and 'Folly') chapters. In this passage some of the most recurrent terms of 'emotional illness' appear, which are discussed in the glossary and the relative chapters: folly-*kuang* (狂), mind-will-*zhi* (志), constraint-*yu* (郁), knotting-*jie* (结), draining-*xie* (泄), inverse *qi-qini* (气 逆), and pathogens-*xie* (邪). East stands for Wood-Liver. See also Chapter 15 for the discussion on spirits as 'projections of the internal aspects'.

All the damages and deficits, all are due to alcoholic beverages, sexual activity, fatigue, emotions-*qiqing*, and eating. These can injure the *qi* first and if the *qi* is injured this will reach the *jing*, or they can first injure the *jing* and if the *jing* is injured, this will reach the *qi*. However, *jing* and *qi* in man are the *yin* layer, *yin* is the root of the unity of heaven, in all illnesses, if they are strong, there must be a great exhaustion below. The damage that arrives from pathogens due to emptiness befalls the *yin*, the damage of the five organs reaches the kidneys.[22]

The movement of emotions is truly powerful and their fire agitates the *shen* – dynamics which are initially expressed in the first person during the Qing Dynasty: 'All emotions *qiqing* and *wuzhi* when they move are fire and all are capable of disturbing the calmness of my heart.'[23]

Too much thinking damages the spleen and knots the *qi*, but too much studying is a also movement of the *shen* and therefore causes *yang* to rise up, produces heat and consumes *yin*: 'Studying out loud, even if the body is sitting quietly, the *shen* of the heart is in movement, all the movements of the five emotions-*zhi* are *yang*, therefore *yang* mounts and has no restrictions'. Furthermore: 'Studying by repeating out loud, the body is quiet, the heart moves, it is very easy for *qi* to be consumed and *yin* to be dispersed.'[24]

Case Study 5.1

The Dark Tongue

A 32-year-old female semiologist states that the reason for her visit is the fact that her tongue often becomes very dark and that she always has a bitter taste in her mouth.

She is very thin, has intense and spirited eyes, and her gestures are quick and nervous. Even though her lucid intelligence and acute sensibility are immediately evident, she seems to have difficulty speaking and the information comes out in bursts.

Further conversation reveals also flatulence, belching, halitosis, normal bowels but with tenesmus, repeated temporal migraines, and – in the preceding months – tachycardia and stabbing pains in the chest together with a sensation of intense cold in the bones.

She then tells of feeling herself 'on fire, as though there was an internal volcano', and at the same time tiredness due to a sort of 'physical jamming up'.

---

[22] Zhang Jiebin, *Jingyue Quanshu*, 'Xusun' ('Damages from deficit') chapter. 'Alcoholic beverages and sexual activity translate as *jiuse*, in which *jiu* is an alcoholic beverage and *se*, which literally means 'colour', is a euphemism for the erotic environment; regarding the phrase 'yin is the root of the unity of Heaven' a modern comment notes that the unit-one of Heaven also refers to *Yijing*, in which it is said that Heaven, the number one hexagram, generates water: *tian yi sheng shui* (天一 生 水).
[23] He Mengyao, *Yibian* ('Fundamentals of medicine').
[24] Ye Tianshi, *Lingzhen Zhinan Yian* ('Guiding cases in the clinic', 1766).

Lastly, she speaks of panic crises, beginning about 4 months previously following stressful family events and now ever more frequent and destabilising, these manifest 'in sudden waves, with a sensation of total disorientation, like an internal slow-down, with violent pains like punches to the stomach'. There have never been similar episodes in the past, but insomnia and agitation have always been her companions.

She has trouble falling asleep and staying asleep, she awakens too early, is very thirsty, has absolutely no appetite and eats in a disorderly fashion. Her menstrual cycle is generally normal, but with pain and the presence of clots, while her last menstruation came early.

The tongue is without freshness, the colour is a dull, dark red, with a very dry, thick dark yellow coating that becomes almost black at the root; the pulse is rapid, strong and tense.

Diagnosis
Extreme agitation of the *shen* from excess heart, liver and stomach fire.

Therapeutic principles
- Eliminate fire and calm the *shen*.
- Harmonise the Heart, liver and stomach.

Treatment
The treatments, which initially should have followed one another in close succession, were in fact dictated by the schedule of the patient, who works a long way from Milan and is unable to continue the therapy with other colleagues.

The first 4 treatments are 2–3 days apart; the 5th and 6th are given after an interval of 2 weeks; the 7th, 8th and 9th after another 2 weeks and the 10th and 11th 2 months later.

First treatment:
- Ren-15 *Jiuwei*, ST-36 *Zusanli*, ST-44 *Neiting*, GB-34 *Yanglingquan*, LIV-2 *Xingjian*.
- Ren-15 *Jiuwei* to activate the *qi* at the level in which the knotting is felt the strongest and to calm the *shen*.
- LIV-2 *Xingjian*, fire point of the liver and ST-44 *Neiting*, water point of the stomach, to purify the fire of liver and stomach.
- GB-34 *Yanglingquan* and ST-36 *Zusanli* to help regulate the *qi* of wood and earth.

Second treatment: the tongue coating has improved, but the levels of agitation and emotional instability are still very high.
- EX-HN-3 *Yintang*, Ren-17 *Shanzhong*, Ren-4 *Guanyuan*, LIV-3 *Taichong*, KI-3 *Taixi*, SP-3 *Taibai*.
- EX-HN-3 *Yintang*, REN -17 *Shanzhong*, Ren-4 *Guanyuan* to calm the agitated *qi* by drawing it downward through the points of the three *dantian*.
- LIV-3 *Taichong*, KI-3 *Taixi*, SP-3 *Taibai* to nourish the root through the *yuan* points of the *yin* channel of the foot.

Third treatment: the patient seems more self-contained, she says that she feels more herself, 'but still on the edge of a cliff, with a sensation of fear that becomes physical, and a sensation that is just as physical of difficulty in finding myself, because I don't know where I am or how to find myself'.

- EX-HN-3 *Yintang*, Ren-15 *Jiuwei*, Ren-6 *Qihai*, HE-5 *Tongli*, KI-4 *Dazhong*.
- EX-HN-3 *Yintang*, Ren-15 *Jiuwei* and Ren-6 *Qihai* to regulate *qi* and transform the accumulations.
- HE-5 *Tongli*, – together with KI-4 *Dazhong* – to put reconnect water and fire and bring down the excess from above through the *luo* points of the heart and kidney.

Fourth treatment: she is again very agitated, having had a number of attacks of great fear accompanied by violent abdominal spasms.

- EX-HN-1 *Sishencong*, LIV-2 *Xingjian*, ST-44 *Neiting*, P-6 *Neiguan*.
- EX-HN-1 *Sishencong*, LIV-2 *Xingjian* and ST-44 *Neiting* to calm the serious agitation of the *shen* and eliminate fire through the four points above and the two *ying*-spring points below.
- P-6 *Neiguan* to calm the *shen* through the *luo* point of the pericardium, which acts on the abdomen.[25]

Fifth treatment: in the 2 weeks that have gone by the attacks of fear have been decidedly less devastating. The patient had a headache only once, premenstrually. The signs of fire on the tongue and pulse are less extreme. She says that in the last treatment – after the stimulation of EX-HN-1 *Sishencong* – she felt a pure sensation of pain over the loss of her mother. She is happy because in the hours and days that followed she yawned continuously, something that she had not been able to do for a long time.

- EX-HN-1 *Sishencong*, Du-26 *Renzhong*, Ren-4 *Guanyuan*, KI-3 *Taixi*.
- EX-HN-1 *Sishencong*, Du-26 *Renzhong* and Ren-4 *Guanyuan* to regulate communication between *yin* and *yang* by acting on three areas: one very *yang* point at the top, the passage between *Dumai* and *Renmai*, and the *yin* of the abdomen.
- KI-3 *Taixi* to act on the source of water and fire.

Sixth treatment: for the first time, the patient feels significantly better.

- EX-HN-1 *Sishencong*, Du-24 *Shenting*, Ren-4 *Guanyuan*, HE-7 *Shenmen*, SP-6 *Sanyinjiao*.
- HE-7 *Shenmen* and SP-6 *Sanyinjiao* to tonify *qi* and blood.

Seventh, eighth and ninth treatments: in the two intervening weeks there have been no attacks of terror. A sort of general contraction of the body remains, which does not correspond to either a state of alarm or one of weakness, but is rather 'as though the body was frightened to death'. She is relieved because she no longer feels so overcome by internal catastrophes, she manages to breathe with her abdomen and to yawn, she no longer has such violent abdominal spasms or headaches and she eats a little more. Every once in a while dull periumbilical pains reappear, liquid and burning diarrhoea, strong thirst, and insomnia. The menstrual cycle was

---

[25] The P-6 *Neiguan* point is often suggested together with Du-20 *Baihui* or Du-26 *Renzhong* for maniacal, hysterical cases or for dementia (for example, in the Qiao Wenlei seminar at MediCina, November 1997, and a comparison can be made with the usage proposed by Jin Shubai in Chapter 20).

25 days, with moderate dysmenorrhoea. The tongue has a more lively appearance, the coating is light yellow, less dry but still thick and greasy, and the pulse is less tense, but still rapid. The following points are retained:

- Du-20 *Baihui*, EX-HN-3 *Yintang*, Ren-6 *Qihai* or Ren-4 *Guanyuan* to regulate and lower *qi*.

  Furthermore, the following points are alternated:
- Ren-12 *Zhongwan*, ST-36 *Zusanli*, ST-44 *Neiting*
  and
- GB-34 *Yanglingquan*, GB-41 *Zulinqi*, LIV-3 *Taichong*

to tonify the *qi* of the middle *jiao*, release heat and dampness, regulate and circulate the *qi* of wood.

In these ten days of treatment she has had a series of 'regurgitation of anger, like something deeply knotted which gets released and is difficult to handle, but it is better to feel it rather than to pretend it does not exist'. This fury is felt in the muscles and tendons, which are 'stretched out'.

The intestinal symptoms of dampness-heat have been resolved. Neither episodes of panic nor symptoms of depersonalisation have been repeated. The tongue coating is less thick and dry.

The patient spontaneously comments that after acupuncture treatments she always feels very well. Her general sensation is that the treatments are liberating, and at times she has the distinct sensation of sparse electrical shocks or heat coming out from her hands, which is interesting – especially considering that she does not appear to me to be very open to suggestion and has little interest in the more mystical aspects of the bodily experience.

Tenth and eleventh treatments: at a distance of 2 months, the patient says that she no longer feels 'that physical and mental clench, that sense of death, that sense of precariousness'. A generalised sensation of physical tension remains, especially in the neck and jaws, and also internally, owing to which, for example, she often does not feel hunger. Sensations of internal heat, thirst and a bad taste in the mouth are still frequent.

She often has trouble falling asleep and the sleep itself is not very restful and is without dreams. When she sleeps little, her stools are hard with difficult evacuation. Her menstruation had arrived early, and was sparse and moderately painful.

The tongue is no longer dry and dull although it is still too red, and the coating no longer has a grey-brown-blackish colour, but it is still thick and yellow.

The pulse no longer seems to have those beats that banged against the fingers like hammering, and it is finer, but still hard.

The format of the last treatments is maintained, with the use of P-7 *Daling* to release heat, regulate stomach *qi* and activate liver *qi*.

Comments

The changes in the tongue testify to the various developments: the passage of the most dangerous phase is indicated by the disappearance of the blackish colour, a sign of fire burning the *yin*, from the coating, and by the more lively and fresher aspect of the tongue body. The excess of heat is still evident in the scarlet colour and the dullness, but these are not such extreme, worrying characteristics.

The other signs and symptoms also show that the imbalance is still significant: there is still an excess of heat and an unresolved stagnation of *qi*, the probable origin of the problem.

We remind the reader that yawning can be a symptom of kidney emptiness,[26] since the kidney is used to bring *qi* down.

The acute crisis in which the patient felt she was 'going mad' and which corresponds to fire blazing upward and phlegm starting to manifest itself, seems to have passed: in this case the use of acupuncture rendered possible the containment of the phase in which the *shen* is very agitated by the fire and muddled by phlegm formation.

Her transition to a less precarious state of balance is another task.

In these cases in which the *shen* oscillates and lacks root, the first encounter with the patient assumes even more importance than usual.

Reserve and restraint are probably characteristics of this woman, but her extreme initial difficulty in relating her story, this sort of reticence, seems to be a way for her to communicate to me how dangerous are the events that are occurring.

The practitioner's response needs to recognise this truth, but resist using wording that attempts to negate its importance; there is simultaneously a need to perceive its destructive potential but avoid being overcome by it.

Follow-up

After an interval of 1 year, I know through indirect sources that there have been no serious relapses, but that a more or less strong agitation remains a characteristic of her life.

---

[26] Regarding kidney deficiency and yawning, see also the discussion on *zangzao* in Chapter 9 on classic syndromes.

Agitation and Restlessness-*Fanzao*

6

The term *fanzao* (烦躁), 'agitation and restlessness', refers more to a symptom than to an illness or syndrome. It is a combination of internal restlessness and external agitation: *fan* (烦) corresponds to being irritated, bothered, disturbed and impatient; whereas *zao* (躁) refers more to a physical agitation, for example in the limbs, due to which the person cannot remain still.[1]

This term had already appeared in the *Neijing* when describing pathological syndromes of the kidney channel, amongst which we find both the symptom 'annoyance to the heart' and other manifestations of a state of restlessness such as 'One is hungry but does not desire to eat and cannot see clearly, the heart is as though it was suspended, like when one is hungry; if *qi* is insufficient then there is easy fright, with the heart alarmed as though one were about to be captured'.

In the *Neijing*, *fanzao* is also a symptom that accompanies other, more physical, signs when the balance of seasonal *qi* is altered – for example, when excess fire damages the heart and agitates the *shen*;[2] when earth is invaded by wood it is weakened and cannot control water; when earth is in excess it invades and weakens water, which in turn cannot rise to balance the sovereign fire; when water is in excess it invades the heart and cold dominates.[3]

---

[1] The character *fan* (烦) is formed of 'fire' and 'head'. In modern Chinese *mafan* is used to say 'what a bother!' The character *zao* (躁) is the same as the one in *zangzao* (臟 躁): it contains the radical 'foot' and therefore the idea of movement, but it is also a homophone of *zao* 'dry', whose root is 'fire'. The meaning is specified in various texts: The Han Dynasty dictionary *Shouwen Jiezi* states: '*Fan*, pain from heat in the head'; the *Cengyun* ('Additonal rhymes') by Mao Huang of the Southern Song Dynasty, states: '*fan* means *men* (闷) (bothered, bored)'; the *Huainan Zhushu* says: '*zao* means *rao* (躁) (to disturb, bother, molest, inopportune)'.
[2] Relapses of *shaoyang*, when heat is about to arrive [...] there is heat in the Heart and *fanzao*'. 'Revenge of the *shaoyin*, there is bothersome heat internally, *fanzao*, rhinorrhoea and sneezing'. In: *Suwen*, Chapter 74.
[3] In: *Suwen*, Chapter 69, we find: 'If, during the year, Wood is in excess, wind *qi* circulates, Earth-Spleen is invaded by pathogens and one takes ill with diarrhoea and unformed faeces, lack of appetite, a heavy body, *fan*'; 'If, during the year, Earth is in excess, rain and humidity spread, Kidney water receives pathogens and one becomes ill from heaviness and *fanzao*'; If, during the year, water is in excess, then cold *qi* spreads, pathogens damage the heart and one takes ill from a hot body, *fan* in the heart, *zao* and palpitations'.

Zhang Zhongjing identifies the *fanzao* symptom in various pathologies such as: (a) lung diseases with oedema; (b) consumptive illnesses with empty fire; (c) blood stasis with hidden heat; (d) *yang* deficiency, for example after diarrhoea, when *yang* is reconstituted, or when purging in a cold illness, in which *yangqi* is already weak and cold *yin* accumulates internally, which can generate heat if it stagnates; (e) jaundice from dampness-heat.[4]

AETIOLOGY

Fanzao is essentially a symptom linked to heat and internal fire, which distress the heart and disturb the *shen*.

The *fanzao* symptom manifests itself in many conditions of chronic emptiness in which heat and fire develop through various pathogenic processes:

- residual heat which has not been completely resolved
- *yin* deficiency with fire that agitates in a disorderly fashion
- consumption of liquids by empty heat
- extreme fatigue with exhaustion of *qi* and excess fire
- accumulation of *yin*-cold and internal heat
- stasis of blood.

Sun Simiao developed the theory of *yin* agitation (*yinzao* 阴 躁), in which restlessness, even though it is a sign of heat, derives from a emptiness of *yin*. This emptiness, in fact, creates the conditions for initiating a great fullness of *yin*, in which *yang* remains floating on the surface and disturbs the heart. This is therefore a case of false heat and true cold with contradictory signs; for example, the body shows signs of cold that do not, however, appear in the kidney pulse, while simultaneously signs of heat such as restlessness-*fan* are present internally: 'The *yin* pulse is not choppy, while on the contrary the body is cold and internally there is *fan*.'[5]

Li Dongyuan takes up Sun Simiao's reflections on *yin* agitation, *yinzao*, in which the symptoms are similar to external heat illnesses, but in reality are due

---

[4] In: Zhang Zhongjing, *Jingui Yaolue* ('Prescriptions of the golden chamber') we find: 'If there is distension in the Lungs, coughs and *qi* rising, *fanzao* and short breath, floating-*fu* pulse, it is due to water under the heart' (Chapter 7); 'In exhaustion due to emptiness (*xulao* 虚 劳) there is empty *fanzao* and inability to fall asleep' (Chapter 6); 'The illness is similar to a case of heat, with *fanzao*, sensations of fullness, dry mouth and thirst, but the pulse does not suggest heat, it is called 'hidden *yin*' and is caused by blood stasis' (Chapter 16); 'After diarrhoea, if *fan* reappears and the epigastrium feels soft under pressure, it is empty *fan*' (Chapter 17); '*Fanzao* with sensations of heat in the centre of the Heart, one cannot eat, sometimes vomits, has jaundice from alcohol, [...] *fanzao* and inability to fall asleep, is found when there is jaundice' (Chapter 15).

[5] Sun Simiao, *Qianjin Yaofang* ('Invaluable prescriptions for emergencies'). Tao Hua, of the Ming Dynasty, takes up this discussion on *yinzao* in which internal signs of *yin* such as abdominal pain or a deep pulse are present together with *fan*: 'Internally and on the surface there is no heat, but only *fan*, in general one does not wish to see light, at times there is abdominal pain, the pulse is deep and thin'.

to heat striking from the inside (*neishang rezhong* 内伤热中) as, for example, in those cases in which 'one desires to sit in mud: in this case it is *yang* which was exhausted first, it is a case of *yinzao* from true cold and false heat'.

The 'Tract on the Spleen and Stomach' places the accent mainly on the role of stomach *qi* in producing true *qi–zhenqi* and in regulating and protecting its various functions. If stomach and spleen *qi* weaken, its normal physiological movement upwards cannot happen and the upper regions are occupied by *yin* fire, producing respiratory symptoms, restlessness, thirst and various heat symptoms and signs. Food *qi–guqi* cannot participate in the production of gathering *qi–zongqi* and this compromises its transformation into nutritive *qi–yingqi* and defensive *qi–weiqi*. There is then insufficient *yangqi* to defend from external pathogens. We find, in fact:

> *Yin* fire which attacks above, then there is superficial breathing and short breath, heat and *fan*, headache, thirst and flooding pulse. Spleen and stomach *qi* slide downwards and therefore food *qi* cannot ascend. This means that the command of the birth of the spring is not executed, therefore there is no *yang* to defend the nutritive *qi* and the defensive *qi*, one cannot stand wind and cold, and has cold and heat. All this following an insufficiency of spleen and stomach *qi*.[6]

In particular, according to Li Dongyuan this process by which *yin* fire, heat and *fanzao* are produced can result from fatigue in people who practise intense meditative methods.

Internal diseases with fear of cold, in which cold causes immediate illness, are also related to anomalies in the ascending and descending movements of *qi*. 'The nutriments enter the stomach, nutritive *qi* rises upward to go to the heart and lungs and nourish the original *qi–yuanqi* of the upper *jiao*, the skin and the interstices-*couli*.' If instead the nutritive *qi* does not ascend but slides downward 'Heart and lungs do not receive, there is no *yang* in the skin, due to which one loses the external protection of nutritive *qi* and defensive *qi*, the *yang* layer between skin and hair is weak; just contact with wind and cold, or staying in a *yin* and cold place or without sun, causes one to become unwell'.[7]

---

[6] Li Dongyuan, *Piweilun* ('Treatise on the Spleen and Stomach'), '*Yinshi Laojuan Suoshang Shiwei Rezhonglun*' ('The damage of nutriments and fatigue start as heat in the centre') chapter. A modern comment explains: 'Even if the case is complicated, the pathological mechanism can be fundamentally summarised in three aspects: Spleen and Stomach *qi* deficiency, excessive vigour of *yin* fire, anomalies in the rising and descending mechanism'. In: Qi Peiran, *Zhongyi Mingjia Xueshuo* ('Theories of famous doctors of Chinese medicine'), 1992, p. 159. See also Chapter 5 on heat for a discussion on the role of heat and *yin* fire.

[7] Li Dongyuan, *Neiwai Shangbian Huolun* ('Treatise on Differentiating in the Confusion Among Damages from External and Internal Causes'), Bianhanre ('Differentiate between Cold and Heat') chapter. We remind the reader of the normal movements of *yin* and yang: 'Pure *yang* exits from the clear orifices above, turbid *yin* exits from the lower orifice. Pure *yang* spreads to the interstices-*couli* (腠理), turbid *yin* goes to the five organs, pure *yang* fills the four limbs, turbid *yin* is shunted to the six bowels, these are the normal movements of rising and descending'. In: Li Dongyuan, *Piwei Xuzi Jiuqiao Butonglun* ('With Spleen and Stomach in Deficit, the Nine Orifices are not Smooth Flowing')

The elaboration of *yinzao* is later studied and developed further precisely because it refers to complex and insidious cases. Wang Ketang, the great clinical physician of the Tang Dynasty, specifies, for example: 'If there is only *zao* and no *fan* it is generally a case of cold; body and limbs cannot remain still. [...] If one stays naked and does not want to put on clothing, or if one sits in a tub, this is external heat and is generally non-rooted fire, therefore in reality it is cold'.[8]

The Jin and Yuan Dynasty theories which attribute a crucial importance to heat particularly underline the relationship of *fanzao* with internal and external fire, due to which cases with 'agitation, *fanzao*, disturbances with sensations of heat, and restlessness, are all due to the fire pathogen, which acts as master, permeating the internal and the external' and 'if heat is in excess externally the limbs are restless, if heat is in excess internally the *shen* and *zhi* are agitated'.[9]

According to Li Dongyuan:

> When fire enters the lungs there is *fan*; if it enters the kidneys there is *zao*, in both cases it is in the kidney since the paths communicate with the mother lung, but mostly *fanzao* is an illness of heart fire. The heart is the sovereign fire; if fire is exuberant metal melts, water is consumed, fire stands out in isolation, lungs and kidneys together produce *fanzao*. Furthermore, the spleen channel connects to the centre of the spleen, the heart channel starts at the centre of the chest, from the encountering of these two channels comes heat-dampness, which generates *fan*.[10]

The consumption of liquids also easily causes *fanzao*: 'Following sweating, diarrhoea, cholera, vomiting, since there is a great loss of liquids, the organs dry out and there is empty fan. This is because *yin* is insufficient to balance *yang*, *yangqi* is relatively in excess; therefore there is empty heat and fan.'[11]

Further mechanisms that can give rise to *fanzao* are empty blood, owing to which the heart loses its nourishment and the *shen* has nowhere to reside, or stasis of blood, which produces a very specific circumstance, described by Wang Qingren: 'If the body is cool externally and inside the heart there is heat this is called 'lantern illness', on the inside there is a stasis of blood; if not even the smallest things are forgiven, this is stasis of blood; a normally calm person who becomes irascible after the beginning of an illness, this is stasis of blood.'[12]

---

[8] Wang Ketang, *Zhengzhi Zhunsheng* ('Standards for Diagnosis and Treatment').
[9] Liu Wansu, *Suwen Xuanji Yuanbingshi* ('Aetiology Based on Plain Questions').
[10] *Dongyuan Shishu* ('The Ten Books of Dongyuan'), attributed to Li Dongyuan.
[11] Dai Sigong, *Zhengzhi Yaojue* ('Principles of diagnosis and treatment').
[12] Wang Qingren, *Yilin Gaicao* ('Corrections of the errors of medical works'). This illness is called *denglongbing* referring to Chinese lanterns, which are cool outside, but have the heat of the candle inside.

Case Study 6.1

Fire and Agitation

Since acupuncture is a system that acts on the *qi*, it is important to understand in the most direct way possible what alterations of *qi* have occurred.

Alterations in the movement or quality of *qi* correspond to specific sensations, but their direct perception is generally lost, since we all tend to engage in conceptual interpretation in one way or the other. As was noted in Chapter 2 regarding the emotions and the movements of *qi*, it is fundamental that physicians have direct experience of these aspects, so that they may lead the patient to perceive them also. Most patients are not accustomed to expressing emotions verbally or perceiving their internal sensations, so it is therefore up to us as practitioners always to keep this difficulty in mind and to refine our own sensitivity so that we may find a way to draw closer to the patient.

The nature of patient–practitioner relationship is an extremely delicate one: it is quite easy to overlay our own hypotheses, expectations and interpretations and in this way to negate the information given by the patient. It is obviously necessary to translate what we are told by patients into our own frame of reference, but this should happen only secondarily. First of all, the patient must be enabled to state his awareness of the situation in his own terms of reference, and with his own words. If we want to use elements of his account to draw attention to a path of association, it is useful to use the patient's own words rather than ours, and furthermore to facilitate his story by repeating his own phrases rather than framing our own direct questions.

The following brief interchange in an initial conversation with a patient is an example of what we have just described regarding the patient's description of suggestive symptoms.

A 45-year-old male colleague, with a specific psychiatric and psychoanalytical grounding, mentions that he suffered some years earlier from a form of anxiety and depression, which had been successfully resolved through analysis and medications.

As an adult he was diagnosed with a type of progressive congenital disease with metabolic sequelae that can seriously damage various organs. He had borne this condition with great courage and intelligence, continuing to care for his children, to work and to live, but in the previous few months had been feeling very poorly and has become afraid that the suffering will prove more than he can handle.

In his story, the colleague inserts a number of interpretative hypotheses regarding his depression as an expression of narcissistic anger about which I do not comment or remark, asking instead:

'What kind of depression?'

'Today is going well, for the first time after a long period, usually ten minutes after I awaken it is as though it activates itself.'

'Do you feel that there is more physical sensation in any particular area?' (I vaguely indicate the belly, chest, throat and head.)

'At the sternum.'

'And what is it like? Can you describe the sensation itself?'

'I have considered it at length, and concluded it is set in motion when I take serotonergics.' (He continues by referring to the relationship between taking the medication and specific symptoms.)

'Yes, however, this is already an explanation, but what do you feel is actually happening?'

After a silence: 'If I am working, I have to go out for a short walk, I cannot remain still, it is an activation'.

[The classical description of *fanzao* flashes in my mind.] 'And you said that it was a sensation mainly in the sternum…'

'Yes, behind the sternum'.

'Is it a sensation of activation and agitation also there?'

'Yes, it is as though I can absolutely not remain still.'

'If you had to describe it, is it more hot or cold?'

'Hot – actually the first thing that came to mind when you asked me was 'fire'.'

At this point, the description of the symptom is so clear as to render any comment superfluous. The job of integrating this manifestation with the other symptoms and signs, understanding the significance, delineating a diagnosis, elaborating a hypothesis of treatment, and acting on *qi* with effective stimulation remains, but all this makes sense only if it has a root from which to take the directions.

This type of sensitivity is often willingly cultivated by the patient and can be of great help, albeit while being cautious not to exaggerate its importance. In this case, for example, during the eighth treatment the colleague says that the needles on the head (Du-19 *Houding*, Du-20 *Baihui*, and Du-21 *Qianding*) did not have the same effect of 'drawing something out' that they had had on the previous occasion.

Insomnia

7

Night-time, the time of darkness and rest, is the moment when *yin* embraces and nourishes *yang*, which withdraws inwardly and settles down.[1]

Alterations in this period of calm and sleep derive from, and are expressions of, a deep imbalance in which *yin* is compromised: 'When one lies down and does not sleep the organs are injured, if *jing* has a place to reside it is calm.'[2] The organs, which are the site of *yin*, are therefore injured; *jing*, the most dense and deep form of *qi*, has lost its residence; *shen*, the most subtle expression of *qi*, no longer has roots and wanders restlessly.

Sleep has a close relationship with *shen* and an alteration in the quantity or quality of sleep is one of the most frequent and significant symptoms of 'emotional illnesses'.

One sleeps poorly when the *shen* is not at peace, whether agitated owing to excess of fire or restless because it no longer has a place to reside owing to deficiency of blood or *yin*.

As Zhang Jiebin says: 'Lack of sleep may be present in many diseases; nevertheless, you need to understand only two things: sleep has its roots in *yin*, and *shen* is its master, if *shen* is at peace then there is sleep, if *shen* is not at peace then there is no sleep. The reason it is not at peace is either because pathogenic *qi* disturbs it or because *yin* is insufficient.'[3]

Disturbed sleep is the nocturnal equivalent of restlessness during the day.

The *hun*, which accompanies the *shen* and which becomes agitated and wanders when liver blood is deficient, also has an important role in sleep and dreams: 'The liver stores the blood, the heart circulates it. When it is in movement, then blood moves in all the vessels; when it is in a state of calm, then blood returns to the liver.'[4]

---

[1] This is also mirrored in the physiological circulation of defensive *qi weiqi*, which: 'during the day circulates twenty five times in the *yang* and during the night circulates twenty five times in the *yin* (*Lingshu*, Chapter 18).

[2] *Suwen*, Chapter 46. The same phrase is repeated by Huangfu Mi, in *Jiayijing*: 'When one lies down and does not sleep the organs are injured, the emotions-*qing* [do not] settle, sleep is not calm' (Book 12, Chapter 3) and by *Yang* Shangshan in *Huangdi Neijing Taisu*: 'When one lies down and does not sleep the organs are injured, *jing* is consumed, there is no peace' (Chapter 3).

[3] Zhang Jiebin, *Jingyue Quanshu* ('Prescriptions of the golden chamber'), 'Bumei' ('No Sleep') chapter. 'Pathogenic *qi*' during the Ming Dynasty referred to patterns which we define today as 'of Fullness'.

[4] *Suwen*, Chapter 10, which later adds: 'When man rests blood returns to the liver; the eye receives blood and can see; the foot receives blood and can walk; the palm receives blood and can squeeze; the hand receives blood and can grasp'. See also the discussion on *shen* and *hun* in Chapter 3.

DESCRIPTION

In today's Chinese texts, insufficiency of sleep is defined by the modern term *shimian* (失 眠) (literally, 'loss of sleep') or *bumian* (不 眠) (literally, 'not sleeping'), while the corresponding classic term, which is no longer in use, is *bumei* (不 寐) (literally, 'not sleeping') or also *budewo* (不 得 卧) (literally 'not being able to remain lying down').

The principal criteria for defining primary insomnia in modern psychiatry are: 'A. The predominant complaint is difficulty in initiating or maintaining sleep, or non-restorative sleep, for at least 1 month' and 'B. The sleep disturbance (or associated daytime fatigue) causes clinically significant distress or impairment in social, occupational or other important areas of functioning'.[5]

The definition of insomnia therefore encompasses difficulty in initiating sleep or maintaining it (initial or intermittent insomnia), premature awakening and the sensation that sleep has not been sufficiently restoring, but it does not quantify the number of hours slept.

The traditional Chinese medicine definition is very similar, but some emphasis is also placed on the symptom of 'too much/too little dreaming'.

We will not enter here into a discussion on dreaming, which is more relevant to the practices of various Chinese meditative traditions, but confine our treatment to the general clinical environment, in which dreams may be defined as 'excessive' when they are perceived as such. This is mainly a question of quality: dreams can be very vivid and deviate into nightmares (from liver and gall bladder fire, but also from heart and gall bladder *qi* emptiness), or they can follow one another without interruption and be perceived by the patient as very tiring because they seem too real, as though there were no respite from the activities of the day.

The stories of many patients and the underlying patterns of insomnia can be recognised in the following description given by Zhang Jiebin:

> There can be fright and alarm, or fear and apprehension, or a feeling of being bound, or with no reason one thinks a great deal and in a disordered fashion. One can even go the whole night without having slept, or one sleeps but continually awakens, and this is because *shen* and *hun* are not at peace. [...] Thoughts, apprehension, and fatigue injure heart and spleen leading to an emptiness of *qi* and a sinking of *jing,* causing arrhythmia and palpitations and failure to sleep.[6]

---

[5] DSM-IV, 1994, p. 557. According to the Diagnostic and Statistical Manual of Mental Disorders, in order to arrive at a diagnosis of insomnia it is also necessary that it does not occur exclusively during the course of another sleep disorder or another mental disorder, and that it not be due to the effects of substance use or to an underlying medical condition.

[6] Zhang Jiebin, *Jingyue Quanshu,* 'Bumei' ('No sleep') chapter.

AETIOLOGY ACCORDING TO CLASSICAL TEXTS

The imbalance manifested in the alteration of sleep can originate from an excess condition that agitates the heart or from a deficiency as a result of which the *shen* is not sufficiently nourished.

> In the absence of pathogenic *qi*, if one does not sleep it is due to an insufficiency of nutritive *qi* in the heart. Nutritive *qi* governs the blood; if blood is empty it cannot nourish the heart, if the heart is empty then *shen* cannot maintain its residence. [...] If the seven emotions-*qing* strike internally and *qi* and blood are injured and consumed, if fear and apprehension injure the kidney, if fright and fear injure the gallbladder, if *jing* is exhausted then the *shen* has nowhere to settle and one does not sleep.[7]

Insomnia therefore acknowledges aetiological patterns of both excess (fire, phlegm) and deficiency (emptiness of blood, *yin*, *qi*).

Forms of insomnia from emptiness in their various guises are the most frequent.

Insomnia due to a condition of deficiency is described in the *Neijing* – for example regarding the process of exhaustion of *qi* and blood that occurs with ageing: 'In the aged, *qi* and blood weaken, muscles and flesh dry out, the paths of *qi* become choppy, the *qi* of the five *zang* organs clash, nutritive *qi* declines, and defensive *qi* is driven inward, therefore during the day one is not alright and at night one does not sleep.'[8]

In particular, empty blood is a cause of insomnia; the blood needs to return to its storage organ, the liver, at night, but if blood is insufficient the *hun* cannot rest there and wanders during the night.[9] Emptiness can either follow fullness of fire that has consumed *yin* and blood, or be the consequence of *qi* and blood consumption in a serious illness.[10]

The most serious patterns of insomnia from fullness are mania-*kuang*, in which the symptom 'lack of sleep' recurs constantly in various descriptions. If these patterns of phlegm-fire which obscure the portals of the heart are

---

[7] *Ibid.*

[8] Lingshu, Chapter 18. 'Not alright' is the translation of *bujing*; in this case *jing* refers to both physical force and mental lucidity. 'Choppy' translates *se*, the same term that is used for the pulse of blood stasis. The same phrase is repeated in the *Neijing*: 'In the aged, *qi* and blood weaken, muscles and flesh are not humidified, nutritive *qi* and defensive *qi* are choppy-*se*, therefore during the day one is not alright and at night does not manage to sleep'. A *yang* deficiency can also have consequences on sleep: 'In the aged there is a *yang* deficiency and they do not sleep. In: *Zhenzhi Yaojue* ('Principles of diagnosis and treatment'). See also the discussion on *fanzao*, restlessness and agitation, in Chapter 6 and the discussion on heat in Chapter 5 regarding this mechanism.

[9] 'The liver stores the blood, the blood is the abode of the *hun*.' In *Suwen*, Chapter 8. Also: 'At night during sleep the *hun* returns to the liver, if the *hun* is not tranquil there are many dreams'. In: Tang Zonghai, *Zhongxi Huitong Yijing Jingyu* ('Essentials of confluent traditional Chinese and Western medicine'),Wuzang Suocang ('That which is conserved in the five organs') chapter.

[10] 'After a serious illness the *zangfu* are still empty, nutritive *qi* and defensive *qi* are not yet harmonised, one has heat and cold, [...] therefore one does not sleep.' In: Chao Yuanfang, *Zhubing Yuanhou-lun* ('Treatise on causes and symptoms of disease', 610).

extreme and relatively rare, lesser conditions in which a full fire prevails that agitates the *shen* are certainly less so.

Other patterns of fullness derive from the attack of external pathogens, which can establish themselves at the *yangming* level or penetrate to the more internal, *yin* levels of nutritive *qi* and blood and affect the consciousness.[11]

Insomnia can also be a direct result of emotions that injure the heart, of *qi* constraints which produce heat or of an accumulation of phlegm which disturbs the portals of the heart.[12]

In those texts that attribute a pre-eminent role to heat in emotional disorders, it is said: 'If one cannot sleep there is heat and restlessness, suffocated constraint internally, and *qi* cannot spread freely'.[13]

However, Zhang Jiebin also takes into consideration fire, constraint and phlegm accumulation as a cause of agitation of the *shen* and relative insomnia: 'There are many cases in which one does not sleep owing to phlegm and fire which disturb and create disorder; the *shen* of the heart is not calm, because of an excess of thought and apprehension, burning fire and phlegm constraint'.[14]

Phlegm can derive from a deficiency in the transforming and transporting functions of the middle *jiao* causing the liquids to condense, from a constraint and knotting of *qi*, or from heat that develops from emotions or improper diet and which thickens the liquids.

It is important to remember that it is often essential to nourish, even if there are some signs of fullness of fire and phlegm:

> An excess of fatigue and thought lead to consuming of blood and liquids, *shen* and *hun* have no master, therefore there is insomnia. Even when there is a little phlegm and fire it is not necessary to attend to them; all you need to do is cultivate and nourish *qi* and blood. Once *qi* and blood have recuperated, all the symptoms regress spontaneously. If we deal with everything at once, treating in a disorderly fashion or by cooling, the illness will become more difficult to cure, until it produces an exhaustion of *shen* and becomes incurable.[15]

EVALUATION ACCORDING TO THE MODALITY OF PRESENTATION

As with any symptom or pathological pattern, the aetiology, symptomatology, therapeutic principles, and treatment must be established and included

---

[11] 'If pathogens establish themselves in man the eyes do not close and one does not sleep [...] You must tonify the insufficiency, drain the excess, regulate full and empty to render the pathways smooth flowing and expel the pathogens.' In: *Lingshu*, Chapter 71.
[12] 'One does not sleep [...], this is pathogenic *qi* from an emptiness in the five zang organs which overflows into the heart, if there is anguish and ire in the heart, they hide their *qi* in the gall bladder.' In: Wang Huayin, *Taiping Shengui Fang* ('Taiping sacred remedies').
[13] Liu Wansu, *Suwen Xuanji Yuanbinshi* ('Aetiology based on plain questions').
[14] Zhang Jiebin, *Jingyue Quanshu*, Bumei ('No sleep') chapter.
[15] Zhang Jiebin, *Jingyue Quanshu*, Bumei ('No sleep') chapter.

in a differential diagnosis. The various patterns, particularly the presence of signs and symptoms and the treatment rationale, are discussed in Chapters 10 and 11 on general clinical practice, while we take into consideration here only those elements regarding sleep in particular.

If the frame of reference is simplified so as to make easier the process of formulating and evaluating the insomnia, this also necessitates a rigidification of the complexity of clinical reality; the following relationships between the expression of a disorder and TCM syndromes should therefore be considered only as an initial approach.[16]

Emptiness of Heart Blood and Spleen *qi*

Intermittent insomnia

Sleep is light, interrupted by frequent awaking, in which there are often obsessive thoughts.[17]

This is the typical pattern of deficiency of *qi* and blood, weakened by situations which are emotionally overtiring or which are fraught with protracted fatigue.

The classic syndrome of empty heart and gall bladder *qi* with timidity, palpitations, and a state of apprehension and alarm corresponds to a severe emptiness of *qi* and causes sleep interrupted by dreams that awaken in fear.

Heart and Kidney do not Communicate (Heart Fire Due to Empty *yin*)

Initial insomnia

Insomnia is generally accompanied by agitation and restlessness (physical and psychic); besides which there may be dreams that disturb the sleep.

---

[16] To underline how complicated a diagnosis can be, we quote Sun Simiao, who recognises various pathogeneses starting from the pulse: cold-emptiness of the stomach, heat-fullness of the spleen, cold-emptiness of the spleen, and fullness of the heart and small intestine. 'If at the right barrier-*guan*, the pulse shows empty *yang* this is the stomach channel, if the patient feels cold in the legs and cannot sleep this is empty cold of the stomach; if at the right barrier *yin* is full this is the spleen channel, if there is restlessness and one cannot sleep it is full heat of the spleen; if at the right barrier *yin* is empty this is the spleen channel, if one suffers from liquid diarrhoea and cannot sleep it is cold emptyness of the spleen; if the left carotid artery pulse-*renyin* has both *yin* and *yang*, the heart and small intestine channel are both full and one cannot sleep because stomach *qi* does not transport and there is fullness of water and grains.' In: *Qianjin Yaofang* ('Invaluable Prescriptions for Emergencies').

[17] In the more serious version, there is difficulty in falling asleep since the spleen does not produce *qi* and blood, and the *shen* therefore has no abode (sporadic difficulties in falling asleep when very tired belong to the same pattern). We remind the reader that conventional medicine relates a difficulty in falling asleep more to anxiety and premature awakening more to depressive disorders.

The difficulty in falling asleep derives from a *yang* that cannot enter into the *yin* of the night since the latter is insufficient to contain the former and give it an abode and rest.

Fire from empty *yin* can also manifest itself as a simple impulse to being active in the nocturnal hours.

Liver Fullness (*Qi* Constraint or Rising of Liver *Yang*)

Premature awaking

Awaking is sudden and conclusive because the *yang* of the day prevails over the *yin* of the night; activity prevails over rest.

This pattern generally derives from a fullness caused by stagnation and constraint of *qi*, or from a rising of *yang* due to an emptiness of *yin*.

If, instead, the premature awaking follows an already interrupted and non-restoring sleep and brings with it the immediate appearance of thoughts and worries, then it is more probably a case of empty spleen and heart.

Heart, Stomach and/or Liver and Gall Bladder Fire

Agitated sleep

Sleep is extremely agitated, often accompanied by nightmares.

As a 'pure' pattern of fullness this is of limited duration and typically is seen in people who already have some heat present, which is then intensified by emotive or dietary factors.

The total pattern varies depending on the involvement of the various organs.

This type of insomnia also appears in pathological fevers when heat has penetrated to the blood, or in serious cases of phlegm-fire, which disturbs the *shen*.

Fullness of the *Yangqiaomai*

Total absence of sleep

Insomnia due to the lack of communication between the *yin qiao* and *yang-qiaomai* is accompanied by a sensation of being totally awake and very far from falling asleep. It can present itself at the start of the night or after an initial bout of sleep. As it is fullness of *yang*, it is often accompanied by signs of heat.

The *Neijing* speaks of this interruption of the continuity between *yin* and *yang* in the chapter on great disorders and refers to it as *yang* that does not enter *yin*, becomes full and produces excess in the *yangqiaomai* and emptiness of the *yinqiaomai*: 'If defensive *qi* does not manage to enter *yin* and is held back by *yang* then *yang* becomes full, the fullness of *yang* provokes a fullness in the *yangqiaomai*, *yang* no longer enters *yin*. Then *yin* is empty, the eyes cannot close'.[18]

NOTES ON TREATMENT

The choice of points depends on the therapeutic principles that follow the specific differential diagnosis, discussed in Chapters 10 and 11 on clinical practice.

We note here only some specific elements that can support the treatment of insomnia.

Moderate stimulation of dorsal points is useful in chronic insomnia. 2 mm permanent needles may also be left in place on the points BL-15 *xinshu*, BL-44 *shentang* and Du-11 *shendao* to calm the heart, and BL-18 *ganshu* and BL-47 *hunmen* to pacify the liver.

Three points are generally used bilaterally to induce communication between the *yin qiao* and *yang qioa* vessels: disperse the confluent point of *yangqiaomai*, BL-62 *shenmai*, open the point where the two channels meet BL-1 *jingming* and tonify the confluent point of *yinqiaomai*, KI-6 *zhaohai*.

The use of just these three points focuses the needles' action specifically on regulating the passage from *yang* to *yin*.

Extra points with specific action on sleep are EX-HN-14 *yiming*.[19]

EX-HN-3 *yintang*, a point that calms the *shen*, opens the portals of the heart and transforms phlegm is also often used in cases of insomnia.

Ancillary methods like ear acupuncture therapy, cranial acupuncture, and the wrist–ankle technique are generally supportive in cases in which the response to treatment is not satisfactory, but the technique of using seeds on ear points, stimulated by the patient, is often useful as a front-line treatment.[20]

---

[18] *Lingshu*, Chapter 80. The same explanation is repeated in the *Jiayijing* (Book 12, Chapter 3). In cases of insomnia from imbalance between the two, C. Chase also suggests dispersing *Yang Qiao* and nourishing *Ying Qiao* with intradermal needles of metal or zinc in BL-62 *Shenmai*, and of gold or copper in KI-6 *Zhaohai*. Seminar at MediCina, May 1998.

[19] *Anmian* 1 (a medial point between SJ-17 *Yifeng* and GB-20 *Fengchi*) and *Anmian* 2 (a medial point between TB-17 *Yifeng* and EX-HN-14 *Yiming*) are not recognised in the standardisation of the WHO (1991) but are often used in any case, especially the first one (also called simply *Anmian*). EX-HN-14 *Yiming* is found 1 *cun* behind TB-17 *Yifeng*.

[20] For a discussion on these various techniques, see Chapter 12 on methods of stimulation.

In ear acupuncture therapy Shenmen is the principal point for calming the *shen* and can also be used as the only ear point. In accordance with the diagnosis, points such as Heart, Liver, Brain, Spleen, Kidney, Endocrine, Subcortical, Sympathetic, Ear apex, Gall bladder and Stomach may be chosen. The seeds should be pressed 30 times or for one minute both during the day and before retiring.

In cranial acupuncture the areas along the median line which are used in neuropsychiatric disorders are generally chosen, especially MS-1 (from Du-24 *shenting*, for 1 *cun* downward) and later MS-5 (from Du-20 *baihui* to Du-21 *qianding*). Electrostimulation may be applied, mostly with continuous waves, and medium intensity and frequency.

The wrist–ankle technique can be a good method in those cases where it is preferable that the sensation of arrival of *qi* not be too strong, or when the stimulation of a permanent needle is considered important, or if other techniques have not met with success. The point of choice is Upper-1 (on the ulnar edge of the ulnar flexor tendon of the carpus, two finger widths from the wrist crease) and also Upper-5 (on the median line of the dorsal side of the forearm, two finger widths from the wrist crease).

Moxa in its various forms accompanies the basic formulation of the acupuncture and is used to tonify or warm, but also as a 'small fire that calls up the big fire'.

Bleeding is used mainly for eliminating full heat, but also empty heat. In general, bleeding is done on points higher up on the head or on the back, or the *jing*-well points.

Internal practices, herbal remedies and *tuina* are beyond the scope of this discussion, but their role is fundamental. Besides the more elaborate and complex forms of these methods, simple *qigong* exercises, careful attention to diet and use of medicines and self-massage techniques are of great help.

TREATMENT ACCORDING TO SOME CONTEMPORARY AUTHORS

A number of hypotheses of treatment drawn from important modern clinical practitioners are presented here.

Wang Leting: 'A Method for Calming the *Shen* and Stabilising the *Zhi*'[21]

The text indicates this method, called *anshen dingzhi fa*, especially for 'insomnia caused by fear, with palpitations and a non tranquil mind-*shenzhi*'.

[21] Born in 1894, Wang Leting was the director of the Acupuncture Department of the TCM Hospital of Beijing and was published for the first time in 1983. These indications are drawn from his book, edited by Niu Yunduo, *Jinzhen Zaichuan* ('Transmissions of the experiences of Wang Leting 'golden needle'),1994, p. 15-16 and p. 86. The text *Golden Needle Wang Leting* (Blue Poppy Press, 1997) translates interesting parts of his work of 1984, but these parts on insomnia do not appear in it.

It is specified that the *shen* is restless because it is without an abode because of emotional factors that cause fear and abnormal movements of *qi* and *shen*, imbalance of the organs, and disorders of *qi* and blood.

The following therapeutic principles are defined: nourish the *yin*, benefit the *qi*, put heart and kidney in communication, calm the fright, stabilise *zhi*, harmonise the centre and calm the *shen*.

Basic treatment includes:

- Du-24 *Shenting*, GB-13 *Benshen* to calm the *shen* and tranquillise the heart;
- Ren-12 *Zhongwan*, Ren-6 *Qihai*, ST-25 *Tianshu* to calm the *shen* and stabilise *zhi*. These four points, called 'the four gates' (*simen*), are very effective for apprehension, fear and anxiety;
- HE-7 *Shenmen*, SP-6 *Sanyinjiao* to benefit *qi* and blood;
- P-6 *Neiguan* in cases of constraint and liver *qi* stagnation;
- KI-3 *Taixi* in cases of empty liver and kidney *yin*;
- LIV-3 *Taichong* in cases of excess liver *yang* above.

In a previous chapter dedicated to insomnia the following are suggested as fundamental points:

- HE-7 *Shenmen*, SP-6 *Sanyinjiao*

  as well as:

- Du-20 *Baihui*, EX-HN-3 *Yintang*, GB-20 *Fengchi* in cases of dizziness;
- P-6 *Neiguan*, LIV-3 *Taichong* in cases of liver heat attacking above;
- BL-18 *Ganshu*, BL-23 *Shenshu*, KI-3 *Taixi* in cases of empty liver and kidney *yin*;
- BL-15 *Xinshu*, BL-18 *Ganshu* in cases of heart blood insufficiency;
- BL-62 *Shenmai*, KI-6 *Zhaohai* in cases of lack of communication between *yin* and *yang*;
- Ren-12 *Zhongwan*, ST-36 *Zusanli* in cases of stomach *qi* disharmony;
- BL-47 *Hunmen*, BL-42 *Pohu* in cases of excessive dreaming.

  According to the clinical patterns:

- Thought injures the heart and spleen: HE-7 *Shenmen*, P-6 *Neiguan*, HE-5 *Tongli*, SP-6 *Sanyinjiao*;
- Liver and gall bladder heat: GB-11 *Touqiaoyin*, P-7 *Daling*, LIV-2 *Xingjiang*, GB-43 *Xiaxi*, HE-7 *Shenmen*, SP-6 *Sanyinjiao*;
- Empty and cold gall bladder: GB-44 (+ moxa);
- Stomach disharmony: Ren-12 *Zhongwan*, ST-36 *Zusanli*, HE-7 *Shenmen*, SP-6 *Sanyinjiao*:
  - Ren-11 *Jianli*, SP-44 *Gonsun* in cases of bad digestion,
  - ST-25 *Tianshu*, ST-44 *Neiting* in cases of abdominal distension and borborygmi,
  - TB-6 *Zhigou*, ST-37 *Shangjuxu* in cases of constipation,
  - LIV-13 *Zhangmen*, P-6 *Neiguan*, LIV-3 *Taichong* in cases of liver *qi* constraint and knotting.

He Puren: 'Clinical Cases of Insomnia'[22]

Heart and kidney do not communicate:

- difficulty or impossibility in falling asleep, vertigo, ringing ears, hot flashes, nocturnal sweating, heat in the 'five hearts' (palms and soles), lack of memory, abundant dreams, weak knees and lower back, spermatorrhoea or continuous erections (strong-*qian yang*).

Empty heart and kidney:

- easy awakening and difficulty in falling asleep, many dreams, dull colouring, asthenia, short breath, difficulty in speaking, palpitations, bad memory, lack of appetite, loose stools.

Stomach heat which produces fire:

- big appetite with difficulty in transforming foods, difficulty in falling asleep, restlessness, dry mouth and tongue, a feeling of weight on the chest, epigastric closure, languor and continuous hunger, constipation or foul smelling stools.

Constraint due to liver and gall bladder heat:

- agitated sleep, easy sudden awakening with fright, many dreams, fullness in the ribs, bitter taste in the mouth, red eyes.

According to the clinical pattern, points may be chosen such as: BL-15 *Xinshu*, BL-23 *Shenshu*, Ren-12 *Zhongwan*, P-6 *Neiguan*, ST-36 *Zusanli*, etc.

Case Study 7.1

A 54-year-old woman has been suffering from insomnia for the last year. She is tired and worried about her job, takes Western medications to sleep, but they are now no longer effective and at times she does not sleep for the whole night. She has many dreams, nightmares, is confused and restless, irascible, and impatient, has lumbar pain, weak knees, asthenia, dark and scanty urine, and constipation. She is menopausal, her face and lips are red, the tongue is light red with a light coating, and the pulse is deep and rapid.

---

[22] Born in 1926, He Puren received the qualification of 'Famous physician' *mingyi* in 1990 after directing the Acupuncture Department at the TCM Hospital of Beijing. He is particularly noted for his use of needles, fire (scorching needles) and bleeding: starting from the preposition that all illnesses derive from stagnation and constraint of *qi* he uses these methods with the aim of opening the passages to activate *qi*. The clinical cases presented here are taken from *Zhenjiu Santongfa Linchuan Yingyong* ('Clinical usage of the three passage methods of acupuncture and moxibustion'), Beijing, 1999, p. 61-64.

Diagnosis

Excessive worries and thoughts; heart and kidney do not communicate; the heart *shen* lacks nourishment.

Therapeutic principles

Re-establish the communication between heart and kidney, nourish the heart, and calm the *shen*.

Treatment

- BL-15 *Xinshu*, BL-23 *Shenshu*.

Daily treatment, tonifying with rotation, for 30– 40 minutes.

After the first treatment the dreaming has diminished; after three treatments she falls asleep more easily and the dreaming is further diminished; after five treatments she falls asleep well, no longer has dreams and the sleep is tranquil and restoring; after ten treatments the insomnia has disappeared and the other symptoms have improved.

Case Study 7.2

A 35-year old woman has suffered from recurring insomnia for a number of years. She has trouble in falling asleep and her sleep is interrupted, even though she uses Western medications, and the condition worsens with tiredness and tension. Aside from this, the following are also present: asthenia, cold limbs, good appetite, constipation, scarce and late menstruation, dull colouring, pale lips, pale tongue, white coating, deep, thin and weak (*wuli*) pulse.

Diagnosis

Empty heart and spleen; *qi* and blood deficiency; the heart *shen* lacks nourishment.

Therapeutic principles

Regulate heart and spleen, tonify *qi* and blood, nourish the heart and calm the *shen*.

Treatment

- Ren-12 *Zhongwan*, P-6 *Neiguan*, ST-36 *Zusanli*

Treatments on alternating days, tonification with rotation, for 30 minutes.

After two treatments sleep has improved; after five treatments she falls asleep easily, dreaming has diminished and is less vivid, she is less tired; after eight treatments her sleep is deep and with few dreams, she feels more physical and mental energy, she is less cold in the limbs, and the constipation has improved; after ten treatments sleep is good and the other symptoms have improved.

Case Study 7.3

A 31-year-old woman has suffered from insomnia for 6 months. Her trouble in falling asleep appeared following an argument in the family, she uses Western medications, is restless, has a dry mouth, constipation, white tongue coating, and a tight and slippery pulse.

Diagnosis

Exhaustion of *yin*, consumption of liquids, liquids do not ascend to the higher regions and heart *shen* lacks nourishment.

Therapeutic principles

Benefit *yin* and calm the *shen*.

Treatment

- TB-4 *Yangchi*.

Daily treatment, balanced method, 30 minutes.

After three treatments she feels well, falls asleep easily but her sleep is not deep, her mouth is less dry; after six treatments sleep is good, the mouth is no longer dry, the constipation has improved; after ten treatments her sleep is tranquil and bowel movements are regular.

The insomnia in this case started after an argument – in other words a disturbance of *qi*, which causes a loss of proper flowing in the *Shao yang* and a deficiency of liquids. *Shao yang* is the 'fulcrum', anger and constraint cause the lack of fluidity in the fulcrum, hand *Shao yang* and foot *Shao yang* communicate; if *Shao yang* does not flow then liquids are not moved forward regularly from the *San jiao* and this causes a lack of peace for the *shen*, and insomnia.

TB-4 *Yangchi* is chosen because it is the source-*yuan* point of *San jiao*, it stops thirst, produces liquids and humidifies, aids the distribution of the *San jiao*'s liquids.

Gao Lishan: 'The six points of sedation'[23]

This combination (*zhenjing liuxue*) is suggested for painful pathologies, wind patterns, palpitations and mental illnesses (*shenzhibing*). The latter may have diverse aetiologies: accumulation of dampness in the spleen and stomach originating phlegm which obscures the portals of the heart; emotions that cause constraint of the liver; emptiness of the heart and spleen due to which the heart lacks nourishment; heart fire which inflames and agitates the *shen*;

[23] Gao Lishan, a physician at the Guanganmen Hospital of the TCM Academy of Beijing, has published four books which compile his experiences. This discussion on insomnia is drawn from *Zhenjiu Xinfei* ('Notes on the heart in acupuncture and moxibustion'), 1997, p. 264.

improper diet with stomach and spleen disharmony. Possible illnesses include, for example, neurosis, depression, anxiety and nervous breakdown. The heart loves tranquillity; if there is tranquillity the *shen* is gathered and stored internally; therefore the following points for calming the *shen* may be used:

- ST-36 *Zusanli*, HE-7 *Shenmen*, LI-20 *Yingxiang*
- + ear points: Heart, Lung, Shenmen.

Shen is tranquillised using the following principles: harmonise the stomach, nourish the heart, and purify the lung.

Zhong Meiquan: 'Use of the 'plum-blossom' needle'[24]

It is necessary to examine the areas along the sides of the spinal column, from the neck to the sacrum, and discover points and zones which present alterations such as contractions, fibrosity, raised areas or pain under pressure and treat them with the 'plum blossom' needle. The medial side of the leg is also examined and eventually treated.

Method

The individual points: treat 20–50 times, on an area with a diameter of 0.5–1.5 cm.

On the sides of the spinal column: work along 3 lines, respectively at 1, 2, and 3–4 cm from the column, from above to below, 3 times.

On the head: work along a 'net' of lines, a number of times.

Upper abdomen: work along 8–9 vertical lines, and 4–5 lines across the body.

Groin: work along the line that passes from the iliac crest to the pubic bone, 2–3 times.

Legs: work along the medial side, from the knee to the medial malleolus, 3–4 times.

Frequency

Generally the treatments are on alternate days; a cycle consists of 15 treatments, after which 15 days of rest follow.

Technique

Loose wrist, medium power; if possible perform treatment in the evening before retiring.

---

[24] Zhong Meiquan, also a physician at the Guanganmen Hospital of the TCM Academy of Beijing, specialised in the use of techniques with the hammer. These notes are drawn from *Zhenjiu Linzheng Zhinan* ('Clinical guide for acupuncture and moxibustion') edited by Hu Ximing, 1991, p. 234.

Specific points

- Empty heart and spleen: ST-36 *Zusanli*, Ren-12 *Zhongwan*, P-6 *Neiguan*, HE-7 *Shenmen*, SP-6 *Sanyinjiao*.
- Liver constraint and *qi* stagnation: GB-20 *Fengchi*, LIV-14 *Qimen*, SP-6 *Sanyinjiao*, Ren-12 *Zhongwan*, Du-14 *Dazhui*, EX-HN-3 *Yintang*.
- Heart and kidney do not communicate: Du-14 *Dazhui*, Du-20 *Baihui*, HE-7 *Shenmen*, SP-6 *Sanyinjiao*.

Case Study 7.4

Insomnia as an After-Effect of Old Anxieties

A 22-year-old male student suffering from persistent insomnia is sent to me by a colleague.

He informs me that he has been a hypochondriac and very anxious for a number of years, and has suffered from panic attacks with strong agitation, vertigo, and crises in which he felt depersonalised. He has been in analysis for 4 years and these symptoms seem to have been relieved, but a fairly serious insomnia remains.

The insomnia consists of difficulty in initiating sleep, at times accompanied by an anxiety he perceives as a retrosternal oppression: a knot like 'an octopus'. When the tardiness of sleep interferes with his studies too much, he takes tranquillisers, whose effectiveness is, however, variable.

He studies a lot, eats too much and in an erratic fashion (already overweight, he has gained eight kilograms in the last year), bowel movements tend to constipation, he suffers from periorbital headaches which started after having taken an exam and from allergic asthma in the spring. His colouring is white; he has an appearance of flaccidity.

The patient's tongue has a wide central crack which does not reach the tip, the tongue body is a bit small and a light retraction at the centre of the tip produces an indentation in the continuity of the curve, the colour is dark red, dull, the coating is white, the sublingual vessels are slightly yellow.

The pulse is deep, and thin with respect to his physique.

Diagnosis
Knotting of *qi* with internal heat, especially in the stomach; spleen *qi* and heart blood emptiness with accumulation of dampness and phlegm.

Therapeutic principles
Regulate *qi*, clear heat, tonify the spleen, and transform phlegm, which obscures the portals of the heart.

Treatment

Seven treatments: biweekly, with the last ones at intervals of 3 and 6 weeks.

First treatment:

- Du-24 *Shenting*, EX-HN-3 *Yintang*, Ren-18 *Yutang*, Ren-15 *Jiuwei*, Ren-6 *Qihai*, HE-7 *Shenmen*, SP-3 *Taibai*.

The combination of points on the *Du* and *Renmai* regulates the movement of *qi* drawing it downward when it agitates above:

Du-24 *Shenting* and EX-HN-3 *Yintang* calm the agitation of the *shen* and transform the phlegm, which obscures the portals of the heart.

Ren-18 *Yutang* is chosen on the base of the location of the feeling of anxiety; like Ren-17 *Shanzhong*, it regulates and descends *qi*.[25]

Ren-15 *Jiuwei*, *luo* point of the *Renmai*, activates and regulates *qi*; Ren-6 *Qihai* brings it down.

The *yuan* points of the heart and spleen, HE-7 *Shenmen* and SP-3 *Taibai*, calm the *shen* while nourishing blood and *qi*.

The following are maintained:

- Du-24 *Shenting*, EX-HN-3 *Yintang*, Ren-6 *Qihai*.

The other points used in the first treatment are alternated with:

- Ren-17 *s*, Ren-13 *Shangwan*, SP-4 *Gongsun*, P-6 *Neiguan*.

Ren-18 *Yutang* is substituted by Ren-17 *Shanzhong* because already after the second treatment the 'knot' has become a lighter and more diffuse sensation of vague oppression in the chest.

Ren-15 *Jiuwei* is alternated with Ren-13 *Shangwan* to regulate and bring down stomach *qi*.

The SP-4 *Gongsun* and P-6 *Neiguan* couple regulate the urgent ascending of *qi* in the *Chong mai* and activate *qi* in cases of constraint with manifestations at the emotional and dietary levels.

After the second treatment, with the exception of one night, the patient has invariably slept well, even close to taking exams, owing to which during the fifth treatment I decide to pause treatment for an interval of 3 weeks.

During this period, he has slept without problems and there is some qualitative improvement in the sleep, thanks to which he arises feeling more rested and notes that he has faced this exam with greater equanimity. The tongue has a more normal colour, while the sublingual area remains unchanged. The pulse is a bit rapid, but it is no longer so deep and thin.

Comments

Stagnation, constraint and knotting of *qi* create internal heat, which consumes spleen and heart *qi*. The insufficiency of spleen *qi*, which was probably a constitutional tendency in this young man, favours the accumulation of dampness and the heat fosters its thickening into phlegm, which obscures the portals of the heart.

---

[25] The classical prescriptions in which Ren-18 *Yutang* is indicated for perversely rising *qi* and agitation of the heart may be found in *A Manual of Acupuncture* by P. Deadman and M. Al-Khafaji (2001).

We recall here that the conditions of *qi*, blood, and organs may be seen on the tongue, while there are no direct signs of the *shen* there; the state of the *shen* does however manifest itself in the fresh or not very vigorous appearance of the tongue body. In this case, the colour of the tongue was red owing to internal heat, but dull; the small tongue and the indentation in the tip (which generally indicates empty blood) revealed the scanty nourishment of the heart in its role of abode of the *shen*. The sublingual yellow indicated turbid dampness in the stomach.

The fact that after the treatment there was more consistency in the pulse indicates an improvement in the *shen*.

The basic treatment of the *Ren* and *Dumai* is focused on regulating the disorder in the flow of *qi*, which has great relevance in manifestations like anxiety and insomnia.[26]

The confluent point couple of *Chong* and *Yin Wei Mai* generally shows itself to be useful for regulating *qi*, which tends to ascend violently and manifest as panic crises, retrosternal oppression or as a knot in the throat, but also through the difficulty in calming the *shen* in sleep.

Cases where the patient is impelled to eat in order to calm the agitation linked to the heat produced by the constraint of *qi* are frequent: the labour of digestion in the stomach at least temporarily consumes this heat. In these cases, in which the *qi* disorder alters the balance of emotions and eating, and is in turn injured by their disturbance, the two *luo* points of spleen and pericardium are very effective and it often happens that the patient simply no longer feels the necessity to eat continually.

Remembering the earlier case of the frightened woman (see above), in which the use of heart and kidney *luo* points had probably activated the *qi* too early, I preferred instead to initiate the therapy by tonifying the spleen and heart through their respective *yuan* points.

Not all cases are resolved so rapidly and brilliantly, nor is it always easy to make an accurate prognosis.

In this case, for example, tongue and pulse seemed to be indicating a clinical condition and relative need for treatment much more serious than they turned out to be.

Follow-up

After an interval of 6 months the young man has a consolidating treatment. He is very content: he falls asleep calmly and the sleep is restful; he has started being careful with his diet eliminating greasy and fried foods, dairy products and snacks between meals; he is losing weight.

The tongue is still a little red at the tip, but the indentation in the tip has disappeared and the crack is less accentuated. The pulse is the same as 6 weeks' previously.

---

[26] In this regard, compare the comments of Jin Shubai in Chapter 20, the protocols used for General Anxiety Disorder in Chapter 25 and the use of similar combinations in patients with different diagnoses such as cases 5.1, 7.5, 9.2, 9.4, 10.5 and 11.3.

We see each other again after a few months for preventative treatment for the spring asthma.

Case Study 7.5

Difficult Sleep

A 60-year-old woman is suffering from a chronic difficulty in initiating and maintaining sleep, which has worsened over the last two years.

A retired teacher, she is of robust build, has a strong voice, with lively eyes and laughter.

Notwithstanding the use of benzodiazepine and herbal products, her sleep remains irregular and unsatisfactory. 'Ugly thoughts' emerge at night and the lack of adequate sleep also interferes with daily life, owing to which she often finds herself tired and irritable.

The patient is not very thirsty, but feels her mouth is dry, especially at night, and she has a sensation of internal heat. She also has had nocturnal sweating, palpitations, and at times shortness of breath ever since she started the menopause at the age of 40 – at which time she also started to suffer from hypertension.

Bowel movements are regular and appetite is excellent, but eating greasy or spicy foods – which she loves – cause her pain or epigastric heaviness and she is often subject to halitosis upon awakening.

She is on antihypertensive and antiarrhythmia medication for extrasystolic supraventricular arrhythmia.

Her tongue is red without coating, with the tip even redder and slightly pointed.

Diagnosis
Kidney and heart *yin* deficiency, with empty fire that disturbs sleep.

Therapeutic principles
Nourish heart and kidney *yin*, calm the fire and the *shen*.

Treatment
Ten treatments: seven weekly and then twice a month
   These points are alternated:
- BL-15 *Xinshu*, BL-4 *Shentang*, Du-11 *Shendao*, BL-23 *Shenshu*, BL-52 *Zhishi*, SP-6 *Sanyinjiao* (in the first three points 2 mm needles are left in place for 3 days) to nourish heart and kidney and calm the *shen*
   and
- EX-HN-3 *Yintang*, Ren-17 *Shanzhong*, Ren-4 *Guanyuan*, HE-6 *Yinxi*, KI-6 *Zhaohai* to calm the *shen*, nourish heart and kidney *yin* and clear empty fire.
   The following are maintained:

- *Anmian* or ear point *shenmen* to facilitate sleep.
  At times, the following points are used:
- ST-36 *Zusanli* or Ren-12 *Zhongwan* to regulate the middle *jiao* and clear stomach heat.

The patient's reaction to the insertion of the needles is decidedly strong, owing to which not only do I not stimulate them, but in the initial phase I do not even obtain *deqi*.

The response is rather variable, but, all told, she shows some improvement.

The patient alternates nights in which she sleeps eight hours (until 7:00 a.m.) with others in which she sleeps six, which she considers insufficient. After only two treatments, she wakes up only twice a night instead of four to five times, and most importantly she falls asleep again easily, but on a few nights still she is agitated and this bothers her greatly.

After ten treatments, or approximately 3 months, the woman feels she 'has more energy' in the morning, but her mouth is still a little dry at night and the sensation of internal heat remains.

She is sporadically short of breath, but is no longer subject to palpitations or sweating. She also no longer takes tranquillisers and sleeps an average of 7 hours, and her sleep is generally tranquil and resting.

Her tongue is still red and the coating is scarce, the pulse is still irregular, but less rapid and thin.

Comments

The deficiency of heart and kidney *yin* is probably a consequence of a stagnation of liver *qi*, with invasion of earth and transformation into heat in the middle *jiao*. This heat from *qi* constraint has consumed the *yin*, and the fire that now manifests itself as insomnia, palpitations and sensations of internal heat is typical of empty *yin*.

I therefore preferred to focus the treatment on nourishing the *yin* and acting in part on the constraint of *qi*, while concentrating, however, on the regulation of the stomach rather than the liver.

During the first treatments, the insertion of the needles met with sudden and violent screams and it was probably only her implicit awareness of our mutual relationship that kept her from insults and only the good results that convinced her not to stop the treatment.

The empathy that a physician should have with a patient in this case consists in acceptance of the latter's 'hypersensibility' and also use of verbal indications that provide a sort of continuous restatement of the therapeutic relationship – for example, 'I remember that this point was painful for you, I'll massage it first, now tell me if you feel the needle too much. This other point was all right, today I will try to touch it a little more (meaning the *qi*)' – while continuously trying not to be overcome by her furious and offended stare. After a few treatments, things went more smoothly.[27]

---

[27] In this regard, see also Chapter 12 on needle stimulation methods and Chapter 15 on the therapeutic relationship.

Follow-up

Seven months' later the patient returns and states that her sleep had been good until a couple of weeks previously, but that she now awakens every couple of hours, owing to which she takes a half of a tranquilliser pill, often followed by another half and at times yet another half.

Furthermore, she has a sensation of oppression in the chest, frequent palpitations, and recurring epigastric burning sensations two hours after supper. She is in the midst of adjusting her antihypertension therapy because her minimum arterial pressure is again too high.

I prescribe 10 drops of *en*, to be taken regularly and at a decreasing dosage (in effect, it is suspended after 1 month, as the dosage is decreased by two drops per week).

This second cycle of treatments also consisted of ten treatments, with the same frequency as the preceding one and the choice of points was also similar, but also anticipates the use of HE-5 *Tongli*, Ren-15 *Jiuwei* or Ren-14 *Juque*, in relation to the palpitations, the arrhythmia of the pulse and the gastric disturbances.

The insomnia, palpitations, and epigastric pain were resolved, the pulse remains arrhythmic, the pressure is now under control. The patient is evaluating various opportunities that will help her develop her creative talents.

Case Study 7.6

Can't Close His Eyes

A 53-year-old male public transport driver, tells me that he has always slept little (approximately 5 hours per night), but that in the last year the situation has got worse and he now awakens after 2 to 3 hours of sleep with the feeling of being completely awake. He falls asleep again only after having taken a tranquilliser, which he substituted in the last month for a hypnotic drug; in this way, he sleeps 5 to 6 hours, but not always.

The insomnia does not appear to be accompanied by other relevant symptomatic manifestations.

There is an underlying full and heat condition, which is evident in his colouring, his voice and his general appearance. The patient defines himself as being warm, has a good appetite and is a bit overweight, but digestion, bowels and urination are regular and there are no other disturbances beyond rare episodes of frontal–temporal headaches.

The tongue edges and tip are redder with a greasy, slippery white coating that has a light yellow tint.

The pulse is full and tight at the left barrier-*guan* position.

Diagnosis

Heat in heart, stomach and liver. Fullness in *yangqiaomai* and lack of communication between *yin* and *yang*.

Therapeutic principles

Clear heat, activate communication between the *Ying qiao* and *Yangqiaomei*.

Treatment

Six treatments: weekly, with the last one after an interval of 2 weeks.

First treatment:

- BL-62 *Shenmai*, BL-1 *Jingming*, KI-6 *Zhaohai*
- Ear point *Shenmen* with 'permanent' seed.

BL-62 *Shenmai*, called 'the chimney of ghosts', Guilu by Sun Simiao, calms the heart, the *shen* and internal wind; BL-1 *Jingming* calms wind and clears heat; KI-6 *Zhaohai* nourishes *yin* and liquids and clears heat.

The combination of these three points acts on the communication and balancing of *Yin* and *Yangqiaomai*.

Five days later the patient mentions that he has slept well. He arose to urinate but fell asleep again immediately. He also slept about an hour in the afternoon when he had no work.

Afterwards treatment is repeated, alternating it with:

- HE-8 *Shaofu*, KI-2 *Rangu*, BL-1 *Jingming*, in the third treatment
  and
- P-7 *Daling*, LIV-2 *Xingjian*, ST-44 *Neiting*, BL-1 *Jingming* in the fifth treatment.

The earth point of the pericardium and the spring-*ying* points (fire points on the *yin* channels and water points on the *yang* channels) clear heat.

A combination focused on the water–fire axis is alternated with one that is more aimed at clearing heat at the *zangfu* level.

In any case BL-1 *Jingming* is maintained as representative of the passage between the two channels, *Yinqiaomai* and *Yangqiaomai*.

Comments

Since the excess of heat seems to essentially flow into *Yangqiaomai* filling the *yang* and compromising communications between the two *qiao*, I chose to act firstly at this level, putting off an eventual regulation of these organs until later.

I started on the left, the *yang* side, stimulating the confluent point of the *Yangqiaomai* in dispersion to 'push and unlock' the fullness of *qi*, next needling the meeting point BL-1 *Jingming* with the intent-*yi* to 'open' the passage and lastly stimulating the confluent point of the *Yin Qiao Mai* in tonification to 'summon' *qi*. I repeated the same sequence on the right.

We recall here that BL-1 *Jingming* has a strong significance with respect to *yang*, also because of the fact that the branch of the *Dumai* that goes up to the head, penetrates the brain, re-emerges at Du-16 *fengfu* and descends along the sides of the spinal column emerges here.

In needling BL-1 *Jingming* does not require any stimulation of the needle; nevertheless the insertion must not be too superficial. Even more important, it should not be forced; however if the point and the direction of the needle are correct the insertion will find no resistance and a needle of 1 *cun* enters easily.

Follow-up

After an interval of 1 month I see the patient again: pulse and tongue have not changed but he sleeps well without a need for pharmacological therapy and his awakening to urinate is now only sporadic; he sleeps a little in the afternoon if he is at home.

After fearing that he was losing his strength due to ageing, he now feels that he has returned to his normal state; in other words he has a lot of energy even though this is a period of intense work.

It will now be fundamental for him to understand which lifestyle habits should be modified in order to avoid such excess of heat in future.

Mental Health Conditions–*Diankuang*

8

Classical texts generally refer to the more severe mental conditions by the term *diankuang* (癫狂), which in modern Chinese medical literature is often used when speaking of 'schizophrenia'.[1] In effect, the term *diankuang* is used as a blanket term for the various mental illnesses of psychiatric interest that concern a loss of ability to comprehend the meaning of everyday reality and to behave in an autonomous and responsible manner.

> The breaking out of *kuang* is mostly an illness of heat; one goes up high and sings, undresses and walks around, seeing water jumps in, curses and swears, shouts death threats, words are unstoppable, the tongue is as though covered with thorns, one drinks without respite, phlegm colour is shiny, the face as though swollen by fire. At times, one may take a knife and kill people, or when seeing someone in authority showers him with insults, one does not recognise relatives, one does not recognise his own children, on seeing water one becomes happy, on seeing food one becomes angry, one is agitated as if having just seen a ghost.[2]

Western terminology on serious psychiatric pathology has changed over the course of history, just as it varies between different cultures. The term 'schizophrenia', which was coined by Bleuler in 1911 to designate a class of endogenous functional psychoses with a slow and progressive course, underlines the elements of dissociation and fragmentation. This absence of cohesion between the various aspects of the personality comprises not only distortion of the usual associations in the logical–causal procedures of thought, but also loss of the connection 'between idea and emotive resonance, between content of thought and behaviour, between sentiments, actions and desires'.[3]

---

[1] *Jingshen Fenlie Zheng* (精 神 分 裂 症) is the modern translation of the Western term 'schizophrenia'; in fact, *fenlie* has the same meaning as the Greek *schizein* 'divide, break, cleave, split'.
[2] Chen Shiduo, *Shishi Milu* ('Secret notes from the stone chamber'), 'Lihun' ('Departing *Hun*') chapter.
[3] F. Giberti, and R. Rossi, Manual of Psychiatry, 1983, p. 273. Bleuler ascribed the principle characteristic of schizophrenia specifically to the scission and to associative disorder in contrast to Kraepelin, who was the first to distinguish endogenous psychosis in premature dementia and cyclothymia (or manic–depressive psychosis), but who considered schizophrenic disorder essentially as a progression towards dementia.

In the DSM-IV definition, schizophrenia must have at least two of the following symptoms: (a) delusions, (b) hallucinations, (c) disorganised speech, (d) grossly disorganised or catatonic behaviour, and (e) negative symptoms (to wit, dulling of affectivity, alogia, lack of willpower); besides which, it must be accompanied by a substantial social or affective dysfunction; it must be in existence for at least 6 months with active phase symptoms present for at least 1 month; schizoaffective and mood disorders with psychotic manifestations must be excluded; it must not be due to the effects of substances or a general medical condition.

Diankuang has been translated as 'calm madness and agitated madness' or 'depressive–manic state'.

Examination of the character shows that the ideogram *kuang* (狂) is composed of the radical 'dog' (犬) and the phonetic part *wang* (王) 'ruler'. The character as a whole is translated as: (1) 'crazy, mad, senseless', (2) 'wild, furious, violent, unrestrained', (3) 'arrogant, overbearing', or (4) 'madness'.

In modern Chinese, *dian* (癲) exists only in combination with other characters – for example, in *fengdian* (瘋 癲) 'mad' or *dianxian* (癲 痫) 'epileptic'. The character is composed of the radical *ni* (which appears in many ideograms relating to diseases and cures) and the phonetic part *dian* (癲), which can mean: (1) 'to be startled', (2) 'to fall', (3) 'to destroy', (4) 'top', or (5) 'top of the head'.[4]

In classical Chinese medical literature the descriptions and terminology have also undergone changes over time. The term *diankuang* appeared for the first time in the *Shangshu* and has always been associated with madness, disorder and overturning.[5] In classical medical thought there are, however, similar conditions called by different names; for instance we also find the terms *dianxuan*, *fengdian* and *fengxie*, *fengxuan* and *dianxie* next to *diankuang*.[6] In particular, the concepts of *dian* and *xian* (癲痫) (which corresponds to 'epilepsy') overlap, for example in sayings like: 'above 10 years of age it is *dian*, below 10 years of age it is *xian*'[7] or this description by Sun Simiao: 'In the beginning the patient appears to be dead, then he has loss of urine, (the

---

[4] *Kuang*, Karlgren p. 454, 1298; *dian*: Karlgren p. 1194.

[5] 'Weizi' chapter. The *Shangshu* text, also called *Shujing* ('Classic of documents'), is one of the six Confucian classics catalogued at the beginning of the Han Dynasty and gathers material attributed to the oldest antiquity, from the times of the mythological emperors up to the Zhou.

[6] Composed of *dian* (癲), *xuan* (眩), 'vertigo'; *feng* (风) 'wind', *xie* (邪) 'pathogens, perverse'. Respectively in: Zhang Zhongjing, *Jingyue Yaolue* ('Prescriptions of the golden chamber', 20); Chao Yuanfang, *Zhubing Yuanhoulun* ('Treatise on causes and symptoms of diseases' 610); Sun Simiao, *Qianjin Yaofang* ('Invaluable prescriptions for emergencies', 625).

[7] Caho Yuanfang, *Zhubing Yuanhoulun* ('Treatise on causes and symptoms of diseases' 610). Epilepsy (from the Greek *epilambanein* 'to be caught by surprise') is a symptomatic neurological pattern characterised by recurrently flaring crises, whose classic manifestation presents loss of consciousness, spasms and clones, but whose international classification (proposed by Gastaut in 1964) considers over 40 variations. In the absence of the EEG it was also problematic for Western psychiatry to separate madness and epilepsy, which was attributed to supernatural forces in antiquity and the Middle Ages and probably classified for the first time by Paracelsus in 1500.

episode) is resolved in a short time', which seems to be a description of an epileptic-type crisis.[8]

During the Ming Dynasty the definition of *diankuang* was revised to emphasise the specific symptoms, so that we find statements such as: '*Dian, xian* and *kuang* are different things, they are not the same thing with different names, the *Lingshu* also puts *dian* and *kuang* in the same chapter but describes them separately, the treatment is different, and *xian* is yet another thing'.[9]

DESCRIPTION

From the description of the *Huainanzi*, a Daoist text of the same period as the *Neijing*, in which '*kuang* is abnormal disorder', up to a dictionary of the recent Qing Dynasty, which defines *kuang* as 'abnormal happiness and laughter, over-turning and disorder', the essential feature that characterises *kuang* is 'disorder' – a term that refers to a disordered state of things generally, and also one beyond social rules and perceptive or emotive logic.[10]

Conditions where there is a consistent detachment from reality are attributed to *diankuang*, in which the mood is seriously at odds with reality; perception, thought and behaviour are profoundly altered and the rules of social conduct are abandoned.

Whereas *kuang* alludes more to a manic condition and psychotic symptoms of a 'productive' nature – such as delirium, hallucinations, violent behaviour and disorganised speech, *dian* rather refers more to a state of apathy or dementia and negative psychotic symptomatology with psychological withdrawal, lack of willpower, dulling of affectivity and mental torpor.

These extremely suggestive classic descriptions reveal a state in which the need for sleep is diminished, moods are persistently abnormal, there is inflated self-esteem, excessive involvement in pleasurable activities, psychomotor agitation, verbosity, and improper behaviour: these symptoms are all listed under 'manic episodes' according to DSM-IV and correspond to numerous classical Chinese descriptions, physical signs such as bowel movements, thirst and the colour of the face are also considered to be of great relevance.

---

[8] Sun Simiao, *Qianjin Yaofang* ('Invaluable Prescriptions for Emergencies', AD625) Book 14, 'Fengdian' chapter. Zhang Jiebin specifies: In *dian* and *kuang* illnesses the root is different, when a *kuang* disease arises, madness and disorder develop progressively and it is difficult for them to be resolved later. In contrast, in *dian* diseases, one suddenly stiffens and falls, in bursts. In *kuang* diseases one is usually vigilant and quite angry; in severe *dian* diseases one is dazed, exhausted and quiet'. In: *Jingyue Quanshu* ('Jingyue's complete works', 1640), 'Diankuang' chapter.

[9] Wang Ketang, (*Liuke*) *Zhengzhi Zhunsheng* ('Standards of diagnosis and treatment in six branches of medicine', 1602), 'Diankuangxian Zonglun' chapter.

[10] Respectively in the 'Zhushu' chapter of the *Huainanzi* (a Daoist text of the same period as the *Neijing*) and in *Zheng Zitong* ('General explanation of the correct names'), a section of the *Kangxi Cidian* ('Kangxi dictionary', 1710) dictionary.

The *Neijing* dedicates a specific segment to *diankuang* and in the *Nanjing* we read: '*kuang*, one rests very little, is not hungry, considers himself a saint, believes himself to be wise, presents himself as a noble, laughs in a mad manner, wants to play music and sing, and walks madly with no rest'.[11]

A description according to which in a state of *kuang* 'one sings and laughs, or is sad and cries, is in a hurry, considers himself a saint, remains awake and cannot sleep, can eat but does not expel urine and faeces'[12] is attributed to Hua Tuo, and the following pattern described by Sun Simiao is similar: 'In *kuang* the eyes are kept closed, the face is red, the mouth is open wide, one drinks without limit, talks much and without respite, sings or cries, laments or laughs, gets undressed, wanders day and night, insults and swears without measure'.[13] Zhang Jiebin reiterates the essential feature saying that 'in *kuang* diseases one often remains awake, is irascible and violent.'[14]

It should be noted that a hypomanic state in which exaltation, aspects of grandiosity and psychomotor acceleration occur can deteriorate into displays of asocial behaviour (to the point of having dishevelled hair – a sign of complete disregard for social convention), self-damaging behaviour or that dangerous to others, up to signs of real delirium; '*kuang* is violent madness, in a light form one feels superior, and loves to sing and dance; when it is serious, one undresses and walks around, does not avoid water and fire, and furthermore desires to kill people. [...] That which one sees, hears, says, does, is all mad; in a very serious case one talks of things never seen or heard in normal life and of five coloured *shengui*.[15]

In *dian* the features are often mixed – including mood changes, incoherent behaviour and discourse, and distorted perception, but also relevant are dulled responses, impoverished affective and cognitive behaviour, and deterioration as far as dementia.

The description of *dian* as: 'at times the person sings and laughs or is sad and cries, laments, is offended, some stay awake and cannot sleep, others sleep and cannot stay awake, at times cannot speak, its sounds are obscure' goes back to Hua Tuo.[16] Sun Simiao notes that 'there can be silence, much talking, singing, crying, lamenting, laughter, continuous sleep, or even sitting and eating faeces in the cesspool, one undresses, wanders day and night and swears without stopping'.[17]

[11] *Nanjing*, Chapter 59. *Xian* (仙) is the Chinese 'wise man-saint', therefore the phrase approaches our 'he thinks he is Napoleon'. See the discussion on treatment further ahead, for the translation of the passage in the *Suwen*, Chapter 22.
[12] *Huazhi Zhongzhangjing* ('Treasured classic of the organ of the centre'), Chapter 15, a text attributed to Hua Tuo, but probably a work that goes back to the Six Dynasties period (317–618).
[13] Sun Simiao, *Qianjin Yifang* ('Supplement to invaluable prescriptions for emergencies', AD682). In cases of *kuang*, manic behaviour, going up high and singing, undressing and running, Sun Simiao suggests the ST-40 Fenglong point.
[14] Zhang Jiebin, *Jingyue Quanshu* ('Jingyue's complete works', 1640), 'Diankuang' chapter.
[15] Li Chan, *Yixue Rumen* ('Introduction to medicine', 1575). *Shengui* (神鬼) means spirits and ghosts of all types, to signify visual and auditory hallucinations.
[16] Hau Tuo, *Huazhi Zhongzhangjing* ('Treasured classic of the organ of the centre'), Chapter 15.
[17] Sun Simiao, *Qianjin Yaofang* ('Invaluable prescriptions for emergencies'), 'Fengxuan' chapter.

As in *kuang*, there is therefore also 'disorder' in *dian*: an uncontrolled emotionality, disorganised behaviour, and a giving way of the sense of reality are described. The loss of contact with the surrounding world is exemplified by the lack of adherence to social norms: one swears or 'with *dian* one is not normal [...] the heart is unhappy and speaking has no order' – in which the phrase 'speaking has no order' describes speech that is not only incongruous, but also an expression of true madness.[18] 'Order' in fact, is a translation of the term *lun* (伦), which means 'logic-principle', but also refers to the ordering of human relations based on the Confucian ethic.

There is also, however, in *dian* an aspect of mental deterioration, the following description of which recalls the dementia praecox of Kraepelin – in other words the classical psychiatric definition of 'schizophrenia simplex' or the 'disorganised form' of present terminology: 'In *dian* there can be mania-*kuang* or idiocy; one sings, laughs, is sad, cries, is as though drunk, like an idiot, discourse has a head but no tail, one does not distinguish between dirty and clean, nor does he heal with the passing of months or years'.[19]

The dissociative aspect can be seen in the hallucinations, for example in the situation where the subject sees his own double: 'One feels as if all of a sudden his body divides into two people, but only he himself sees the other'.[20]

AETIOLOGY

Yin and *Yang*

The early medical texts attribute the origin of the condition to a failure of the dynamic between *yin* and *yang*: The dominance of one over the other becomes a source of serious pathology.

The *Neijing* speaks about *diankuang* numerous times, attributing *kuang* to a *yang* disease and *dian* to a *yin* disease – for example, when the Emperor asks about the origins of this pathology as follows: 'Those who fall ill with *kuang* and anger-*nu*, from where does there illness come?' Qi Bo answers: 'It originates from *yang*'.[21] External pathogens, whose penetration produces effects varying in both type and seriousness, can also be the cause of *diankuang* diseases, for which if 'the pathogens enter the *yang* there is *kuang*, [...] if the pathogens enter the *yin* there is painful obstruction *bi* (痹), if they conquer the *yang* then it is *dian* disease'.[22]

---

[18] Li Chan, *Yixue Rumen* ('Introduction to medicine').
[19] Wang Ketang, *Zhengzhi Zhunsheng* ('Standards for diagnosis and treatment'), 'Diankuangjian' chapter.
[20] Chen Shiduo, *Shishi Milu* ('Secret notes from the stone chamber'), 'Lihun' ('Departing *Hun*') chapter.
[21] *Suwen*, Chapter 46.
[22] *Suwen*, Chapter 23. The same concept is repeated by Sun Simiao: 'When wind enters the *yang* it is *kuang*, when it enters the *yin* it is *dian*. In: *Qianjin Yaofang* ('Invaluable Prescriptions for Emergencies'), 'Fengdian' ('*Dian* wind') chapter.

The *Neijing* also cites emotions as being an important cause of *diankuang*, for instance great fear-*kong*, anguish-*you* and tedium-*ji*, or great euphoria-*xi*.[23]

The same concept of imbalance between *yin* and *yang* is expressed in the *Nanjing*: 'Double *yang* is *kuang*, double *yin* is *dian*, if the *yang* departs one sees ghosts-*gui*, if the *yin* departs the eyes cannot see'.[24] This 'doubling' of *yin* or *yang*, and so the relative increase in importance of one aspect compared with the other, has often been mentioned in pulse examination.[25]

In a modern text 'double *yin*' is explained in the following way: 'The *Neijing* and *Nanjing* place emphasis on the aetiological mechanism beginning with invasion by external pathogens, believing that the origin of *dian* is due to an overlapping of two *yin*, as is stated in the *Nanjing* that 'double *yin* is *dian*'. By *yin*, the following is meant: (1) cold pathogenic *qi* of a *yin* type, (2) a *yin* nature, or (3) the *yin* vessels, channels and *zang* organs. *Yin* governs the calm; if *yin* pathogens invade people who have an empty *yang* type of constitution or who are easily subject to internal accumulations of cold, dampness and liquid phlegm, or who have a reserved, retiring and silent personality, these pathogens enter the *yin*. Then the two *yin* overlap and overcome the *yang*, *yin* becomes preponderant and *yang* weakens, and this leads to the establishment of the *dian* pattern.'[26]

In this passage, Zhang Zhongjing attributes *dian* and *kuang* to a weakness of the *yin* and the *yang* respectively, also introducing the concepts of *hun* and *po* disorders and 'the separation of *jing* and *shen*':

---

[23] *Suwen*, Chapter 22.

[24] *Nanjing*, Chapter 20. 'Double' is the translation of *zhong* (重) 'heavy' and *chong* 'repeated, copied, doubled' (Weiger p. 120K, Karlgren p. 1270); 'departs' is the translation of *tuo* (脱), which means 'flesh' (the radical is *rou* (肉) 'flesh'), depart, leave, omit, escape, free oneself from' (Karlgren 1138).

[25] For example, Ding Deyong (1062) comments the passage thus: 'Double *yang* is *kuang*, that is if the pulse/vessels-*mai* (脉) is floating, slippery and long, and also full and rapid, one speaks in a mad manner of great affairs, thinks of himself as being high-ranking and a saint, passes the limits [of propriety] and removes his clothing. The affirmation 'if *yin* departs, the eyes become blind' means that one suddenly loses the ability to see, therefore the text speaks of blindness and in this case blind stands for emptiness. Double *yin* is *dian*; in this case *dian* stands for falling-*jue* (蹶).
The commentator Yu Shu also refers to the *qi* of the pulse: 'The opening of the *cun* position is called *yang*. A *yang* appears here which is [increased] three times, therefore the text speaks of 'double *yang*'. The resulting illness is *kuang* and madness. One perceives oneself as high-ranking and a saint, goes up to high places and sings, undresses and runs around, insults others uncaring whether they are relatives or strangers; then we speak of madness. The *chi* position is called *yin*. A double *yin* appears here in the vessel, therefore we speak of madness; the resulting illness is called *dian*. This is to say that one falls down, keeping the eyes closed, without reawakening, and when *yin* reaches the maximum then *yang* returns. For this we speak of *dian*. Man is provided with *yin* and *yang*, if *yin* and *yang* are balanced the entire organism is regulated. Here the *yin* is lost and only the *yang* is vigorous. The five *zang* organs pertain to *yin*, the five *zang* organs store and transmit *qi* and blood. They furnish nourishment above to the eyes; if *yin* departs the *qi* of the five *zang* organs cannot give nourishment to the eyes and the eyes become blind and cannot see. Therefore it is said 'when *yin* departs the eyes become blind'.
Chang Shixian (1510): '*Yang* in both *chi* (尺) and *cun* (寸), this is 'double *yang*'. *Yin* in both *chi* and *cun*, this is 'double *yin*'. *Kuang* is a *yang* illness, *dian* is a *yin* illness. Ghosts pertain to *yin*, one sees them when *yang* departs. The eyes are the essence of *yin*, they become blind when *yin* departs'.

[26] Li Qingfu and Liu Duzhou, *Zhongyi Jingshen Bingxue* ('Psychiatry in Chinese medicine'), p. 11.

> The pathogens weep, *hun* and *po* are not tranquil, blood and *qi* are scarce, if blood and *qi* are scarce this pertains to the heart, if heart *qi* is empty the person is apprehensive, closes his eyes and wants to sleep, dreams of going far away, *jing* and *shen* separate and disperse, *hun* and *po* move disruptively, if *yinqi* weakens this is *dian*, if *yangqi* weakens this is *kuang*.[27]

Pathogens can therefore penetrate if there is a disharmony between full and empty, and an emptiness of *qi* and blood. If the pathogens accumulate in the *yang* there is *kuang*; if instead they penetrate the *yin* then *dian* is produced.

> *kuang* disease is due to pathogenic wind, which enters and aggregates in the *yang*. [...] The liver stores the *hun*; if sadness and sorrow move the centre they injure the *hun*; if the *hun* is injured there is *kuang*, folly-*wang* (王) and absence of lucidity [...] and all this is caused by an emptiness of blood and *qi*, due to which the pathogenic wind strikes.

In the case of *dian*, however:

> It is caused by an emptiness of blood and *qi*, due to which the pathogens enter the *yin* channels. If blood and *qi* are scarce in man the heart is empty, *jing* and *shen* depart and disperse, *hun* and *po* flow in a disorderly fashion, in this way the pathogenic wind can strike, the pathogens enter the *yin* and there is *dian* disease. [...] Man is born with *qi*, *yin* and *yang*, the pathogenic wind enters and aggregates with the *yin* and this becomes *dian*, *yin* with respect to *yang* can be empty or full; when it is empty the pathogens aggregate and *dian* manifests itself.[28]

Emotions and Heat

Medical thought of the Jin and Yuan periods emphasised the prevalence of emotional factors in the aetiology of *kuang*, and attributes the pathogenesis to an excess of fire deriving from them.

Liu Wansu, who is considered to have first formulated the theory based on the centrality of heat as a pathogenic element, explains how madness derives from the loss of the *zhi* of the kidney, whose water is exhausted by the excess of fire. If fire is already full, the element which precedes it cannot discharge its excess into it and settle down: it is therefore anger, the emotion of wood, that most easily fills up and originates madness:

> Anger is the emotion of the liver, if fire is full it attacks metal and cannot calm wood, therefore if the liver is full there is much anger and it becomes *kuang*.

---

[27] Zhan Zhongjing, *Jingui Yaolue* ('Prescriptions of the golden chamber', 220), Chapter 11.
[28] Chao Yanfang, *Zhubing Yuanhoulun* ('Treatise on causes and symptoms of diseases', 610), 'Fengdianhou' and 'Diankuanghou' chapters.

That which comes from the five emotions is always heat, therefore *kuang* manifests itself following the five emotions, but especially after anger. [...] If the heat of the heart is excessive then the water of the kidney is exhausted; there is a loss of *zhi* and madness.[29]

Li Dongyuan's teacher, Zhang Yuansu, elaborates on this excess of fire, which weakens water, and the mental disorder deriving from it:

Folly-*wang* from emptiness, the fire is *yang* therefore on the outside it is pure and light and on the inside it is turbid and dark; it governs movement and disorder, therefore if heart fire is in excess kidney water weakens and *zhi* is not concentrated, there are hallucinations in seeing and hearing, one asks himself and answers himself; this is an alteration of *shen* and *zhi* and it is like seeing spirits and ghosts.[30]

Li Dongyuan continues the discussion by underlining the consequences at the level of the spleen and stomach:

If heart fire is vigorous it can provoke a fullness of the mother wood–liver, when wood–liver is vigorous and unites with the power of fire it is afraid of nothing and flows with folly-*wang*, therefore spleen and stomach suffer it. If there is much anger it is wind and heat which enters into earth–centre, one can see madly and hear madly, it causes a mad heart, at night one dreams of dead people, the four limbs are full and blocked, with spasms, and all this is the pathogenic [effect] of the excessive vigour of wood–liver.[31]

Phlegm

Heat and fire easily associate with phlegm, which knots in the chest obscuring and obstructing the *xinqiao* (心 窍), the portals of the heart. In particular, Zhu Danxi develops the argument for the following aetiology: '*Dian* is when *shen* does not maintain its residence.' The reason is identified in the fact that 'heat accumulates in the heart channel' and that this 'in the majority of cases is due to knotted-*jie* phlegm between heart and chest' because 'the phlegm obscures

---

[29] Liu Wansu, *Suwen Xuanji Yuanbingshi* ('Aetiology based on plain questions', 1182), 'kuangyue' ('Madness') chapter. 'Madness' in this case is the translation of *kuangyue* (狂 越), in which *yue* means 'go beyond'. See also Chapters 5 and 6 on heat and *fanzao* for a discussion on the relationship between the emotions, heat, consumption of *yin* and organs, imbalance of the water–fire axis and the relative manifestations of confusion and disorder.

[30] Zhang Yuansu, *Yixue Qiyuan* ('Origin of medical science', 1186).

[31] Li Dongyuan, *Piweilun* ('Treatise on the spleen and stomach', 1249). ' Seeing madly and hearing madly' is the translation of *wangjian wangwen* (妄见 妄闻), in other words, visual and auditory distortions or hallucinations. The character *wang* (妄), which in modern Chinese means 'absurd, unreasonable', is also used in medicine to describe the disordered movement of blood in the vessels (its composition – the radical 'woman' plus the phonetic part *wang*, which means 'to go away, to finish' – can allude to an event that is decidedly out of the ordinary).

the heart's portals.' This fire and its transformation in phlegm can be attributed to emotional pathology: 'The fire of the five emotions-*zhi* originates due to the constraint-*yu* of the seven passions-*qing* and becomes phlegm.'[32]

In this account a great underlying emptiness – and not external pathogens or possession by spirits and ghosts – is the precondition whereby fire and phlegm can injure the *shen*, which in this way loses its abode:

> Heart fire is vigorous, *yangqi* is in excess, the *shen* does not maintain its abode, phlegm and heat accumulate causing such consequences that when a sick person sees, hears, speaks, and acts in an unreal manner it is said that this is due to a *shengui*, whereas instead it is due only to an extreme emptiness of blood and *qi*, insufficiency of *shen* and *zhi*, excessive phlegm which obstructs; in this way the *shen* is confused and agitated, therefore it is not due to spirits and ghosts.[33]

Zhang Jiebin also underlines the role of emotions in altering the movement of *qi*, therefore producing fire and the relative thickening of phlegm, which condenses in the chest and obstructs both the channels and the portals of the heart.

> Due to an excess of emotions-*qingzhi* the *qi* is injured and fire accumulates, the excess of heat generates internal wind, the union of wind and fire condenses the phlegm which sticks to the *tanzhong*, in this way one loses the custody of one's own *shen* and there is *dian*. … The *dian* disease comes about mainly from *qi* and phlegm, when there is converse movement of *qi* and when phlegm stagnates it can accumulate, closing the channels and obscuring the portals of the heart.[34]

It is interesting how nineteenth century knowledge of the evolution of schizophrenia is translated in terms of *dian* and *kuang*. 'In *diankuang*, with continuous weeping and laughing, singing and cursing, [...] *qi* and blood condense in the brain, the *qi* of the organs and bowels is not connected, it is as if being in a dream.'[35] In particular, texts from the beginning of the 1900s tend to take into account both Chinese tradition and Western knowledge. For example, this description details the transition from the violent symptoms of a *kuang* syndrome to a *dian* pattern, with the typical characteristics of psychic and mental deterioration:

---

[32] *Danxi Xinfa* ('Danxi's experiental therapy', 1481). Before him, Zhang Zihe affirmed: 'Phlegm obscures the portals of the heart'. In: *Rumen Shiqin*, 1228. Dai Sigong (1324–1405) returns to the same concept saying that '*diankuang* is caused by the constraint of the seven emotions'. In: *Zhenzhi Yaojue* ('Principles of diagnosis and treatment'). The pathogenesis of *dian* is also placed in relation to phlegm, which obscures the heart's portals during the Qing Dynasty: 'Heart fire is obfuscated by phlegm and cannot release itself'. In: Chen Shiduo, *Shishi Milu* ('Secret notes from the stone chamber', 1751).
[33] Li Chan, *Yixue Rumen* ('Introduction to medicine', 1575).
[34] Zhang Jiebin, *Jingyue Quanshu* ('Jingyue's complete works', 1640), 'Diankuang' chapter.
[35] Wang qingren, *Yilin Gaicao* ('Corrections of the errors of medical works', 1830).

> Due to an excess of worry heart *qi* becomes knotted and does not spread, consequently phlegm also thickens and becomes knotted, if an excess of apprehension is added then heart *qi* is consumed internally and originates hidden internal heat, phlegm is condensed by the heat, its stickiness becomes even stronger, the heat is engulfed by the phlegm, phlegm and fire cannot be released and resolved, they therefore fill up and overflow completely obstructing all the portals and the *luo* channels which establish communication between heart and brain, and this is the reason why the *shen*'s light is confused.[36]

It continues by stating that in the beginning there is only a light veil of *dian* and the phlegm-fire is not yet strong, but when it later accumulates the latter becomes violent and *kuang* breaks out. In the passage to the more chronic phase the *shen*'s confusion is at its peak, with diminution of awareness, and thought and worrying: the stagnating phlegm becomes irremovable, but there is no longer any fire to nourish the *kuang* and so the pathology transforms into one of *dian*.

TREATMENT

Phlegm blocks communications with the outside world, confounds the clearness of discernment, and impedes the integration of emotions.

The therapeutic principle therefore consists of purging phlegm, the fundamental pathogenic element of *diankuang*, which obscures the portals of the heart and obscures the *shen*.

In general, especially in *kuang*, it is also necessary to eliminate fire, which agitates violently.

Furthermore, it is necessary to calm and stabilise the *shen*, and depending on the state of the individual's *qi* it is often necessary to harmonise the liver, regulate the stomach, tonify the middle *jiao* or nourish the *yin*.[37]

Neijing

In the 'Diankuang' chapter, the *Neijing* proposes a treatment that specifies the channels, but not the individual points: 'In the initial phase of *dian* disease, one is at first unhappy, the head is heavy and sore, the eyes look upwards and are reddened, there is restlessness of the heart (*fanxin*); its signs may be observed

---

[36] Zhang Xichun, *Yixue Zhongzhong Canxilu* ('Records of traditional Chinese and Western medicine in combination', 1924), 'Zhidianfan' chapter.
[37] Diagnosis and treatment in TCM are discussed in Chapter 10 on patterns of fullness, a number of clinical exemplifications are mentioned in the contributions of Jin Shubai (Chapter 20) and Zhang Mingjiu (Chapter 19). Only the more articulated classical treatments are mentioned here.

on the face.[38] The bladder, stomach, spleen and lung channels are chosen, and when the colour changes one concludes (the acupuncture).

When *dian* disease crises start, one moans for no reason. The large and small intestine channels should be observed; treat the right side if the left is stiff and the left if the right is stiff and when the colour changes, conclude.

When *dian* disease crises start there is stiffness and then pain in the spinal column. The bladder, stomach, spleen and small intestine channels should be examined and when the colouring changes one should conclude. To treat *dian* it is often necessary to live with the patient in order to observe which points to choose.

When there is a crisis one should observe which channel is ill and perform bleeding. The blood that is removed should be stored in a squash and when the moment of breaking out of the crisis occurs the blood will move. If it does not move, use 20 cones of moxa on *Qionggu* ('extreme bone', another name for Du-1 *Changqiang*).

In the initial phase of *kuang* disease first one feels sad, forgets things easily, angers easily, and there is often fear; the predisposing causes for this are worry and boredom. To treat it, use the lung channel [in some versions it is *shou tai-yang*] and large intestine channel and when the colouring changes, conclude. Afterwards, use the spleen and stomach channels.

When a *kuang* crisis starts one sleeps little and there is no hunger, one feels saintly, superior to others, one deems oneself a wise man, considers oneself a noble, one easily insults other people, and does not pause day or night. This should be treated with the large and small intestine, lung and heart channels, under the tongue.[39] If vigour is observed, one takes all of them, otherwise not.

If there is mad joyfulness, fear, much laughter, a tendency to sing, to move in a disorderly fashion and without pause, then this is caused by fright. To treat it, use the large and small intestine and lung channels.

Kuang with visual hallucinations, auditory hallucinations, and a tendency to shout from fright, is caused by scarce *qi*. To treat it, use lung, large and small intestine and spleen channels and the two points of the head at the two cheeks.

Kuang with great hunger, a tendency to see ghosts and to laugh, but that does not manifest itself on the outside [Yang Shangshan interprets: 'The disease does not manifest itself in front of other people'], is due to a great euphoria-*xi*. To treat it, use the spleen, bladder and stomach channels and then the lung and small and large intestine.

---

[38] *Yan* (颜) 'face' originally defined the area of the forehead, between the eyebrows, corresponding to the heart. *Hou* (候) means 'examine, observe the signs' (*zhenhou* [症候] is the clinical pattern). 'Restlessness of the heart' is the translation of *fanxin*.

[39] According to the commentator Wang Bing, these are the two points where the artery beats under ST-9 *Renying* (*Suwen*, Chapter 59), while the majority believe that this refers to Ren-23 *Lianquan*, even if this is a point on the *Ren Mai*.

In recent onset *kuang*, in which these symptoms have not yet appeared, first use *Ququan* [LIV-8] on the left and right where the artery beats; 'if it is vigorous then it can be cured with bleeding in a short time, if it does not heal then it must be treated according to the 20 cone moxa method at the coccyx.'[40]

Gui Points

In his 'Ode on the 13 *gui* points of Sun Zhenren', Sun Simiao proposes a series of points 'for *diankuang* disorders caused by the one hundred pathogenic factors'.[41]

The significance of these points and the specific sequence are probably linked to practices for nourishing life, of which Sun Simiao was a great advocate. The 13 points are:[42]

Guigong	Ghost palace	Du-26 *Renzhong*
Guixin	Ghost faith	LU-11 *Shaoshang*
Guilei	Ghost fortress	SP-1 *Yinbai*
Guixin	Ghost heart	P-7 *Daling*
Guilu	Ghost chimney	BL-62 *Shenmai*
Guizhen	Ghost pillow	Du-16 *Fengfu*
Guichuang	Ghost bed	ST-6 *Jiache*
Guishi	Ghost market	Ren-24 *Chengqiang*
Guicu	Ghost cave	P-8 *Laogong*
Guitang	Ghost hall	Du-23 *Shangxing*
Guicang	Ghost store	Ren-1 *Huiyin*
Guitui	Ghost leg	LI-11 *Quchi*
Guifeng	Ghost seal	*Haiquan* (extra point under the tongue).

Other similar combinations were codified afterwards, of which the one suggested by Gao Wu for *dian* conditions is famous. In this prescription, four points – Du-24 *Shenting*, ST-17 *Ruzhong*, GB-34 *Yanglingquan*, and LIV-2 *Xingjian* – are substituted for BL-62 *Shenmai*, Du- 23 *Shangxing*, LI-11 *Quchi*, and *Yumentou/Yinxiafeng*.[43]

---

[40] *Suwen*, Chapter 22.

[41] *Sun Zhenren Shisan Quixie Ge* ('Ode on the 13 *gui* points of Sun Zhenren'). In: Sun Simiao, *Beiji Qianjin Yaofang* ('Invaluable prescriptions for emergencies', 625). The same formula is found in the *Zhenjiu Dacheng* ('The great compendium of acupuncture and moxibustion', 1601), Chapter 9.

[42] The *Guicang* points correspond to Ren-1 *Huiyin* and used to be called *Yumentou* in women and *Yinxiafeng* in men. According to some commentators, *Guixin* was LU-9 *Taiyuan* and *Guili* was P-5 *Jianshi* or P-8 *Laogong* (see P. Deadman, M. Al-Khafaji, *A Manual of Acupuncture*, 2000, p. 51, in this respect).

[43] '*Dian*, in the beginning there is much worry and the intelligence becomes progressively more turbid. The patient can go days without speaking or speak in an incoherent manner. Apathy, thought, sadness, bitterness, oppression, unmotivated weeping and laughing, and lack of appetite. Tongue with a greasy coating, deep and slippery pulse or wiry and slippery.' From: *Xuqiufu Guibing Shisanxue Ge* (In: Gao Wu, *Zhenjiu Jiuying*).

Odes from the Yuan and Ming Dynasties

Specific indications for *dian* and *kuang* are found in various other works:

- '*Kuang*, one jumps and runs, Ren-13 *Shangwan*, HE-7 *Shenmen*.'[44]
- In an attack of *kuang* use HE-3 *Shaohai*, P-5 *Jianshi*, LI-11 *Quchi*, SI-3 *Houxi*, GB-1 *Sizhukong*, KI-7 *Fuliu*, treating these points you will have great success. In *dian* use HE-7 *Shenmen*, Du-26 *Renzhong*, P-5 *Jianshi* and 'HE-7 *Shenmen* specifically treats dementia of the heart; Du-26 *Renzhong* and P-5 *Jianshi* eliminate mortal *dian*'.[45]
- '*Shuigou* [in other words, Du-26 *Renzhong*] and P-5 *Jianshi* treat perverse *dian*.'[46]
- 'HE-7 *Shenmen* eliminates dementia of the heart.'[47]
- 'Du-26 *Renzhong* is the best point for treating *dian*, there is not even any need for the thirteen *gui* points.'[48]
- 'HE-7 *Shenmen* treats *dian* in particular, to better reach it, turn the bone of the hand.'[49]
- 'In *dian* disorders Du-12 *Shenzhu* and GB-13 *Benshen* are indispensable.'[50]

Case Study 8.1

The Woman Overcome by the Waves

The patient, a 63-year-old female, seems physically very worn-out, even if a glow of great interior depth is still visible: She walks with difficulty as a result of a series of hip surgeries, is overweight, and her face is subject to sudden contractions.

The woman is feeling decidedly not well: she says that she has pains all over, but especially during the last five months she has felt as though her head 'is splitting' and she spends hours with ice on her head.

She attributes the cause of all this to electromagnetic waves, like those from the ever more invasive cellular phone booster masts, which are beginning to multiply rapidly. These 'microwaves', which she says are 'frying' her, which she is in the process of fighting against through letters to the press, are concretely felt by her, vary in various zones of the city and modify their intensity in the space of seconds.

---

[44] *Baizhenfu* (In: Gao Wu, *Zhenjiu Jiuying*).
[45] *Zabing Xuefage* (In: Gao Wu, *Zhenjiu Jiuying*).
[46] *Linguangfu* (In: Xu Feng, *Zhenjiu Daquan*).
[47] *Tongxuan Zhiyaofu* (In: Dou Hanqin, *Zhenjing Zhinan*).
[48] *Xihongfu* ('Xi Hong was a famous acupuncturist during the Song Dynasty. In: Xu Feng, *Zhenjiu Daquan*').
[49] *Yulongge* (In: Wang Guorui, *Bianque Shenting Zhenju Yulongjing*).
[50] *Baizhenfu* (In: Gao Wu, *Zhenjiu Juying*).

They are particularly present in certain places, for example in her apartment, owing to which she is presently living in a residence hotel. One of the two rooms in my studio is also unusable (by chance, the first few times I had always received her in the same room).

She is very tired, her breathing is laboured, and at this point it is almost impossible for her to keep up with her interests, both cultural and material.

The patient declares that she has had this 'geopathic sensitivity' for 20 years, but that only lately has it caused her pain. This pain diminishes when she takes a tranquilliser, but the patient rejects any suggestion of a more structured pharmacological treatment or psychotherapeutic support.

Her tongue is red, with many cracks and without any coating, the pulse is thin, rapid and very deep.

During the first treatment she weeps and sobs after the insertion of the needles, while during treatment with the hammer she belches noisily without interruption.

Diagnosis
Very dense phlegm-fire that obstructs the *jingluo*, obscures the portals of the heart and consumes *yin*.

Therapeutic principles
Clear fire, transform substantial and insubstantial phlegm, activate *qi* and blood, and nourish the *yin*.

Treatment
Weekly treatments for 6 months, for a total of 25 treatments.

The points that I utilise most frequently are chosen from:
- Du-20 *Baihui*, GB-18 *Chengling*, Du-24 *Shenting*, BL-5 *Wuchu*;
- P-7 *Daling*, HE-7 *Shenmen*, SP-6 *Sanyinjiao*, KI-4 *Dazhong*, KI-3 *Taixi*, KI-1 *Yongquan*;
- 'plum-blossom' hammer on the upper area of the back.

For the choice of points the principal references used were the clinical cases of serious psychiatric disorders by Professor Zhang Mingjiu (Chapter 19).

The points on the head act especially on phlegm and fire, the distal points clear fire, activate *qi* and blood and nourish *yin*.

The stimulation with the hammer helps unblock and circulate *qi*.

The specific choice of points during each treatment is related to whether I decide to concentrate on the action of activating or that of nourishing.

During these months the patient progressively reduces the application of ice to her head, starts to think about returning home, begins to attend a number of conferences, no longer weeps during treatments and has stopped belching, she flies to Sicily for a holiday, but the pain is still strong and her perception of reality remains the same. She says that before the therapy her panic was continuous and interrupted by moments of lucidity, while now the situation is reversed.

In the last month, however, the condition began deteriorating again, with a return to symptoms similar to the original ones, though more moderate in degree.

Comments

This case is not presented as a pointer for acupuncture treatments, but rather because it exemplifies the delicacy of these more serious psychiatric conditions and the necessity of specific care. Information on the use of acupuncture in psychiatric cases where there is serious compromise of thought processes is very limited and private practice is certainly not the ideal place for treating these patients, who are in need of much more integrated and multidisciplinary therapeutic support. The therapy plan should also anticipate much more frequent treatment.

Unfortunately, the factors that have caused the deterioration in the last month are also unclear. I can only surmise that, at the point that the patient started to become aware of her deep depression, my response was inadequate. In fact, only after 5 months of treatment did the patient start referring to personal events such as a recently interrupted relationship after having gone through a period in which she maintained that she 'did not want to stir things up' in her history, while over that same period she was steadily becoming more aware. She continued for example, to insist that there were too many waves in her house, but also said that she could not return there because it made her 'too sad', or spoke of having 'passed through the house to check things out and the harp was out of tune' – truly sad.

This clinical episode, however, offers a starting point for a number of reflections on the therapeutic relationship, and in particular the question of 'abstinence'. This concept was central to the position that I assumed with respect to my patient's evaluation of reality: I do not agree with what I consider to be her delirious thoughts, but nevertheless I refrain from directly attacking her convictions. (For example, during the 16th treatment she says to me: 'I don't know if you believe in waves, but that's alright, I understand that you have decided to act in another manner'.)[51]

In this case, however, a different problem presented itself since the patient constantly made many comments on the effects of the points chosen; it is always a delicate matter how much and in what manner to take a patient's considerations on this subject into account. In many ways, the patients are our teachers and what they say about the effects of the needles in general, and on individual points in particular, is quite important. Consequently, trusting in their sensitivity, which is often refined over time, can become an integral part of the evaluation of the clinical picture and treatment choices. On the other hand, this can also become a manipulative tool – a way for patients to test both their power and the stability of the therapist. In such cases, the worst response is the one where the acupuncturist deviates from his original intent, changing the choice of points in order to follow the impulses of the patient.

In this specific case I chose to make it quite clear that I took into consideration her comments on the benefits and inconveniences of the points I utilised; to gather these suggestions meant to acknowledge that a healthy side existed and to ally with it.

---

[51] See also the article in which Chase discusses the case of a patient that referred to being subject to astral voyages, where he comments thus: 'I accept my patent's experience without judging it, attempting to remain at the same time sufficiently sceptical to consider a wider picture'. In: C. Chase, *Ghosts in the Machine*, European Journal of Oriental Medicine, vol.1, no.l, 1993.

While the indications of the classics on proceeding in a correct way and on 'maintaining oneself united' corresponded to my abstaining from saying anything about her delirious thinking.

Follow-up

She does not return to continue treatments after the summer break and I lose track of her.

Classic Syndromes: *Zangzao, Bentunqi, Baihebing, Meiheqi*

9

These patterns make their appearance in medical literature mostly after the period in which the first classics were compiled; they are, in fact, defined and described in various chapters of the *Jingyui Yaolue* by Zhang Zhongjing, who also discusses their treatment with various pharmacological prescriptions.[1]

Many authors of various periods and schools later carried out revisions and in-depth studies of these patterns, in particular, with regard to their pathogenic processes.

Modern classification includes these patterns in the category of emotional illnesses, both because of the psychological component of the symptoms and the importance of emotive factors in the development of the pathology.

Chinese texts that also make reference to Western psychology generally attribute these disorders to a somatiform disturbance and classify them as 'hysteria'.[2]

ZANGZAO (脏 躁)

Poorly translated as 'agitation of the organ(s)', according to a contemporary text of clinical psychiatry '*zangzao* indicates a category of pathologies that have the common characteristic of changing emotions'.[3]

---

[1] Zhang Zhongjing, *Jingui Yaolue* ('Prescriptions of the golden chamber's, AD220).
[2] For a number of references in English texts, please see the following articles: *Hysterical Diseases* edited by T. Dey, 1996, from the magazine 'Zhongguo Zhenjiu'; the work by M. Al-Khafaji on *bentunqi*, 1989, and that of Gu Yuehua on *baihe* syndrome, 1992. As has already been noted in the introductory discussion on nosology, analogous assertions can also be found, such as: 'Hysteria pertains to the category of *zangzao, baihebing*, etc.' (Hou Jinlung, *Traditional Chinese Treatment for Psychogenic and Neurological Diseases*, 1996, p. 134).
[3] Li Qingfu and Liu Duzhuo, *Zhongyi Jingshen Bingxue* ('Psychiatry in Chinese medicine', 1989), p. 109.

This term appears for the first time in the chapter titled 'Pulse, symptoms, and treatment of the various diseases of women' in the *Jingui Yaolue*: 'Women with *zangzao* love to be sad, desire to weep, act as though possessed, many yawns and stretches.'[4]

Since the term *zang* indicated all the *zangfu* (organs and viscera) including the *qibeng zhifu*, the extraordinary viscera – brain, marrow, bones, vessels, gall bladder and uterus – there is controversy about which organ the term *zangzao* refers to, but as a general rule classical commentators interpret it in two ways: according to some *zang* indicates the *zizang*, the uterus, while according to others it is the *xinzang*, the heart organ.[5]

As far as *zao* is concerned, the etymological dictionary of the Han Dynasty explains that *zao* means 'restless, uneasy, agitated'.[6] This *zao* is a homophone of *zao* 'dry', with which it shares the phonetic part *sao* – in this case preceded however, by the radical 'foot' instead of the one for 'fire'. The 'foot' suggests movement and therefore agitation, but the idea of dryness from fire is also repeated a number of times in the discussion on its aetiology.

Aetiology

Zanzao disease does not appear in the Neijing, yet modern texts nevertheless quote various passages from it in order to underline how its main symptom of 'being sad, wishing to weep' had already been discussed. In general, the passages already referred to in Chapter 2 on emotions are quoted, taken from the *Suwen* Chapter 5 and the *Lingshu* Chapter 8: 'The sound of the heart is laughter, its emotion is euphoria; euphoria injures the heart; the sound of the lungs is weeping, its emotion is anguish, anguish injures the lungs'; 'If *shen* is in excess one laughs without pause, if it is insufficient there is sadness'; 'In euphoria *shen* is frightened and disperses and is not stored, in worry and anguish *qi* is closed and blocked and does not circulate' and 'If heart *qi* is empty there is sadness, if it is full one laughs without rest'.

Starting with the description by Zhang Zhongjing, the *zanzao* pattern is examined in all the later medical literature, which investigates the causes of its origin and methods of development.

---

[4] Zhang Zhonjing, *Jingui Yaolue* ('Prescriptions of the golden chamber, AD220), Chapter 22. 'Act as though possessed' *ru shen ling suo zuo* is the version that appears in: Wu Jian, *Yizong Jinjian* ('Golden mirror of medicine, 1742) and was adopted in two commented editions of the *Jingui Yaolue* (Li Keguan, 1983 and Liu Duzhuo, 1984), but another variant is also found: 'Act as though it does not come to them' *ru feiji suo zuo* (Li Qingfu, 1989).

[5] The uterus, *nuzi bao* (女子包), 'receptacle of women', is one of the extraordinary viscera. This opinion is expressed, for example, by Shen Jinzhui, in: *Shenshi Zunsheng Shu* ('On the importance of life preservation', 1773) and Yao Zaijing, in: *Jingui Yaolue Xindian* ('Commentaries on the synopsis of the golden chamber', 1732), while according to Wu Jian, for example, it is the *xinzang*, the heart organ, in: *Yizong Jinjian* ('Golden mirror of medicine', 1742).

[6] Xu Shen, *Shuowen Jiezi* ('Explanations of characters and words', 121).

Generally, all the evaluations indicate empty *yin* as the fundamental factor and dryness as a specific sign of this syndrome.

Alternative hypotheses with regards the pathogenesis can be found: in some texts, the action of pathogenic fire, the role of emotions in disturbing the *shen*, or the importance of empty blood, liquids and the *Chong Mai* is accentuated.

A modern text underlines the relationship between blood deficiency, alterations of *qi*, and afflictions of the *shen* and *zhi*:

> If *yin* and blood are insufficient they are not able to moisten and nourish the organs. *Qi*, lacking the containing moistness of the blood, rebels in the higher regions and its excess transforms into heat and fire. *Qi* does not counterbalance the external pathogen, so wind can penetrate and transform easily into fire, and wind and fire nourish each other reciprocally. Empty *qi* and blood influence the *shen* of the heart above and cause sadness and weeping, while they act on the *zhi* of the kidney below producing yawning and stretching.[7]

This all occurs more easily in women, because the female body is *yin* and its root is blood:

> *Zangzao* is considered by some as an emptiness of blood in the uterus with invasion of wind and transformation in heat. In *zangzao* from empty blood the internal fire disturbs the *shen*, which is not calm. The symptoms 'to be sad, desire to weep, act as though possessed' are in reality signs of an empty disorder; they also appear in the *Jingui Yaolue*, where they are mentioned in heart pathologies and described as emptiness of *qi* and blood. As for the numerous yawns and frequent stretching, the classics say that 'in kidney illnesses one stretches and yawns a lot, the complexion is black'. The five emotions produce fire, the movement of fire involves the heart, injures the *yin* of the organs and lastly reaches the kidney.[8]

In these cases the *shen* is unable to root itself and even the smallest emotions injure it producing disorders, whereas if *qi* is vigorous and the *shen* is lively its functions are healthy and it can easily resist the changes due to emotions:

> For *zang* the heart is intended; if the heart is calm it can contain the *shen*, if it is injured by emotions the *shen* is agitated, disturbed, restless. Therefore if 'one is sad and has a desire to weep' it is the *shen* that is unable to govern the emotions; if one 'has the appearance of one who is possessed' it is the heart that does not allow clarity of the *shen*, in other words there is a loss of *zhi*, and there is *diankuang*.[9]

Other comments which tend to underline the central role of fire in the parching of the organs make reference to the fact that the word *zao* 'dry, dryness' is a homophone of *zao* 'restless, agitated' and add:

---

[7] Li Qingfu and Liu Duzhou, *Zhongyi Jingshen Bingxue* ('Psychiatry in Chinese medicine', 1989), p. 109.
[8] You Zaijing, *Jingui yaolue xindian* ('Personal selection from the *Jingui yaolue*').
[9] Wu Jian, *Yizong jinjian* ('The golden mirror of medicine').

zangzao in women, the *zang* are *yin*; if *yin* is empty the fire conquers it, then there is dryness. The dryness is not just limited to any particular organ; once it is produced it is common to the various patterns. If there are only the symptoms of sadness with a desire to weep and a possessed appearance this means it is manifesting in the heart; if there is stretching and frequent yawning, then it is in the kidney.[10]

In his treatise on disorders of blood, Tang Zonghai refers to the relationship between the insufficiency of stomach liquids – an expression of insufficiency of kidney water – and the dryness of the uterus in order to explain the pattern of *zangzao*, in which women are sad and desire to weep, act as though possessed, yawn often and stretch. In fact, if kidney *yin* is deficient it cannot nourish the blood of the *Chong Mai* and the uterus below, or the lung and heart above:

> If the stomach liquids are insufficient the uterus is parched, there is sadness and a desire to weep, the appearance is as though possessed, there are frequent yawns and stretching. This happens because kidney water is insufficient and the blood of *Chong* is scarce and does not nourish adequately. The water of the kidney regulates the functions of the uterus through the heavenly water *tiangui* below, it constitutes the liquids of the mouth above. In *zangzao*, the lung–metal does not receive the moistening nourishment of the liquids; the lung governs sadness. Yawns and stretching are disorders of the kidney. They are as though possessed because the blood is dry, therefore the heart does not have its liquid and the *shen* is not retained.[11]

Clinical Notes

The Chinese description, though quite brief, shows extreme attention and precision. This clarity in the medical view gives a concrete possibility of recognising the *zangzao* pattern in our modern clinical settings also. The condition corresponds to those cases, certainly not rare, in which the patient presents a series of somatic and psychic symptoms that can be traced back to a period of physical and especially emotional strain that has consumed *qi* and blood.

The classic description essentially considers four elements: the pleasure of being sad, the desire to weep, acting as though possessed, and the numerous yawns and stretching.

Stretching and yawning correspond to the kidney's attempt to bring the *qi* downward where there is emptiness.

---

[10] Tang Zonghai, *Jingui yaolue qianzhu buzheng* ('Commentary and correction of the *Jingui yaolue*').
[11] Tang Zonghai, *Xuezhenglun* ('Treatise on the illnesses of the blood'). The term *tiangui* 天癸 is used in reference to the reproductive function and specifically to menstrual blood, which depend on the kidney *jing*; *tian* means 'heaven' and *gui* is the tenth heavenly trunk, corresponding to the kidney, *yin* water.

It is interesting to note that the character *qian* signifies 'yawn' and also 'lack' and that originally it showed a person with the mouth opened in a yawn.[12] This is a sign of emptiness that seems also to indicate the seriousness of the situation, since gestures such as yawning and stretching in women were probably conceived of only in cases of serious illness. Rather, we would recognise kidney emptiness in other symptoms and signs, such as an extreme tendency to fatigue deriving from the absence of a reserve of *qi* and a deep and pervasive tiredness, which are characteristic of empty *qi*. In general, patients show excessive emotionality and an extreme tendency to weep – unmistakable signs of a *shen* that has lost its 'unity' and no longer controls emotional reactions.

There can be various levels of *yin* exhaustion, but in all cases the *shen*'s residence is clearly injured. The agitation of the organs – whether the internal organs, the heart or the uterus – indicates a profound compromising of the *yin*, and corresponds to a *shen* that separates from matter.

The classic description seems to recognise a type of satisfaction in suffering: it is noteworthy that, in the phrase 'they love to be sad', 'love' is rendered as *xi* (喜), the same word as used for 'joy-euphoria'. The term may express the subtle pathological nuance of this desperation, alluding to a component of pleasure, a gratification in not being well.

It is also said that the patient behaves as though there are spirits or as if her actions are not her own – sayings that criticise the belief in spirits and possession, but at the same time recognise the autonomy of certain types of behaviour with respect to conscious control.

In the clinic these dissociated aspects may manifest more explicitly with the breakdown of the functions of consciousness, memory, identity, and perception, or they may appear in a more surreptitious manner. In the latter cases, and in general more often in our clinical practice, the patients mention that they feel strange, that they do not recognise themselves, that they no longer have control of their feelings or behaviour, or that they feel overcome. There may also be loss of contact with what is happening in external reality, with mental haziness or an overall decrease in emotional activity.

In all these cases, the common denominator is this experiencing of being alien to one's own personality.

BENTUNQI (奔 豚 气)

Translated as the '*qi* of the running piglet', the classic dictionaries explain that '*ben* means to run', '*ben* means to rush', while '*tun* is a piglet'.[13]

---

[12] Wieger p. 99a, Karlgren p. 378.
[13] Respectively in the dictionary of the Han period *Shuowen jiezi*; in the *Cengyun* of the Southern Song period; in the contemporary etymological dictionary *Ciyuan*.

The *qi* of the 'running piglet' was a way of describing the disorderly move-ment of *qi* and the term was not confined to medical language.[14]

A very incisive description reads: '*Bentun* disorder starts in the lower abdo-men, rises and attacks the throat, when it breaks out one feels like he is dying, it returns and then stops; all this derives from fright and fear'.[15]

Contemporary classification includes it mostly among the emotional ill-nesses:

> *Bentun* is often classified among the internal or gynaecological illnesses, but in the clinic it is generally associated with psychic symptoms such as 'it is as though one is frightened by things, afraid of people, with distortions of hearing and sight', furthermore, its upsurges are often related to emotional factors. For this reason it is important to understand its aetiology and pathogenesis also with respect to psychological illnesses.[16]

Aetiology

The various medical schools differed in parts in their description and interpre-tation of *bentun* pathologies.

The term had already appeared in the *Neijing*, linked to serious kidney pathology, with emptiness and cold, and there it corresponds to the accumula-tion of the kidney, one of the five accumulations-*ji*. 'When the kidney pulse is very hurried then there is *dian* disease of the bones, if it is slightly hurried then there is sinking, overturning-*jue*, *bentun*, there is no control of the feet and an inability to urinate and defecate.'[17]

The symptomatology is very similar to that of *chongshan* disorder, 'the her-nia that attacks', which presents a characteristic pain radiating upward that originates from a disorder of the *du mai*, due to which in many of the texts of later periods the two pathologies are considered together in the category *bentun chongqi*.[18]

---

[14] For example we find in Mencio: '*Zhi* is the chief of the *qi*. The *qi* makes it strong, if we nourish it directly and we do not damage it then it is fine, if we can not control our *zhi* then we damage our *qi* and we have *bentun*.'

[15] Zhang Zhongjing, *Jingui yaolue*, Chapter 8.

[16] Li Qingfu and Liu Duzhou, 1989, p. 113.

[17] *Lingshu*, Chapter 4. The other four accumulations-*ji* are: *feiqi* – liver, *fulian* – heart, *piqi* – spleen, *xiben* – lung. The *dian* illness of the bones, *gudianji* (骨 癲 疾), is severe because it is localised in depth: Zhang Jiebing in the *Leijing* says: '*Gudianji*, the illness is deep down in the bones'.

[18] 'In the *Du Mai* illnesses the illness rises from the abdomen and attacks the heart with pain, one can not urinate nor defecate, it is called *chongshan* (冲 山).' In: *Suwen*, Chapter 60. *Du Mai*, which also has a front branch, it originates in the kidney; 'hernias' translates *shan*, a pathology characterised by acute abdominal pain and difficulties or a failure at the intestinal and urinal level (different texts talk about *wushan*, 'five hernias', or *qishan* 'seven hernias').

The *Nanjing* returns to the concept of *bentun* as an accumulation of the kidney and describes its manifestations of violent, sudden and unexpected ascending of *qi*. These disorderly movements of *qi* are referred to the control-*ke* cycle of the five *zang* organs, almost as though they bounced the pathogenic *qi* back and forth between them, causing it to accumulate and suddenly break out:

> The accumulation-*ji* of the kidney is called *bentun* it starts in the lower abdomen and ascends to underneath the heart; it is like a piglet. Sometimes it goes up, sometimes down, without a specific moment in time […]. The illness of the spleen transmits to the kidneys, the kidneys have to transmit it to the heart, but in the summer the heart is in the position of sovereign, the sovereign does not accept pathogens, the kidneys therefore want to return them to the spleen, the spleen does not want to accept them, therefore they remain, and knot as accumulations.[19]

The first specific classic on acupuncture returns to the explanation in the *Nanjing* and defines the clinical pattern and possible treatments: 'The pain travels to the genitals, one cannot urinate, there is abdominal distension and pain, the mouth is stiff and one cannot speak, loins and lower abdomen are stiff and painful, there is pain and bother in the heart, one is hungry but cannot eat'; '*Bentun* with a distended and hard upper abdomen, pain that travels to the genitals, inability to urinate, the testicles pull, Ren-7 *Yinjiao* is the primary point'; '*Bentun* with *qi* that ascends, distended and painful abdomen, stiff mouth and inability to speak, swollen penis with pain that radiates to the waist, Ren-5 *Shimen* is the primary point'; '*Bentun* with cold which enters the lower abdomen, Ren-4 *Guanyuan* is the primary point'; '*Bentun* which ascends to attack the heart, in serious cases one cannot breathe, or short and wheezing breath, there is *jue* like a corpse, Ren-3 *Zhongji* is the primary point'; '*Bentun* with abdominal swelling, LIV-13 *Zhangmen* is the primary point'; '*Bentun* with *qi* that goes up and down, LIV-14 *Qimen* is the primary point'; '*Bentun* with the testicles that withdraw upwards and re-enter, pain in the penis, ST-29 *Guilai* is the primary point'.[20]

The 'Pulse, symptoms and treatment of *Bentun* and diseases of *qi*', chapter of the *Jingui Yaolue* is dedicated to this pathology, where it is treated as a disorder of *qi* and two main sources are identified for it. The origin can be fear or a fright, which produce a fundamental change in the movements of *qi*, owing to which it rises suddenly and with such violence that one feels like he is dying. The other possibility consists of an incorrect treatment, which further depletes an already weak *yang*, due to which the water yin cannot be transformed by the *yang* and it rises to invade the heart.

---

[19] *Nanjing*, Chapter 56; see also Unschuld, 1986, p. 501 e 507.
[20] Huangfu Mi, *Zhenjiu Jiayijing* ('The systematic classic of acupuncture and moxibustion'), book 8, Chapter 2. Recalling the passage from the *Nanjing* it states: 'The spleen illness transmits to the kidney, the kidney wants to transmit it to the heart, the heart gives it back, it refuses the pathogens so that they remain and knot themselves causing accumulation.'

The first case is described thus: '*Bentun* disorder starts in the lower abdomen, rises and attacks the throat, when it breaks out one feels like he is dying, it returns and then stops, all this derives from fright and fear. *Qi* rises and attacks the chest, there are abdominal pains and alternating heat and cold, the indication is *bentun tang*'.[21] The text continues, providing indications for treatment including various prescriptions according to its evolution.

The prescription is actually directed at the liver, whose role is, in fact, highlighted by later commentaries, that specify:

> The kidney is injured by fear, *bentun* is a disease of the kidney, the pig is an animal of water, the kidney is the organ of water. Kidney *qi* moves internally, attacks the throat, like a running pig, for this reason it is called 'running piglet'; there are also cases where the origin is a liver disorder because kidney and liver have common origins in the lower *jiao* and the *qi* of both of them ascends conversely.[22]

The other aetiological factor taken into account by the *Jingui Yaolue* is an incorrect treatment that damages the *yang*, with water–*qi* ascending:

> If after sweating one uses the smouldering-*shao* needle to induce sweating again, if the area around the needle catches cold and becomes red and raised, in this case there will be *bentun*, with *qi* that rises from the lower abdomen to the heart. One must use a moxa cone on the swelling and treat it with *Guizhi jiagui tang*. [...] If after causing sweating there is a sensation of palpitations–pulsations under the umbilicus, this is *bentunqi*, which is about to break out, and it must be treated with *Fuling guizhi ganzao dazao tang*.[23]

A modern commentary explains:

> We are speaking here of a case where the physician after having caused sweating, forces sweating once again by using the hot-*wen* needle method and in this way induces a large opening of the pores; however, if defensive *qi* is not solidly contained, wind-cold invades from the outside. If after sweating one causes further sweating, heart *yang* becomes empty and if heart *yang* is empty the water pathogens of the cold *yin* of the kidney in the lower *jiao* use the strength of external cold and rise upwards to 'lay siege' to heart *yang*. Then *bentun* manifests itself. Treatment with excessive sweating permits the invasion of wind-cold in people who already have latent water and liquids present

---

[21] Zhang Zhongjing, *Jingui yaolue*, Chapter 8. The prescription contains herbs to purify the heat, harmonise the liver, nourish the blood, harmonise the stomach and bring the *qi* downwards (for a punctual discussion on the syndrome and on the corresponding prescriptions see also the article by M. Al-Khafaji, *Running Piglet Qi*, 1989).

[22] You Zaijing, *Jingui yaolue xindian* ('Personal selection from the *Jingui yaolue*').

[23] Zhang Zhongjing, *Jingui yaolue* ('Prescriptions of the golden chamber', AD220), Chapter 8. The burning needle or 'fire needle' *huozhen* is used with a quick needling and today it is mostly employed in treating *bi* illnesses with cold in the bones. In the chapter on *taiyang* illnesses in the *Shanghanlun* we find the same direction: 'When the pathogens wind-cold settle in the *taiyang* channel, one must solve them by using the sweating method'.

in the lower *jiao* and damages the *yang*. In this condition, heart *yang* cannot descend to warm and transform kidney water and every time that *qi*-water attempts to invade upwards, the *qi* and water collide and there is a pulsation under the umbilicus, which is an early sign of *bentun*.[24]

In successive periods *bentun* continues to be considered in the category of '*qi* diseases' and the emotional aspects of the aetiology, already introduced in the *Jingui Yaolue*, are detailed above all:

> *Bentun* [...] starts from fright, fear, anguish, worry [...] Fright and fear injure the *shen*, the heart stores the *shen*, anguish and worry injure the *zhi*, the kidney stores *zhi*. If *shen* and *zhi* are injured they move the *qi* with accumulation in the kidney and the *qi* goes down and up and moves like a running piglet which runs in a disorderly fashion [...] When *qi* ascends to the heart, the heart jumps internally, it is as though one is frightened or terrorised by somebody, when eating there is retching, there are sensations of fullness of air in the chest, *kuang*, dulling and instability, alterations in speaking and seeing. [...] If *qi* is full and pushes the heart there are disturbances and disorders below the heart, one does not wish to listen to the sound of voices, the episodes alternate with remissions, at times it disappears and at times it reaches its peak, breathing is short, hands and feet have *jueni*, there are internal disturbances, knotting and pain, dry retching, this is *bentun* from anguish and worry, when examining the pulse one feels it arrive beating with vigour.[25]

Tang Zonghai returns to the two possible causes of liver and kidney *qi* conversely rising and emptiness of kidney *yang* with ascending *qi*–water, including them in his observations, which in any case tend to place the role of blood in evidence.

In the first case, he highlights the role of *qi* and liver fire, which attack upwards starting from an agitation of liver and uterine blood; in the second he describes the process whereby the cold *qi* of the kidney which cannot be transformed by an excessively deficient *yang* rises through the *Chong Mai*, the sea of blood.

> If liver and uterine blood are not calm then liver fire ascends conversely, this is *bentunqi* which rises and it is liver *qi*. [...] 'Liver and kidney are in communication, *yi* and *gui* have the same origin, liver and kidney *qi* together tend to move perversely upward, in this case it is *bentun* that starts from liver pathogens and the inversion of its wood–*qi*, therefore it ascends and attacks the chest.' And: 'If

---

[24] Li Qingfu and Liu Duzhou, 1989, p. 115. We speak of heart *yang* because in the prescription *guizhi* (Ramulus Cinnamoni Cassiae) is increased, which liberates the outside and specifically reinforces the heart *yang*. A tet of the Ming period explains: 'If there is a kidney accumulation the external cold pathogens attack the lower *jiao* and move it. It is like the running of a water pig because the real *qi* is empty on the inside, the water is knotted and does not disperse and the *qi* crashes into it.' In: Xu Xun, *Dongyi baojian* ('The precious mirror of medicine', 1611).

[25] Chao Yuanfang, *Zhubing yuanhuolun* ('Treatise on the origin and symptoms of illnesses', 610) section *Qibing zhuhou* ('All the symptoms of the illnesses of the *qi*'), chapter 'Bentun qihou'.

kidney *yang* is not able to transform water the *qi* of the cold water flows conversely following the *Chong Mai* to the chest and lungs, in other words, it enters the heart, and this is *bentun* of kidney *qi* that lays siege to the heart.'[26]

To complete the picture, we also note interpretations from more recent periods in which attempts to tie in with Western anatomy–physiology are apparent, for example: 'The origin of *bentun* disease is in the fouled *qi*/air of the intestine, it comes from the gases produced by the fermentation of residual materials inside the stomach and intestines'.[27]

Clinical Notes

Bentun disease can be caused by an incorrect treatment that depletes an already weak *yang*, permitting a cold pathogen to penetrate into a subject that already has an excess of *yin*, water and cold in the lower *jiao*.

Nevertheless in general, in modern clinical practice, emotions are the prime cause of *bentunqi*, this 'running about' of *qi*, as though it were an assault by a pig – a domestic animal that can become wild and dangerous.

The condition has many similarities with panic attacks.[28] The panic attacks start suddenly and are of short duration, often lack precipitating factors, and resolve themselves spontaneously. The patient has a sense of imminent danger and an urgency to flee. The emotional tension and unbearable terror obstruct proper thought processes and action and may be accompanied by feelings of depersonalisation and unreality. Neurovegetative disturbances are also present, such as excessive sweating, nausea and abdominal disorders, palpitations, shortness of breath, sensations of suffocation in the throat, tightness in the chest, numbness, trembling, shivers, flashes, dizziness and a faint feeling.

The original description in the *Jingui Yaolue* acknowledges its outbreak and spontaneous resolution, the terror and sense of death that accompany the attack, the symptoms of tightness in the throat and chest, the abdominal pain, and changes in temperature. Slightly later descriptions also include retching, loss of clear thinking, loss of perception of reality and perceptive

---

[26] Tang Zonghai, *Jingui yaolue qianzhu buzheng* ('Comment and correction of the *Jingui yaolue*'). *Yi* and *gui* mean liver and kidney, they are the two heavenly trunks corresponding respectively to the *yin* wood and *yin* water.

[27] Cao Yingfu (1851–1914), *Jingfang shiyanlu* ('Experimental researches on classical prescriptions').

[28] Some clinical suggestions with reference to the trigrams of the *Yijing* can be found in the article by G. Morelli and E. Rossi, *L'Attacco di Panico: zhen, il drago dal profondo si lancia verso il cielo* ('The panic attack: *zhen*, the dragon which from the depths glides to the heavens'), 1995. The criteria for the diagnosis according to conventional psychiatry can be found in Appendix B for the classical description of *bentunqi* see the above quotes from Chapter 8 of the *Jingui yaolue* ('Prescriptions of the golden chamber', AD220), and of the 'Bentun qihou' of the *Zhubing yuanhuolun* ('Treatise on the origin and symptoms of illnesses', 610).

distortions, numbness and a faint feeling. In all cases, an emotional origin is acknowledged.

Panic attack disorder tends to become chronic, and concomitant disorders such as states of diffuse anxiety, hypochondria, lack of self-esteem, and substance abuse are frequent. A tendency to amorality and foreboding often prefigure phobic avoidance behaviour, which interferes with normal social and occupational life.

The effort to dominate fear and panic through thought, which attempts to foresee and govern all possibilities, corresponds to earth dominating water in the control-*ke* cycle. Maintaining this balance over time in the presence of a pathological condition of excess of one of the five elements, however, implies a rigidifying of the structure, a continuous increase in the energy necessary and a growing vulnerability. In effect, avoidance behaviour is a defence, which however, turns out to impair normal life.

BAIHEBING (百 合 病)

Bai means 'one hundred', *he* means 'reunion, meeting', and *bing* signifies 'illness'.

The term *baihebing* also appears for the first time in the *Jingui Yaolue* by Zhang Zhongjing, who explained: '*baihe* disease is so named because the one hundred vessels originate from a single root, the illness reaches all of them.'[29] The name of the disease, therefore, derives from the fact that it involves many channels; since all the 'one hundred vessels' of the body originate from the same source, if the source becomes ill, all the vessels become ill.

Other writers, however, maintain that the name comes from the classic remedy used to cure it: 'In *baihe* disease one uses *baihe*, it already had the name *baihe* in ancient times, because this one single medicine is used to cure it, and for this reason it took its name.'[30]

Whatever the origin of the name, *baihebing* indicates a clinical pattern with few physical signs, but instead strange alterations in behaviour regarding vital areas of living (food, rest, activity). In his description, Zhang Zhongjing notes that even though it is connected with febrile diseases, it seems to be an illness of the *shen* and the consciousness. A condition in which the presence of a continuous swing from one thing to its opposite is outlined, intentions and possibilities are counterposed, they seem to be patterns of heat or cold, but in fact, are neither.

---

[29] Zhang Zhongjing, *Jingui yaolue* ('Prescriptions of the golden chamber', AD220), Chapter 3.
[30] Wei Nianting, *Jingui yaolue benyi* ('The original meaning of the *Jingui yaolue*). *Baihe* is the Bulbus Lilii, which nourishes the lung and heart *yin*, humidifies the lung and stops the cough, purifies the heart and calms the *shen*.

Intention-*yi* desires to eat but cannot, one remains in silence, desires to remain lying down, but cannot stay supine, desires to walk, but cannot, at times enjoys food and drink and at others cannot stand even their smell, it is like heat, yet there is no heat; it is like cold, yet there is no cold; the mouth is bitter, the urine is red, no drug can cure it, if one takes medicines there is vomiting and diarrhoea, it as though it is an illness of the *shen* and the consciousness-*shi*, while the body and form are as normal, the pulse is small and rapid.[31]

Aetiology

Baihe disease derives from empty lung and heart *yin* with heat. It may have various origins: it can break out following a febrile disease, when *yin* and blood have not yet been reconstituted and the residual heat which consumes liquids has not been extinguished; or in cases of excess thoughts and preoccupations which injure the heart; or furthermore when there is constraint of emotions owing to which fire is produced, which dries outs the liquids. Internal heat then accumulates in the hundred vessels:

Whatever the cause of the disease, the pathological pattern must always be lead back to the heart and lung, since the heart stores *shen* and governs the blood vessels and the lung houses *po*, governs regulation and looks out on the hundred vessels. If residual pathogens smoulder after a disease and cloud the heart and lung, or if the constraint of emotions produces heat which disturbs the *shen* and *po*, one arrives at a situation where *qi* and blood are no longer governed, the clarity of *shen* is obscured, *shen* and *zhi* are in disarray, the hundred vessels lose nourishment.[32]

The original description in the *Jingui Yaolue* relates *baihebing* to febrile diseases, both in initial and in advanced stages, and the commentators specify:

The heat pathogens spread, are not contained in the channels, their *qi* wanders without coming to a standstill, therefore the illness also comes and goes without coming to a standstill, but the fact that it is a case of heat is testified to by the pulse, mouth, urine and stools [...]. This disorder is found mostly before and after febrile diseases. If it manifests before the disease it is a case of *qi* heat which moves first, if it manifests 4 or 5 days after the disease, or after an interval of 20 days or a month, it is a case of residual heat that did not go away.[33]

---

[31] Zhang Zhongjing, *Jingui yaolue*, Chapter 3. The sentence 如有 神识之 疾 *ruyou shenshi zhiji* 'like an illness of the *shen* and conscience' in some versions has a different character 如有 神灵 者 *ruyou shenling zhe*. It then becomes 'like having spirits', from which derive the presentations of sympomatological frames in which we find elements of trance, possession or mental vagueness.
[32] Li Qingfu and Liu Duzhou, 1989, p. 123.
[33] You Zaijing, *Jingui yaolue xindian* ('Personal selection from the *Jingui yaolue*').

Later, in any case, a correlation is evident between its emergence and a depletion of *qi* and *yin* caused by heat pathology becoming chronic owing to complications, lack of treatment, or incorrect treatment: '*baihebing* is often caused by emptiness due to a depletion which follows febrile diseases; after a serious illness the body does not recuperate and this disorder follows.'[34]

In the following debate emotions are also specifically introduced as causes of *baihe* disorders: 'Thought damages the spleen, spleen *yin* is injured; *jueyin* fire accumulates in the heart, disturbing the hundred vessels and causing *baihe* disorder.'[35]

Qing Dynasty texts support the theory that interprets *baihebing* as a serious consequence that may follow febrile diseases, but particularly underline the role played by emotional elements in producing *baihe*-type patterns. It is said, for example: 'After serious febrile diseases if *qi* and blood have not returned to their normal balance, this can transform into *bahei* disorder.' But also: 'In people who think a lot without pause, if the emotions-*qingzhi* are not seconded or if fright or unexpected circumstances arise, then the body and the *shen* both fall ill and one can have symptoms of this type.'[36]

Clinical Notes

Baihebing corresponds to a pathological condition characterised by internal heat and a deep distress that interferes with the most natural activities.

If unresolved febrile illnesses initially constituted the main cause of *baihe*, even today the residual heat component is certainly not to be ignored in the aetiology of this pattern, possibly in its most insidious forms, which can be identified with the various types of chronic viral infections, autoimmune diseases, or hidden heat that remains after an antibiotic therapy or is a concomitant of various pharmaceutical treatments.[37]

However, the hypothesis of an emotion-related aetiology continued to gain weight in medical thought over time and became dominant in the modern clinical environment.

In the classical description we find a pattern that is effectively at the opposite pole from the spontaneous and immediate adherence to the unfolding world as exemplified in Daoist thought: the patient would like to eat, rest, speak, or walk, but is unable to do so.

[34] Chao Yuanfang, *Zhubing yuanhoulun* ('Treatise on the origin and symptoms of illnesses', 610).
[35] Zhang Luzhuan, *Zhangshi Yitong* ('General medicine according to master Zhang 1695).
[36] Wu Jian, *Yizong jinjian* ('The golden mirror of medicine' 1742).
[37] See also the report of the seminar in Nanjing in June 1988 by professor Wang Chenhui on the hidden heat, feverish illnesses and AIDS, in: *Fure calore nascosto* ('Fire, hidden heat'), E. Rossi (ed.), 1994.

A condition that is well known to us is depicted with a few strokes – that is, there are no signs of underlying organic illness, 'the body and the form are as if normal', 'it is a disorder of the *shen* and the consciousness'.

The doctor is disoriented owing to the confusion of heat and cold signs and furthermore obstructed in treatment because the patient does not tolerate medicines.

In today's clinical setting we often see patients who seem to be restless and unsatisfied, and we notice this state of diffuse restlessness in their stories; we recognise here the difference between what one desires to do and what one is able to do as referred to in the classic description.

We should recall here, in any case, that *baihebing* is a disorder and not a mood or personality trait; it therefore has a beginning, is defined by precise criteria and produces suffering that is torturously debilitating.

MEIHEQI (梅核气)

The term *meiheqi*, or 'plum stone *qi*', is relatively recent, going back only to the Qing Dynasty: 'In *meiheqi* one has the impression of something blocked in the middle of the throat, it cannot be expelled or swallowed, and has the form of a plum stone.'[38] However, the disorder had been described similarly in the *Neijing* where the sensation of an extraneous body in the throat was called 'obstructed throat' (*houjie* 喉介) and essentially the same concept appears throughout the medical literature as 'roast meat' (*zhirou* 炙 肉).

It is specifically taken into consideration by Zhang Zhongjing in the chapter on women's disorders, before the discussion on *zangzao*: 'In women if there seems to be a bit of roast (*zhiluan* 炙 脔) in the throat, the indication is *Banxia houpo tang*.'[39]

Aetiology

The source of the sensation of obstruction in the throat is attributed to phlegm that rises to the throat and accumulates there. 'When there is a sensation of a bit of roast meat in the throat, it is a case of knotted phlegm which bonds to *qi* and is transported upward by it, accumulating in the throat, and it has the shape of a bit of roast meat.'[40]

---

[38] Long Xin, *Gujin yijian* ('Ancient and modern medicine reflections, 1589') The term also appears in the text by Wu Jian, *Yizong jinjiang* ('The golden mirror of medicine', 1742) and since then it has been commonly used.
[39] Zhang Zhongjing, *Jingui yaolue*, Chapter 22. The prescription contains herbs that move the *qi*, untie the knots, bring the *qi* downwards, transform mucosities.
[40] Chao Yuanfang, *Zhubing yuanhoulun* ('Treatise on the origin and symptoms of illnesses', 610).

The reason for this condensing and knotting is connected to the emotions:

> If euphoria and anger are not regulated, worry and thoughts accumulate, sadness and fear are generated, at times there can be tremors of fright, this leads to an imbalance of *qi* in the organs. [...] The throat is obstructed above, as though there were a bite of roast meat that cannot be swallowed, and all this is a produced by the seven emotions.[41]

A particularly revealing aetiological factor is constraint-*yu*, which if persisting progressively dries out the liquids, knots *qi* and produces phlegm-heat: 'In the seven emotions *qi* is constrained, knots, produces phlegm and saliva, accumulates and agglomerates with *qi*, becomes hard and large like a mass, establishes itself between the heart and abdomen, at times obstructs the throat like a prune stone or cotton, it cannot be expelled or swallowed.'[42]

The relationship between stagnation and knotting of *qi* and alterations of emotions is also returned to later: 'This disorder derives from the knotting of *qi* and the condensing of the liquids by the seven emotions.'[43]

A passage from the Ming Dynasty that relates the stagnation of *qi* and the accumulation of liquids and phlegm in the throat to the lack of determination of the gall bladder is interesting:

> The upper *jiao* is *yang*, it governs correct *qi*, it is important that it be free and flowing since what it fears most is stagnation. If there is stasis, liquids do not flow and there is accumulation in the form of saliva. The gall bladder's ambassador is the throat, the gall bladder governs determination, its *qi* governs ministerial fire, if it is not determined when encountering the seven emotions then fire stagnates and does not spread, if it does not spread then *qi* goes to the throat and phlegm accumulates in the chest, therefore the sensation is that of roast meat.[44]

Clinical Notes

The description of a 'prune stone' corresponds to the globus hystericus of Western psychology. Also called 'oesophageal constriction', it is the sensation of an extraneous body at the level of the pharynx that obstructs the throat and interferes with breathing.

---

[41] Chen Wuze, *Sanyin jiyi bingzheng fanglun* ('Treatise on the three categories of illness causes').
[42] Zhu Hong, *Nanyang huorenshu* (As it is often the case the translation of the title in Italian and English is not easy because of its multiple references: for example in this case Nanyang refers to Zhang Zhongjing, the city of birth, and *Huorenshu*, 'book for the life of the happy man', refers to the way in which Hua Tuo had defined the *Shanghanlun*).
[43] Wu Jian, *Yizong jinjian* ('The golden mirror of medicine').
[44] Gong Xin, *Jingui yuhanjing* ('Hidden treasures of the *Jingui*' 1589).

Case Study 9.1

A Possessed Appearance

I already knew this 30-year-old woman, a television production assistant, because I had treated her in the past for dysmenorrhoea, and when she calls me I hear a note in her voice that alarms me.

A few days earlier she had had an experience that greatly frightened her: she suddenly felt like she was going to faint, she was dizzy and had difficulty in breathing, vomited and was overcome by great tiredness and an 'empty-headed' sensation.

She seems very tired; she weeps as she tells me that she feels like she no longer has control over anything. She is coming out of a period of emotional and occupational trauma, is afraid of her own death and of those dear to her, she fears that she has been infected by 'mad cow' disease or that she has a brain tumour, she sees herself as pale, others tell her that she looks ill (in fact, she has lost a number of pounds in weight, as had already happened previously, since she has difficulty in digesting food and therefore eats little).

There have been no further episodes of what appear to have the characteristics of panic attacks, but the dizzy spells continue especially in the morning, together with a sense of instability.

She feels exhausted, cannot concentrate on her work, her thoughts are unravelled, she feels a deep sadness, does not understand what is going on and feels overwhelmed by something outside herself.

Furthermore, she suffers from constraint in the chest, her stools are not well formed, she sweats a lot at night but is not thirsty and does not have a dry mouth. Her menstrual cycle is regular with a scanty, dark flow. She does not suffer from insomnia but sees sleep as a type of black hole that she enters from exhaustion.

She has a dull complexion with a drawn face, a slightly pale and swollen tongue, with a wide superficial crack in the centre, and a slightly scanty coating, with no sublingual congestion. The pulse is rapid and wiry.

Diagnosis

Emptiness of *qi* and blood, initial deficiency of *yin* with wind in the higher regions and empty fire that disturbs the *shen*. *Zangzao*?

Treatment

Eight treatments: four after an interval of 2–3 days, two after one of 5 days, and two after one of 7 days.

First treatment:
- GB-20 *Fengchi*, EX-HN-3 *Yintang*, Ren-17 *Shanzhong*, Ren-4 *Guanyuan*, HE-7 *Shenmen*, SP-6 *Sanyinjiao*.

The dizziness and sense of instability regress immediately; this greatly reassures her and interrupts the vicious cycle in which apprehensions and fears consume her strength. She still complains of great tiredness, nocturnal sweating, and stools that are not well formed.

Afterwards, the following points are maintained:

- EX-HN-3 *Yintang*, Ren-17 *Shanzhong*, Ren-4 *Guanyuan*, or Ren-6 *Qihai* to regulate the flow of *qi* and bring it down.

  In addition, the following points are alternated:

- Ren-4 *Guanyuan*, HE-7 *Shenmen*, SP-6 *Sanyinjiao*

  and

- Ren-6 *Qihai*, P-6 *Neiguan*, ST-36 *Zusanli*, SP-3 *Taibai*.

  These are added:

- ST-25 *Tianshu*, ST-36 *Zusanli*, ST-37 *Shangjuxu*.

  GB-20 *Fengchi* was omitted after the disappearance of the signs of wind in the upper regions.

In the course of the first four treatments the situation slowly improves: the patient eats a little more, her complexion and the *shen* of the eyes improve, her emotionality is less extreme. However, she still sweats at night, is physically weak and emotionally fragile, and has had a number of episodes of diarrhoea with liquid, yellow, foul-smelling stools.

An overall improvement is, however, noted in the sixth treatment, with a return to her normal appetite, and increased mental and physical energy in general. Two more treatments are carried out to consolidate the results.

Comments

A case of this type can be included in the *zangzao* pattern: the weeping and symptoms of kidney emptiness corresponding to 'stretching and yawning' in the classic description are present.

In the modern clinic, the traditional symptom of 'possessed appearance' is often classified under hysterical manifestations, but it can also be attributed to the condition which was once generically defined as 'nervous breakdown' and to those states in which, as in this case, the person suddenly appears almost to be the prey of something alien.

The suddenness and violence with which the tiredness and consumption of *qi* transformed into a condition of pervasive fear and loss of lucidity are, in fact, central elements in this pattern.

Since, however, we are speaking of a young woman with a good underlying *qi*, the tonifying of *qi* and regulation of its movement while avoiding dramatic intervention allowed the *qi* to right itself in a short time and restore the balance necessary for self-healing to take place.

Naturally, a discussion concerning the causes that had produced a depletion of *qi* and the eventual need to make changes in lifestyle or internal attitudes is another matter.

Follow-up

After a few months I see the patient again for a twisted ankle. She has started practising *qigong* and has started analysis, which she continues with interest and perseverance.

She still does not feel calm and at times she feels like she is excessively tired, but she has had no further attacks of intense anxiety, she sleeps well, eats with a good appetite, her bowel movements are regular, and she no longer sweats excessively or has feelings of constraint in the chest.

Case Study 9.2

A Young Woman Who Could No Longer Find Herself

A young 30-year-old financial analyst, mother of a 4-year-old girl, is sent to me by a colleague because she is in an intense state of anxiety and agitation.

She tells me of always having a feeling of extreme restlessness; both during the day and at night those moments where she feels 'her heart in her throat' are ever more frequent, with tachycardia, palpitations and laboured breathing, followed by cold sweats and trembling.

When speaking she cannot hold back her tears.

Episodes of unreality and depersonalisation ('I see things as though they are happening in a film', 'I see myself as though from the outside') continue to be frequent, but mainly she is having an identity crisis: she, who had always been an independent, determined, naturally efficient and spontaneously organised person, no longer recognises herself and cannot even manage to do the simplest things.

This situation seriously interferes with her life: she drives with difficulty, going to the supermarket is beyond the limits of her strength; working is impossible (she was forced to request sick leave, which she extended because her attempt to return to work failed immediately). She cannot see friends, nor can she speak with anyone.

She is also subject to strong temporal headaches; she awakens after 2 to 3 hours of sleep and at times does not manage to fall asleep again until around dawn; she hardly eats anything because of nausea, and often vomits; she is very thirsty.

Three days earlier she suspended her intake of the antidepressive medication (paroxetine), which she had started taking 20 days before, although she continues to take a minimum dose of tranquillisers in the evening.

The tongue does not show any particular signs, it is only slightly tooth marked, and the pulse is weak and thin, with a sensation of urgency.

The last few years had been physically and emotionally difficult: she was mourning the loss of her father, she abandoned a study project which she was enthusiastic about to take a not particularly rewarding job, and the situation with the father of her child has always been extremely complex, just as her relationship with her mother continues to be difficult. Only recently, a loving relationship in which she had felt understood and protected had broken down.

In her clinical history was a record of pathologies linked to the gynaecological sphere, related to deficiency and stasis of blood: the use of oral contraceptives since late adolescence (prescribed to treat painful menstruation with a heavy flow), suffering during child birth and early motherhood, and surgery for an ectopia of the uterine wall carried out 6 months ago after continuous spotting for 4 months.

Diagnosis
Bentunqi. Qi disorder generated by *qi* exhaustion and consumption of *yin*, and lack of communication between water and fire.

Therapeutic principles
Restore communication between heart and kidney, tonify *qi,* and nourish blood and *yin*.

Treatment
Ten biweekly treatments, in which the following are alternated:
- EX-HN-3 *Yintang*, Ren-17 *Shanzhong*, Ren-4 *Guanyuan*, HE-5 *Tongli*, KI-4 *Dazhong*, and ear point *Shenmen* with a 'permanent' seed
  and:
- EX-HN-3 *Yintang*, Ren-17 *Shanzhong*, Ren-4 *Guanyuan*, HE-7 *Shenmen*, KI-3 *Taixi*, and ear point *Shenmen* with a 'permanent' seed.

After a few treatments the patient feels that a course of psychotherapy for a few months would be useful. The psychotherapy treatments continue at a biweekly frequency for 4 months until she leaves the country. Her shift to psychotherapy necessitates a change in approach, but does not exclude – at least initially – the use of acupuncture treatment at energetic levels, which therefore continues for the first month.

Except for minor variations, the two combinations of points are essentially unchanged for two reasons: a) the healing process is proceeding well; b) when acupuncture is associated with psychotherapy it is best that the needling treatments are as 'neutral' as possible.[45]

During the first 10 days the symptoms do not change, but during the fourth treatment she says there has been substantial improvement: she has slept well for the first time in the last three months, still has a choking feeling in her throat and 'sinking heart' with cold sweats and trembles, but they only last a couple of minutes.

After two months she starts to use makeup again, wears lighter clothing (it had already been hot for quite some time previously), manages to go to the supermarket, to cook and eat, and she is happy because she feels like she has started thinking again.

Comments
This case can be denoted as a *bentunqi* pattern, both due to the disorder-*luan* in the movement of *qi* and for its aetiology, which can be attributed to fear, anguish and over thinking that have injured heart and kidney.

---

[45] Whichever intervention external to the relation based on the verbal and symbolic level has some 'acting' side (see also the discussion in Chapters 13, 15 and footnote 46 in Chapter 3). The same is true for medical drugs, for which in fact the psychotherapist usually refers patients to a colleague.

The specific symptoms of this patient are also easily overlaid on the classic descriptions. For example, comparing her symptoms with the passage by Chao Yuan-fang, we find this patient exhibits the attack in the upper regions by the running piglet-*qi*, the fright and state of alarm, the leaping heart, the retching, the feeling of fullness in the chest and the laboured breathing, the dulling and sense of instability, the impatience with regards others due to which 'one does not desire to hear the sound of voices', and the flaring-up character of the more violent episodes.

The two prescriptions essentially act on the water–fire axis: the first with the two *luo* points mainly moves the fullness above to nourish the *yin* below; the second with the two *yuan* points tonifies the source of the heart and kidney.

The *Du* and *Renmai* points also move and regulate *qi*. EX-HN-3 *Yintang* is preferred to other *Dumai* points located higher up because there are no strong signs of agitation from fire; Ren-17 *Shanzhong* is chosen because the symptoms in the chest were more serious than those of the digestive system; Ren-4 *Guanyuan* tonifies *yuanqi* but also has an important action on *yin* and blood and anchors upward-moving *qi* below.

This case, in which the initial conditions were apparently quite compromised, was resolved in a relatively short time.

The physical and emotional fatigue had probably caused a disorder of *qi*, which could no longer remain anchored and attacked above in ever closer and stronger waves. Naturally, the *shen* also suffered from this, and was becoming confused and disorderly.

Therefore, regulating the basic movements of *qi* by acting on the two *yin–yang* poles of water and fire enabled the restitution of the patient's own resources.

It was therefore unnecessary to aim the intervention specifically towards the stagnation of *qi*, the emptiness of *yin* and the emptiness and stasis of blood, but only to regulate and reorder the movements of *qi* in order to shift the equilibrium from a situation of disorder and imbalance to a state in which *qi* is able to regain its natural tendency to maintain order. This shift allows *qi* to activate the homeostatic processes that lead to balance in the system, in other words, to restore the dynamics that correspond to a state of health.[46]

The psychoanalytical task mainly regarded the very complex relationship with her real mother and her internal representations, a knot that had contorted her energies and prevented the unfolding of her true nature. It is obviously difficult to say what part this process of recognition, recuperation and integration had in finding and maintaining a creative balance.

Follow-up

Eight months after the conclusion of treatments I call her to wish her a good summer and to find out how she is doing: she tells me that she is still in Paris, will be

---

[46] See also the reflection by Yu Yongxi, who interprets the balance *yin-yang* and the role of *zhengqi* and *xieqi* in the light of the mathematical theory of catastrophe by René Thom. In: *Il modello delle catastrofi a cuspide* ('The cusp catastrophe model'), 1996.

going later to Brittany with a new contract for a job she likes very much, that her daughter is fine, that she herself feels calm and has had no further anxiety crises.

Case Study 9.3

Different Pain, Different Mourning

This case was published in the '*MediCina*' magazine, autumn 1994. It is presented without any alterations, except for a final comment and the updating of the point abbreviations: it therefore shows the continuity and changes in the evaluation and therapeutic approach of a case after an interval of eight years.

The girl sitting in front of me has gestures and smiles left suspended, the string of words comes out only up to a certain point, then the sentence interrupts, brief, it goes no farther. Like a sob, a weeping breath that has a very short course. Lung *qi* is knotted.

The girl says that she always has a cough, cold, fever, and is very tired, that as a child she already suffered from tonsillitis. She also feels a knot under her heart; when she is at home she weeps desperately due to anxiety; her stomach burns, she is nauseous, and cannot eat. She dreams 'too much, it is very tiring', and the persons and events of her dreams 'are too similar to those in reality'. It has been a year since her mother died after an illness that lasted for a year: she can no longer take it. Her father and brother, rarely present, in any case do not speak about it.

I see an injured lung, weak like it had probably been in infancy, and more than anything I observe how a movement of consolidation cannot take place, the one of autumn: I seem to understand, in fact, that closure was missing, that there had not been the necessary pause in life after the death of a loved one. I express all this to the girl, and tell her that it might be as though she had tried not to express mourning; she breaks out in incessant tears (this would be the only time she wept in my presence).

Wood in a control-*ke* relationship of rebellion corresponds to a weak metal.

In the meantime, the girl is telling me that her mother was very good, very present, even overly present; she insinuated herself everywhere.

I think that wood is soft, that the tree and spring offer flowers, but also that liver energy is extremely powerful, and that wind has the dangerous property of insinuating itself everywhere.

The girl says that due to the ever-present thoughts about her mother there is a great disorder in the events of her daily life; there is no actual fragmentation, only a great restlessness, an excess of movement, a perverse version of the lung's function of 'distributing energy in the one hundred vessels'.

It is on this element that we will initiate our task.

Her tongue is slightly pale, with a thin, white coating; the pulse is weak for her age, empty in the deep position.

The principle of treatment will be the tonification of *qi*, focusing the work on the lung.

It is true that there are many signs which point to a stagnation of the liver: the mood swings, the depression with unexpressed anger (but which – she will tell me later – at times explodes with great violence towards those closest to her), the suffering of the *hun*, which manifests both through this difficulty with the dream images and in the impossibility of imagining the future.

There are also the nausea, the episodes of vomiting, the loss of appetite (the sight of food is also decidedly disturbing), the burning pain in the stomach, the tendency to diarrhoea (this element is referred to by her later as a characteristic that she has had all her life): signs of the liver invading the stomach, or better yet a stomach that has been invaded by the liver? In fact, the tongue is not red on the edges, but pale, and the pulse is empty: together with the chronic bowel disorder and the fact that there are no other signs of liver stagnation, these elements point us towards a diagnosis of rudimentary deficiency in the middle *jiao*.

Together with this ancient weakness of earth, the first symptoms she talks about, the very specific impression that I received from the way she presents herself and the fundamental element of mourning caused me to select a treatment to support lung *qi*.

Lung *qi* governs energy, and the girl complains of a great weakness; deficiency of lung *qi* is also indicated by her shortness of breath and pallor; there is coughing because the lung cannot descend the *qi*; the voice is weak because *zongqi* is weak; but also *weiqi* (defensive energy) is deficient, so we find coldness and ease of invasion by external pathogens, with the typical succession of colds and tonsillitis.

In order to act directly on the lung, I use the *mu* point LU-1 *Zhongfu* (which is also the meeting point of lung and spleen), the *shu* point of lung BL-13 *Feishu* and the psychic point of the lung BL-42 *Pohu*.

I tonify the *qi* through Ren-17 *Shanzhong* (which is also the *mu* point of the upper *jiao* and acts on *zongqi* and the lung), Ren-6 *Qihai* (which furthermore tonifies *yuanqi*), KI-3 *Taixi* (*yuan* point of the kidney, the birth of *yuanqi*).

I will also use ST-36 *Zusanli* and SP-3 *Taibai* to tonify the *qi* of earth.

I will also keep in mind the psychic point of liver BL-47 *Hunmen* together with BL-18 *Ganshu* and LIV-3 *Taichong* to move *qi*.

A brief note after an interval of 3 months: we are at the beginning of July, after 12 treatments at a weekly frequency and the total regression of the somatic symptoms, but with an agreement to continue in September because there still seems to be a need for work.

Normally I do not explain the significance of the points, but in June I expressly ask for her impressions and comments on the points used during the year, and in this case it seems interesting for me to bring a useful element into her initial evaluation of the treatment.

She felt BL-13 *Feishu*, BL-42 *Pohu* and the *mu* point LU-1 *Zhongfu* 'very much, they were very strong', 'when I leave I also physically feel that there is less devastation': it does not seem to me that this sensation is necessarily automatic, in my experience the back-*shu* points are not particularly 'strong'. But the fact that LIV-3 *Taichong* seemed to be 'neutral' struck me a great deal more – *Taichong*, to which no one is ever indifferent! – so much so that other patients in whom I had used it to activate 'mental' *qi* flow had commented: 'It causes my thoughts to come increasingly one after the other' or 'The images are much livelier'.

It should be obvious that the points used for a specific purpose should turn out to be 'different' and 'felt more', but it is nice to have a little confirmation.

Comments

I later carried out psychotherapy with this girl for two years, and every 2 or 3 years she pays me a visit: she graduated from university and immediately found a job that interested her, she has had a stable relationship for a number of years, and she has not had important physical or psychological health problems.

This case is an example of a situation that can be attributed to a *baihe* pattern.

The lung signs (*baihe* nourishes lung and heart *yin*, moistens the lungs and stops cough, purifies the heart and calms the *shen*), the pervasive anxiety, and the 'strange things' that characterise Zhang Zhongjing's description of *baihebing* all suggest it. There is the 'heat without there being heat' of the burning in the stomach together with the coldness and pallor, the restlessness due to which she would like to rest but is instead out going around the city day and night, the desire to study but the weakness and recurring illnesses (with relative residual heat), the oscillations from the sadness of her emotions to the excitement of her behaviour.

We certainly find a great pain in the aetiology, with accumulation of thought and knotted emotions, after which the dimming of *shen* and sickness in the body follow.

Case Study 9.4

If Your Throat Is Blocked

A 52-year-old woman requests an urgent appointment for a cervical pain radiating to the head that had appeared suddenly a few days earlier, set off by any movement, including the opening of her mouth and swallowing. This pain is localised on the median line and is not accompanied by dizziness, but she has suffered from a paracervical pain on the right for the last couple of years, which worsens when she turns her head to the left.

She is apprehensive and anxious, suffers from tachycardia and palpitations both during the day and at night, has trouble falling asleep and feels a knot in her throat when he is agitated.

The start of this disturbance, described as 'blockage of the throat', goes back to the period following her second pregnancy 30 years earlier; at times it worsens and now seems to be the element which most bothers and frightens her.

Her face is not particularly tense, but as she speaks she is often on the verge of weeping.

In menopause for 2 years, she is still subject to hot flushes and has had vaginal dryness and a total absence of sexual desire for about a year.

The abdomen is often bloated and the bowels tend to constipation, but she keeps herself regular with proper eating.

The tongue is slightly red; the pulse is thin and tight.

Diagnosis

Acute stagnation of *qi* and blood in the *Dumai*, emptiness of *yin* with empty heat and restlessness of the *shen*, liver *qi* stagnation with *meiheqi*.

Therapeutic principles

Circulate *qi* and blood in the *Du Mai*, move and regulate liver *qi*, nourish *yin* and clear empty heat.

Treatment

Fifteen treatments at weekly intervals, then less frequently, for a total of 5 months.

First treatment:

- GB-20 *Fengchi*, Du-14 *Dazhui*, Du-16 *Fengfu*, SI-3 *Houxi*, GB-21 *Jianjing* (plus cupping).

Second treatment:

- GB-20 *Fengchi*, Du-14 *Dazhui*, EX-HN-15 *Bailao*, HE-7 *Shenmen*, SP-6 *Sanyinjiao*.

Third to sixth treatments: during the third treatment she mentions that she remained calm during an argument at work, and that she had no longer felt the obstruction in the throat, but that she has a persistent light feeling of nausea, which disappears during the following treatments. In the following months sleep improves, palpitations and the knot in the throat do not re-emerge and the abdominal bloating diminishes.

The following are alternated:

- GB-20 *Fengchi*, EX-HN-3 *Yintang*, LI-4 *Hegu*, LIV-3 *Taichong*, GB-34 *Yanglingquan* and:
- EX-HN-3 *Yintang*, Ren-17 *Shanzhong*, Ren-6 *Qihai*, preceded by 'sliding' cups on the upper back.

Seventh to 15th treatments: hot flushes, sweating, dry mouth, vaginal dryness and absence of libido are still present. The main points are:

- GB-20 *Fengchi*, Ren-4 *Guanyuan*, ST-29 *Guilai*, HE-7 *Shenmen* or HE-6 *Yinxi*, SP-6 *Sanyinjiao*.

During the 12th treatment she complains of an acute sacralgia, which regresses after the treatment.

- EX-HN-3 *Yintang* and a contemporary mobilisation of the painful section of the spinal column, followed by Du-3 *Yaoyangguan*, M-BW-25 *Shiqizhuixia*, BL-31 *Shangliao*, BL-32 *Ciliao*, BL-60 *Kunlun*.

During these 3 months the various symptoms of heat due to empty *yin* are relieved.

Comments

It is interesting to note how the symptoms in the throat regressed at the beginning of the treatment course, even if the choice of points during the first treatments was aimed mainly at resolving the acute condition, which was the intense pain in the neck and head.

GB-20 *Fengchi* is, however, a point that is very effective on the downward passage, due to which even if it is not one of the first line points normally used in cases of *meiheqi*, we can imagine that its action would extend to any obstruction at this level, just as Du-14 *Dazhui* removes local obstructions in the channel but also regulates the circulation of *qi* when it rises conversely.

The onset of 'prune-stone' sensation and the palpitations is linked to the second pregnancy, which her husband was against because it was too close to the first one. The woman is basically angry with her husband, whom she does not get along with, but is also worried about a number of choices made by her son, with which she does not agree. With therapy, the underlying attitudes certainly did not change; however, hostility, acrimony and recriminations have diminished.

Nourishment of *yin* is fundamental in this case, to avoid heat from *yin* deficiency joining the heat caused by stagnation.

Follow-up

After the summer break, she says that she feels well, and is content: she had no longer suffered from insomnia, palpitations, and *meiheqi*, the hot flushes have become very sporadic, and she has had pleasant sexual relations for the first time in more than a year.

She also went to visit her terminally ill sister, something which fear had prevented her from doing for months. She finds it important that she was able to remain at her sister's side, even though she had become unrecognisable, without being overcome by suffering and consequent panic reactions.

SECTION III

THERAPEUTIC APPROACHES

CHAPTER 10 PRINCIPAL PATTERNS OF FULLNESS

CHAPTER 11 PRINCIPAL PATTERNS OF EMPTINESS

The chapters on clinical framework are organised according to contemporary Chinese methodology (TCM).

The patterns are defined in relation to differential diagnostic-*bianzheng*, that is through a description of symptoms and signs and of possible aetiopathogenetic processes, from which derive therapeutic principles and selections of points.

I have chosen to organise all the elements within the traditional Chinese diagnostic pattern rather than examining every 'illness' individually, reviewing the differentiation of each one and describing its aetiopathogenesis, clinic and treatment.[1]

In this way I have avoided useless and obvious repetition. Moreover with this systematisation I can better respect a basic assumption of Chinese medicine, that is, the attention to the general unbalanced pattern rather than to the final symptom.

In fact what characterises acupuncture practice is that it recognises, for example, a 'full fire' or an 'emptiness of the spleen *qi*' rather than corresponding to a symptom, such as 'easy fear' or 'panic attack', or dealing with a definition, such as 'depression' or 'anxiousness'.

As in any other pathology, in treating patterns where the psychic component is dominant one must be aware that the symptom is the expression of a complex situation, in which the differential diagnosis is based on a set of signs and symptoms as stated in the ever reconfirmed saying: 'Different illnesses same therapy, same illnesses different therapy'.

I have focused on a few major axes in order to assist practitioners in their daily evaluation and help them to deal with symptoms and syndromes that are often not so straightforward.

In considering that an attempt to be exhaustive would result in multiplication of syndrome descriptions with a consequent blurring of their outlines, I have preferred to highlight some specific pathological cores, trying nevertheless to respect their complexity. I have thus chosen a 'simple' grid that functions as a basis for constructing a more sophisticated definition of all patterns.

In practice I have selected and focused upon those patterns that are more common and essential, not wishing, however, to exclude the possibility of the many other variations.

We recall that: '*yin* and *yang* are the *dao* of the heavens and earth, the grid and net of the ten thousand things, the mother and father of change and transformation, the root and origin of birth and death, the palace hosting the clarity of the *shen*. To treat the illness one must search for its root'.[2]

See the specific chapters on issues of terminology, treatment with internal practices, reflection on emotions and *shen*, discussion on certain aetiopathogenetic concepts, deepening

---

[1] The nosologic problem of reference would remain in any case: certain Western authors choose to translate directly the terms used by contemporary Chinese texts. But these refer to a Western psychiatric classification that is often mixed or which has fallen into disuse. For a more articulate examination on this issue see the discussion on nosography in the methodological premises.

[2] *Suwen*, Chapter 5. We translate here as 'grid' the term *gang* 纲, corresponding to the main rope of the fishing net, that is the principle sustaining the whole, and as 'net' the term *ji* 纪 that suggests the thick connecting structure.

of the semiotics of tongue and pulse, and debate on a number of contemporary applications. Since the text is structured so as to limit repetitions, the work of connecting together information is largely left to the reader.

The syndromes are grouped as a rule into the two categories of 'fullness' and 'emptiness'. I recall that lack and excess do not refer directly to the *shen* but to the *qi* in its various declinations. As a result of different alterations the *shen* can loose the peacefulness of a coherence with the *dao*, that is, the capacity to see clearly, to think, to feel, to learn, to answer, to choose, etc. The clinical patterns respect a structure that presents the following:

- The main lines along which an aetiopathogenetic process develops. These are discussed in the chapters on emotions and movements of the *qi* and on constriction and heat (see Chapters 2, 4 and 5).
- Potential paths along which the illness evolves, grouped according to the involved functional areas. No description of a clinical pattern can propose a perfect correspondence: signs and symptoms are related as the most likely possibilities. We know that in reality they are rarely all present at once, or that they are accompanied by other symptoms that we must consider in order to define the pathology more precisely or to modify our selection of points. A specific examination of the two main aspects of symptomatology can be found in the chapters on restlessness and insomnia (see Chapters 6 and 7).
- Some notes that can help in the recognition and reading of symptoms and signs in contemporary clinical practice.
- The therapeutic principles, which in the practice of acupuncture derive from an accurate evaluation of the actual pattern with its signs and symptoms and from the ability to recognise the form of the alteration of the normal physiology of the *qi*.
- The hypothesis of treatment, based on combinations of points that are chosen following a minimal criterion: a sort of root from which to begin thinking about the variations dictated by the course and manifestation of the pathology.
- A discussion on individual points, which again is to be read as suggestions more than as precise indications. They therefore recur mostly in one pattern: an invitation to feel the quality of the point, to recover its meaning in relation to different patterns. The description of the points, embraces characteristics and main actions; there are also some more specific comments on the psychic component. (I have chosen to leave out indications since they are a direct consequence of functions and they have been already clearly discussed in basic manuals.) The list of these points can be found in Appendix G, while some sets of points are re-proposed for use in specific patterns (points of the pericardium and heart, *shu* points of the back and lateral side of the bladder, *Ren Mai* and *Du Mai* points) in Chapter 13.
- A presentation of the structure of clinical cases, placed largely at the end of those chapters to which they relate more closely, see the initial methodological premises (Introduction).

CHAPTER 12 STIMULATION METHODS
The different modalities for the stimulation of points are grouped into one chapter that considers needle stimulation, classical moxibustion methods, cupping, plum-blossom needles, contemporary techniques such as head acupuncture, electrostimulation and the 'wrist–ankle' method.

CHAPTER 13 NOTES ON A NUMBER OF POINTS WITH DIVERSE APPLICATIONS
Here are collected and compared a number of points that belong to the same channel and that find a wider indication in the disorders of the *shen*.

CHAPTER 14 TREATMENT WITH EMOTIONS IN CLASSICAL TEXTS
Cases of 'treatment with emotions' borrowed from classical literature are detailed. The attention given by tradition to this particular type of therapy confirms an awareness of the fact that acupuncture and medical drugs are not the only therapeutic tools. On the

contrary, in cases where the psychic component is very strong, the intervention must share the same space of the particular illness.

CHAPTER 15 THE SPACE SHARED BY THE PATIENT AND THE ACUPUNCTURIST

These are notes on the space shared by the patient and the acupuncturist. The comments aim to draw attention to a number of resources and difficulties in the practice of acupuncture, to various traps and good features that characterise this type of medicine.

The dynamics of relationship, the location and time of the therapy, the concepts of support, empathy and neutrality are all considered as part of the process towards health. Attention to the therapeutic setting may in fact help to throw light on some dark areas and it can unravel some knots regarding we practitioners, who work here and now with a tool as delicate as acupuncture.

CHAPTER 16 NOTES ON EVENTS RELATED TO ACUPUNCTURE

The movement of the *qi* and emotions following the action of the needles can produce immediate psychic effects. These may sometimes go beyond our immediate intentions. I report here on some examples of this type of response and some comments on the quality of requests for help with which we must deal.

Principal Patterns of Fullness-*Shi*

10

Fullness is always pathological. An abundance of correct *qi* does not constitute *shi*, fullness or excess, which rather invariably implies stagnation, stasis, obstruction, accumulation or the presence of pathogens. In those patterns that touch on *shen* more closely, fullness is mainly composed of a stagnation or obstruction of *qi*, an excess of heat or fire that agitates blood and *shen*, an accumulation of phlegm which obscures the portals of the heart or, lastly, a stasis of blood which blocks its nourishment.

Obviously, there would be no illness if there were not some underlying form of deficiency, but the symptoms that make up these patterns are determined by the preponderance of fullness.

Fullness can range from a simple and frequent difficulty of *qi* in flowing smoothly, with its accompanying symptoms, a more significant or chronic constraint with more serious pathologies deriving from it, up to extreme patterns of phlegm-fire of *diankuang*, with violent manifestations.[1]

STAGNATION OF LIVER *QI*

Aetiology

A stagnation of emotion corresponds to a stagnation of *qi*: all emotions that linger for long periods act on *qi*, obstructing its physiological movement, and, vice versa: *qi* that has difficulty in circulating does not permit the free flow of emotions. Liver *qi* especially suffers from this constraint, given its main role of facilitating the circulation of *qi* generally.

Frustration, unfulfilled desires, repressed fury and resentment are all emotions that are associated with anger and which specifically strike the liver. It is

---

[1] See the explanatory notes in the Section III Introduction regarding the structuring of the two chapters on clinical work.

also true that fullness of liver *qi* generates the internal movement of anger and when it stagnates this manifests as a state of irritability.

Any constraint-*yu* (of *qi*, blood, pathogens and, in particular, the accumulation of heat-dampness) tends in any case to block the flow of *qi*. An emptiness of *yin* or blood, as well as an emptiness of *yang*, can also be causes of stagnation, since the liver's function of circulating *qi* is decreased.

For a more detailed discussion of constraint-*yu*, see Chapter 4.

Evolution

The stagnation of liver *qi* can evolve in various ways:

- transformation into fire which can then be transmitted to the stomach, lungs and/or heart, or which can consume the *yin* with a consequential ascending of liver *yang* and an eventual release of wind;
- attack of its controlled element earth causing an alteration of appetite, digestion and evacuation: one of the most common symptoms is a disharmony between liver and spleen;
- rebellion against its controlling element metal causing chest and respiratory disorders;
- transformation into knotted *qi* with the production of phlegm, which can obscure the portals of the heart;
- stasis of blood because the movement provided by *qi* is lacking.

Clinical Manifestations

- Irritability, unstable moods.
- Mental and physical tiredness, muscular tension, restless sleep.
- Sensations of oppression in the chest, frequent sighing, plum-stone *qi* (globus hystericus).
- Sensations of distension, fullness or pain in the lateral costal region.
- Stomach ailments, belching, acid regurgitation, nausea, appetite disorders.
- Borborygmi, abdominal swelling, altered bowel movements.
- PMS, dysmenorrhoea, excessive or scanty menstrual flow and/or irregular periods.
- Normal tongue with raised–contracted sides.
- Wiry pulse.

Clinical Notes

- The clinical picture can be quite varied, but we should hypothesise stagnation of *qi* when the main symptom is a type of indisposition leading to a 'too full' sensation, to something that is blocked, and manifests as a knot, distension, heaviness, or oppression.
- The correlation of the symptoms with emotionally charged situations or events is evident, at least at the onset of the disorder. In all cases, the relationship between emotions and symptoms should be thoroughly researched in the patient's history, because when the problem continues over time the emergence of symptoms often becomes more casual.
- It should be noted that emotional fatigue can derive from deeply conflictual situations, it can be tied to family relationships or to oppressive work conditions; however, it can also simply appear before an exam, a business meeting, or while waiting for a phone call.
- Stagnation corresponds to a form of internal pressure which can manifest itself in various ways: typical symptoms are a sensation of tightness in the chest for which deep breathing offers temporary relief, or the sensation of a weight in the stomach with poor digestion. A knot may also be felt in the throat, the abdomen is or is felt as swollen (the typical 'distension'-*zhang* of the Chinese texts), the breasts are tense premenstrually and the flow 'has difficulty in getting going'.
- Typically, the symptoms are alleviated when the *qi* moves and this movement can consist of physical exercise as well as deep breathing, belching, or emotional expression.
- Since nothing can pass or flow, everything becomes excessive: the patient may not tell us that he gets angry because by that term he means an explosion of rage, but he easily admits his extreme lack of patience for the words and the habits of the people with whom he has to deal; minor incidents very frequently irritate and bother him.
- With regard to emotions, the stagnation of *qi* can take various forms: there can be a difficulty in the flowing of emotions – which therefore knot and do not dissolve – or else a difficulty in bringing them to the surface, in expressing them, or even an inability to recognise them, or to perceive the corresponding movement of *qi*.
- We should remember that tiredness and fatigue can also depend on stagnation rather than on a deficiency: the patient often describes himself as 'depressed', sighs heavily, would sleep continuously but is not restored by sleeping, complains of a tiredness that is typically worse in the morning and not related to physical effort (which in a case of emptiness would instead aggravate the symptoms, since they exhaust an already deficient *qi*).
- Wood–earth disharmony is frequent, with liver invading the spleen and stomach and causing digestive ailments such as nausea, heartburn, abdominal swelling and bowel disorders. This syndrome often presents with strong

emotional components since 'anger is hard and organs are soft' and they are easily injured.

- Changes in appetite, which in Chinese clinical descriptions consist generally of a lack of appetite, often manifest in the Western world as increased appetite, which can lead to the total lack of control found in eating disorders. Digestion, in fact, increases the work of the stomach–earth, which in this way consumes the excess of liver–wood, providing temporary relief (and, unfortunately, damaging the spleen).
- Premenstrual symptoms of *qi* stagnation are frequent, and are often linked to a deficiency of blood; in fact, in the period between ovulation and menstruation, blood is sent from the heart to the uterus, but if blood is deficient it cannot nourish the liver properly.
- The localised lateral costal pain described in TCM texts often appears in patients as heaviness, or else we may find an area of higher sensitivity or stronger resistance.
- During palpation, we often find a paravertebral muscular contraction by palpating at the level of the back *shu* points between T7 and T10 or in the area around GB-21 *Jianjing*.
- People with *qi* stagnation generally appear to be unhappy and unsatisfied, they complain of never-ending frustrations, suffer from continuous disappointments; and never have what they desire. They often think that they do not receive what they deserve and perceive themselves to be victims of injustice, misapprehension, and mistreatment. It should be noted that lack of satisfaction is also characteristic of restless people who never find peace – materially or mentally – but this kind of agitation is already (in itself) a manifestation of heat or fire.
- It is important that some method of moving *qi* becomes part of daily habits, from a walk after dinner to *qigong* practice.
- The stagnation of liver *qi* easily gives rise to a *qi* disorder in which its normal physiological movement is reversed – that is, *qini*, or *qi* that counter-rises. We also use the term 'topsy-turvy' colloquially when we are in a bad mood.

Therapeutic Principles

Regulate liver *qi* and resolve stagnation.

Treatment Rationale

LI-4 *Hegu* + LIV-3 *Taichong*

This combination is particularly indicated for regulating the movement of *qi* in general – for example, in cases where there is obstruction that manifests with diffuse pain, depressed mood, tiredness or irritability.

In fact, LIV-3 *Taichong* and LI-4 *Hegu* make up the 'four gates' (*siguan*), a combination originally suggested for the pain of obstructive *bi* syndrome because it activates the circulation of all the *yangs*.[2] Their use was later extended to the treatment of various types of pain and other disorders caused by stagnation, because of their specific action in promoting *qi* and blood circulation.

LI-4 Hegu

Yuan point.

Principal actions

–Regulates defensive *qi* and clears the surface of invasion by external pathogens.
–Activates *qi* in its channel and relieves pain, with a particular influence on the head and its orifices.
–Activates *qi* and blood, with a specific action on the uterus.
–Tonifies *qi* and supports *yang*.

LIV-3 Taichong

Yuan and *shu* point, earth point.

Principal actions

–Circulates liver *qi* and pacifies *yang* and wind of liver.
–Nourishes the blood and *yin* of the liver and regulates the lower *jiao*.
–Activates the *qi* in its channel and eliminates heat in the head and eyes.

Notes

Being a *yuan* point, this influences all the functions of the liver and, even if it appears in the classical texts mainly in relation to wind symptoms such as convulsions, it is certainly one of the most frequently used points in contemporary literature and clinical practice for emotional disorders.

It is particularly indicated not only for *qi* stagnation – which can simultaneously be the cause and the result of emotional blockage – and ascending of *yang*, but also for empty *yin* followed by fear and uncertainty (which in turn can express themselves as anger–aggressiveness), or for a deficit of blood in which *hun* fluctuates.

SP-4 Gongsun + P-6 Neiguan

For regulating *qi*, mainly in the middle *jiao* and chest.

---

[2] 'For heat and cold with pain *bi* open the four gates.' In: Dou Hanqin, Biaoyoufu ('Ode to reveal the mysteries'), in which it is said further on that the six *yuan*-source points of the six *yang* channels emerge at the 'four gates'. We also note that LI-4 *Hegu* is one of the 11 original star points of Ma Danyang and that LIV-3 *Taichong* was added by Xu Feng.

In relation to the *Chong mai*, this combination treats cases of digestive, appetite and bowel problems deriving from a stagnation of *qi* or its counterflow (gastralgia, belching, acid regurgitation, nausea, borborygmi, abdominal swelling and alternating bowels).

In relation to the *Yin wei mai*, it treats 'heart pain', oppression in the chest, heartburn and stomach heaviness.

SP-4 Gongsun

Luo point, connecting point of the *Chong mai*.

Principal actions

–Reinforces the spleen and harmonises the middle *jiao*.
–Regulates *qi* and resolves dampness and phlegm.
–Regulates the *Chong mai* and calms the *shen*.
–Regulates the heart and chest and treats abdominal pain.

Notes

Being a *luo* point, it is very powerful in moving *qi* and – like the other *luo* points of the *yin* channels – has a specific effect on emotional disorders.

Earth governs the digestive process, transformation and transportation. The close relationship between spleen and stomach is manifested in the movement of *qi*, with stomach *qi* descending and spleen *qi* ascending. The *luo* point connects the two channels and therefore can be used for balancing the movements of *qi*.

Activation of *qi* is also fundamental in accumulations of dampness, which easily transform into phlegm-heat with obstruction of the portals of the heart and agitation of the *shen*.

P-6 Neiguan

Luo point, connecting point of the *Yin wei mai*.

Principal actions

–Regulates *qi* and opens the chest.
–Moves stagnation of *qi*, blood and phlegm.
–Regulates the stomach and moves down rebellious *qi*.
–Clears heat and calms the *shen*.

Notes

Being a *luo* point like SP-4, it acts on emotional disorders and strengthens its effect when used together.

The pericardium envelops the heart: the *luo* point regulates its rhythm in a physical sense, but also acts on the *shen*, calming and regulating it.

The pericardium channel originates in the chest and reaches the middle *jiao*; the *luo* point treats disharmonies between stomach and spleen and regulates the movement of stomach *qi*.

Being *jueyin* it is related to the liver: the *luo* point also acts on alterations of liver *qi* and the rib area.

GB-20 *Fengchi* + GB-34 *Yanglingquan*

These two points are both located on the *yang* channel of 'wind–wood–spring', the growth phase of *yang* within *yin* – in other words, *yang* at the maximum height of its potential.

This pair of points can be used especially when there are symptoms and signs at a muscular level (tension, contraction, pain) and in particular in the upper regions or in case of headache. It also treats symptoms of fullness or pain in the chest area, respiratory oppression and the constipation that are frequently part of the clinical picture.

GB-20 *Fengchi*

Meeting point of the gall bladder, *San Jiao*, *Yang Wei Mai* and *Yang Qiao Mai* channels.

Principal actions

–Extinguishes external and internal wind and moves *qi*.
–Eliminates liver fire and calms hyperactive *yang*.
–Clears the sense organs and activates *qi* in the channels.

Notes

This point moves *qi* when it is blocked in the upper regions, with symptoms such as pain, tension, rigidity or muscular contraction in the neck, shoulders and upper back.

It brings down the excess of *yang* from the upper regions, so it can be used in cases of empty *yin* with hyperactive *yang*, with symptoms like headache, dizziness and sensations of giddiness and eye disturbances.

GB-34 *Yanglingquan*[3]

Hui-meeting point of sinews, *he* point of the gall bladder.

---

[3] The *luo* point is particularly useful when the stagnation produces genital–urinary disorders (for example, cystitis or genital herpes lesions, whose insurgence is often related to emotional states) and in the classics it is suggested for the stagnation of *qi* in the throat *meiheqi*: 'Use LIV-5 *ligou* for worry and anxiety, a closing of the throat as though obstructed by a polyp'. In: Yang Jizhou, *Zhenjiu Dacheng* ('Great compendium of acupuncture and moxibustion').

Principal actions

–Regulates tendons and joints and harmonises *Shao Yang*.
–Activates *qi* in the channel and moves liver *qi*.
–Eliminates damp-heat from the liver and gall bladder.
–Pacifies hyperactive *yang* and calms wind.
–Supports the determination of the gall bladder.

Notes

This point moves down *qi* when it is blocked in the channel, with an immediate relaxing effect both on the muscles and breathing.

This draining and facilitating action on *qi* also improves bowel movements in cases of constipation.

Being a *he*-union point, it also acts directly on the viscera-*fu* and can be used in cases of empty *qi* in the gall bladder with symptoms of timidity, thought and apprehension.

Other points

• The points on *Renmai* and *Dumai* (see Chapter 13).

It is also important to identify signs of possible evolution and the following points can be useful in treating them.

To clear heat:

• P-7 *Daling*, LIV-2 *Xingjian*.

To tonify the spleen:

• SP-3 *Taibai*, ST-36 *Zusanli*, BL-20 *Pishu*, BL-21 *Weishu*.

To support the lung:

• LU-9 *Taiyuan*, LU-1 *Zhongfu*, BL-13 *Feishu*.

To resolve phlegm:

• P-5 *Jianshi*, ST-40 *Fenglong*.

To move blood:

• BL-17 *Geshu*, SP-10 *Xuehai*.

To promote diffusion and descent:

• LU-7 *Lieque*, KI-4 *Dazhong*.

To move *qi* and bring it down:

• GB-41 *Zulinqi*.

To tonify the liver:

- BL-18 *Ganshu*, BL-19 *Danshu*.

To clear damp-heat in the lower regions:

- LIV-5 *Ligou*.[4]

For disharmony between wood and earth:

- LIV-13 *Zhangmen*, LIV-14 *Qimen*.

To eliminate wind and resolve phlegm in the head:

- GB-13 *Benshen*.[5]

HEART FIRE

Aetiology

Stagnation of liver *qi* can very easily turn into depressive heat and fire, which can then travel to the heart and attack the stomach.

All other types of stasis, accumulation or obstruction that last over time also generate heat and fire, which can easily attack the *shen*.

All emotions (and lifestyles) can turn into fire and damage the heart when they become pathological.

Given its *yang* nature, heat tends to rise upwards, and even when it originates in the middle or lower *jiao* it tends to accumulate in the upper *jiao*, where it disturbs the *shen*.

For a discussion on heat and fire see also Chapter 5.

Evolution

Heat activates the *shen* too intensely and irregularly, exciting and depleting it.

It can transmit to the earth; through stomach fire (see the case of heart fire associated with stomach fire).

---

[4] Both harmonise spleen and liver and regulate the middle and lower *jiao*, but the *mu* point of spleen is more indicated if there is a prevailing weakness of the earth, whereas the *mu* point of the liver is more indicated if the invading movement has its origin in an excess of wood.

[5] This point, whose name *Benshen* recalls the title of Chapter 8 of the Lingshu, classically finds more indication in convulsive pathologies and losses of consciousness of a *yang* type. However, given its action on wind, phlegm and uprising of *yang*, it also treats less extreme cases such as vertigo, headache, and tension and pain in the neck and costal region.

It can transmit to its paired small intestine and through the *jueyin* to the bladder: besides irritability, thirst and signs of heat in the mouth, we find scanty urination with a burning sensation and dark or bloody urine.

It can dry out the liquids and produce phlegm-fire (see the problem of blockage due to phlegm-heat).

It can penetrate into the blood and agitate it, causing leaking from the vessels and bleeding.

Over time, it exhausts the *qi* and damages the *yin*, leading to a pattern of fire due to emptiness of *yin* (see the case of heart *yin* emptiness with empty fire).

It can dry out and consume blood, leading to patterns of empty or stagnant blood (see the pattern of blood stasis and emptiness of heart and bladder).

It can interfere with the regulation of the heart and uterus through the *Bao mai* connecting channel or by disturbing the *Renmai* and the *Chong mai*, with excessive or prolonged menstrual bleeding.

It can penetrate into the level of blood and result in febrile illnesses with confusion and disorders of the consciousness.

Clinical Manifestations

- Irascibility, restlessness, insomnia, and disturbed sleep.
- Palpitations, sensations of tightness or heat in the chest.
- Red face, sensations of heat, thirst or dry mouth, bitter taste, tongue irritations.
- Constipation, dark urine.
- Dermatological manifestations with redness, itching, ulceration.
- Haemorrhages, excessive menstrual flow or persistent spotting.
- Elongated tongue or with a sharp point; long and deep longitudinal cracks; red (fire) or dark red (heat in the blood) colour; red and swollen edges (liver fire), red tip (heart fire); the presence of red spots; a coating that is yellow and greasy (phlegm), dry (deficit of liquids) or almost black (very serious consumption of liquids by fire).
- Full, rapid pulse; depending on the accompanying characteristics it can also be long, slippery, wiry or tight; in very serious cases it can be urgent, hurried, flooding, empty or hidden.

Clinical Notes

- Fire is produced more easily in constitutions with a tendency to heat.
- The typical case is a 'plethoric' patient; but heart fire is not always so evident. It is often a case of constrained-*yu* fire or suffocated-*fou* fire and it can be suggested by even just a few symptoms and signs like a red-tipped tongue.

- Patterns of empty fire are very frequent.
- The irritability of *qi* stagnation can easily be transformed into the irascibility of fire. The upward rising *qi* that blazes with strength can manifest itself as rage, but also as diffuse restlessness, causing impatience, lack of tranquillity and a tendency to be bored and at the same time irritated (characteristics which are not always readily evident).
- It is particularly important to avoid foods of a hot nature, coffee and alcohol (which instead are often consumed as a form of 'self-therapy').

Therapeutic Principles

Eliminate fire, resolve stagnation, and calm the *shen*.

Treatment Rationale

HE-8 *Shaofu* (or P-7 *Daling*) + KI-3 *Taixi*

This combination of points has an important action on the heart–fire kidney–water axis.

It is fundamental to nourish water, because fire can derive from its deficiency, or the fire itself can consume the *yin*, which therefore needs to be nourished, both in the case of its deficiency and as a preventative measure.

The choice of P-7 *Daling* depends on the eventual involvement of the stomach with conversely rising *qi* or the presence of fire. It is also a first choice when there is heat in the blood or when desiring to intervene further in cases of liver stagnation.

HE-8 *Shaofu*

Ying point, fire point

Principal actions

–Eliminates heart and small intestine fire.
–Regulates heart *qi* and calms the *shen*.
–Activates *qi* in the channels.

Notes

It shares the ability to clear heat in the *zangfu* and channels with the other stream-*ying* points.

Its use is not limited to a full type of heat, since it also regulates heart *qi* both in cases of stagnation and in cases of emptiness; it may be used both for fire deriving from obstruction of liver *qi* and also for empty fire.

It possesses a strong action with respect to agitation in all of its expressions (such as mental restlessness, disturbed sleep, emotional hyperactivity, palpitations) and should be kept in mind in many pathologies with somatic expressions but strong psychological components, where the symptoms reveal heat related to states of emotional agitation, for example:

- disorders in urination or of the eternal genitals (fire transmits from the heart to its paired small intestine and through the *Tai yang* to the bladder, for example in recurring cystitis);
- dermatological pathologies (fire that penetrates the blood and manifests on the skin with pruritis sans materia, eczema, rash-like or psoriasis type lesions);
- alterations in menstrual flow (fire that disturbs the *Renmai* and *Chong mai* and agitates the blood, with excessively heavy menstruation or persistent spotting).

P-7 Daling

Shu and *yuan* point, earth point, sedation point.

Principal actions

–Eliminates heart fire and clears the heat in the blood.
–Opens the chest and regulates the stomach.

Notes

Particularly indicated when *qi* rises conversely or fire attacks the stomach. Being *jueyin* it acts on stagnation of the liver (constriction of emotions that transforms into fire).

KI-3 Taixi

Yuan and *shu* point, earth point.

Principal actions

–Nourishes kidney *yin* and drains empty fire.
–Anchors the *qi* down and supports the *jing*.
–Tonifies kidney *yang* and controls the lower orifices.

Notes

To grasp the importance of the diverse aspects of KI-3 *Taixi* we refer the reader to the works of Zhang Shijie (see Chapter 21), who was also called 'Zhang Taixi' specifically for his knowledge and breadth of use of this point.

In any case, we note that KI-3 *Taixi* acts on the channel in its external and internal pathways (*Dumai*, *Renmai*, kidney, bladder, liver, diaphragm, lung, heart, throat and tongue).

As a *yuan*-source point of the kidney it tonifies both its roots, *yin* and *yang*; it nourishes the *yin* of the essence-*jing* and at the same time warms the fire of the *mingmen*.

The action on water also consists of:

- moistening dryness;
- controlling the opening and closing of the lower orifices;
- treating marrow–brain, ears–hearing, bones–teeth;
- nourishing liver *yin*, organ–child, with which it shares the source;
- pacifying urgent uprising of the *Chong mai*.

LIVER FIRE AND STOMACH FIRE

Heart fire is very often associated with liver fire and stomach fire.

Liver Fire

- Often derives from the obstruction and stagnation of *qi* (irritability, indisposition or pain in the lateral costal region, sensations of oppression).
- Disturbs the heart, *shen* and blood (palpitations, restlessness, insomnia).
- Blazes upward (*Shao yang* headaches, reddened eyes, dizziness, tinnitus).
- Invades the stomach transversely (acid reflux, burning or 'empty stomach' sensation).
- Rebels against the lung (chest oppression, dry cough).

LIV-2 Xingjian

Ying point, fire point, sedation point. Drains liver fire and regulates *qi*, subdues liver *yang* and extinguishes wind.

Gall Bladder Points from GB-1 Tongziliao to GB-20 Fengchi

The higher points on the gall bladder channel act on the upward movement of *yang* and on heat. They are chosen according to the location of the symptoms.

- Often results from liver fire transversely invading the stomach or from heart fire that directly travels to the stomach.
- Is easily increased by foods that produce toxic heat.
- Rises and manifests through symptoms and signs on the level of the upper tract of the *Yang ming* channel (irritation or ulceration of the oral cavity, abscesses or inflammations of the gums, temporal headaches).
- Produces heat in the viscera (halitosis, stomach or heartburn, acid reflux, thirst for cold drinks, frequent or excessive appetite, vomiting after eating, constipation).

ST-44 Neitung

Ying point and water point. Clears the heat in the stomach channel, especially in the upper regions and regulates stomach *qi*. It is a first choice if channel signs such as gingivitis, dental abscesses and *Yang ming* headaches continue.

ST-21 Liangmen

Eliminates stomach heat and favours the descent of conversely rising *qi*. It is a first choice if the signs and symptoms mostly involve the stomach in its role as one of the viscera, with *qi* that rises conversely and fire that disturbs digestion.

Notes

In the classic description of the pathologies of the stomach channel we find many 'psychiatric' signs and symptoms, a large number of which coincide with the description of *kuang*, which is also cited among the illnesses of the stomach channels.[6]

- when the illness breaks out one cannot stand the sight of people and the light of fire;
- the sick person cannot stand the sound of beating on wood and if he hears it he is frightened;
- the heart wants to move and jump;
- the sick person prefers to be alone in a house with shuttered windows and doors;
- when the illness becomes severe the sick person wants to climb high and sing, strip off his clothing and run back and forth.

---

[6] *Lingshu*, chapter 10.

Other Points

- Points on the *Renmai* and *Dumai* (see Chapter 13).

  It is also important to treat concomitant situations.
  To nourish *yin* and liquids:

- SP-6 *Saninjiao*, HE-6 *Yinxi*, KI-6 *Zhaohai*.

  To drain fire in the *Tai Yang*:

- SI-3 *Houxi*, SI-7 *Zhizheng*, Ren-3 *Zhongji*, BL-40 *Weizhong*.

  To resolve phlegm:

- P-5 *Jianshi*, ST-40 *Fenglong*.

  To clear heat in the blood:

- BL-17 *Geshu*, SP-10 *Xuehai*, SP-6 *Sanyinjiao*.

  To nourish the heart:

- BL-15 *Xinshu*, BL-44 *Shentang*, HE-7 *Shenmen*.

OBSTRUCTION BY PHLEGM-*TAN*

Aetiology

Phlegm is always pathological and can be produced in the following situations:

- The spleen does not properly perform its functions of transporting and transforming, for emotional reasons (persistent excess of thoughts, worry and sadness), for dietary reasons (improper diet in both quantity and quality), for congenital reasons (deficiency of spleen *qi*), or because it has been invaded by the liver, etc.
- The lung does not perform its function of diffusion and descending or the function of regulating the water pathway.
- The stagnation of *qi* slows down the circulation of liquids.
- Heat or fire, whether full or empty, dries out the liquids (phlegm is also called 'a substantial part of fire' and fire is also called 'a non-substantial part of phlegm').
- Constrained-*yu qi* stagnates-*zhi*, knots-*jie*, accumulates-*chu* and condenses-*ning* into phlegm.

Evolution

- The stagnation of phlegm produces heat, with patterns of phlegm-fire.
- Phlegm can establish itself in any *zangfu*, channel or region of the body.
- The obscuring of the portals of the heart causes more or less serious disorders of the conscience, with tendencies towards psychic withdrawal if associated with cold or more aggressive expressions if associated with heat.

Clinical Manifestations

Called 'with form' (*youxing*) or 'without form' *(wuxing)* because they can be more or less 'substantial', they involve a range of pathologies from mucus in the respiratory tract to obscuring of the portals of the heart.

They can establish themselves in any organ, in the channels, and in all the areas of the body (head, throat, chest, abdomen, limbs) with different symptoms and signs according to the prevalent location:

- sleepiness, insomnia;
- dizziness, headaches, visual disorders, disturbances of balance;
- difficulty in concentrating, poor memory, heaviness in the head, or confusion;
- absence of communication, unreactivity, apathy, psychotic withdrawal;
- convulsive crises, loss of consciousness (if internal wind is also produced);
- sensations of an extraneous body in the throat (*meiheqi);*
- palpitations, feelings of oppression in the chest, mucus in the respiratory tract, sighing;
- stomach heaviness, nausea, digestive difficulties, abdominal swelling;
- sensations of heaviness and swelling, generalised pain, joint pain with deformation;
- numbness, hyperesthesia, partial paralysis;
- lipoma, lymph node enlargement, thyroid nodules;
- gall bladder or kidney stones;
- tongue with greasy yellow coating;
- slippery pulse; depending on the accompanying characteristics, it can also be wiry or short, or in more serious cases knotted.

Phlegm fire:

- interrupted sleep, disturbed by many dreams and nightmares;
- red face, constipation, dark urine;
- agitation, mental confusion (in conversation, action and thought), manic crises, anomalous or violent behaviour, rapid mood swings ('laughter and

crying'), delirium or hallucinations, convulsive crises, loss of consciousness;
- tongue with a greasy yellow coating (dark and dry, especially in the longitudinal crack if fire prevails strongly) swollen tip; presence of the other possible signs of fire;
- rapid, full, slippery pulse; in more serious cases it can also be hurried.

Notes

- Phlegm is a thick, turbid, sticky, heavy substance; characterised by great inertia, it is difficult to eliminate.
- In the clinic it can be perceived as a type of fogginess: the patient himself usually refers to a sensation of physical dizziness or mental fatigue. In other cases, the doctor can reveal a form of dullness not only in the characteristics of the symptoms referred, but also in the patient's way of moving or speaking or in the quality of the pulses.
- When phlegm produces fire the element of agitation is added: in these cases the compromising of the consciousness is manifested with uncontrollable behaviour or delirious conversation and it is characterised by confusion, violence and suddenness. These syndromes can overlap with the syndrome that is classically described as *kuang*.
- Phlegm and dampness have characteristics that overlap in part, but they also have substantial differences. Phlegm, which is always pathological, is the origin of more complex conditions; it produces masses of various dimensions and types, which tend to obstruct the *luo* and obscure the portals of the heart. It is easily transformed into wind and fire; its specific symptoms are dullness and dizziness. Dampness, on the other hand, tends to accumulate in the lower regions, it is more diffuse, does not produce delimited masses and its characteristic signs are heaviness and torpor.
- We should also note that phlegm alone does not produce pain, whereas *qi* or blood stagnation do.

Therapeutic Principles

Resolve phlegm, tonify spleen *qi*, activate *qi*, clear the portals of the heart, calm the *shen* and clear heat if it is present.

Treatment Rationale

P-5 *Jianshi* + ST-40 *Fenglong*

P-5 *Jianshi*

Jing point and metal point.

Principal actions

–Resolves phlegm and clears the portals of the heart.
–Drains fire and calms the *shen*.
–Activates *qi* and opens the chest.
–Regulates *qi* in the upper, middle and lower *jiao*.

Notes

This is one of the main points for treating phlegm, especially when it obscures the portals of the heart. It also removes *qi* stagnation at any level.

ST-40 *Fenglong*

Luo point.

Principal actions

–Resolves phlegm and eliminates dampness.
–Clears the portals of the heart and calms the *shen*.
–Activates chest *qi* and activates *qi* in the channel.

Notes

We can use this point for any type of phlegm accumulation at any level and in particular when it accumulates in the portals of the heart or in the head, throat and chest.

Being a *luo* point it performs an important regulating action on the stomach–spleen pair ('the origin of phlegm'), it acts on the *qi* of the *luo* channel (which reaches the throat) and on the main channel (which meets *Dumai* at Du-24 *Shenting* and at Du-26 *Renzhong*).

It is specifically indicated in various classical texts for the treatment of *diankuang* syndromes.

Other Points

- *Renmai* and *Dumai* points (see Chapter 13).
  It is also important to treat the causes of the formation of phlegm.

To activate *qi*:

- LI-4 *Hegu*, LIV-3 *Taichong*, GB-34 *Yanglingquan*, P-6 *Neiguan*.

  To tonify the spleen:

- SP-3 *Taibai*, ST-36 *Zusanli*, BL-20 *Pishi*, BL-21 *Weishu*.

  To reinforce the lung:

- LU-9 *Taiyuan*, LU-1 *Zhongfu*, BL-13 *Feishu*.

  To promote the diffusion and descent of *qi*:

- LU-7 *Lieque*, KI-4 *Dazhong*.

STASIS OF BLOOD-*XUE*

Aetiology

This can derive from emotional causes, generally following a stagnation of *qi*, heat that dries out the blood or an exhaustion of *qi*. It is, in essence, a pattern that accompanies other pathological alterations when they persist over time:

- *qi* stagnation, which therefore does not move the blood;
- internal heat, which condenses, dries and arrests the blood;
- *qi* and *yang* emptiness, which in turn causes deficient movement;
- emptiness of blood (also due to haemorrhage), which is then insufficient for a proper circulation;
- emptiness of *yin*, due to which there are insufficient liquids to promote a proper flow;
- internal cold, which 'freezes' the blood and slows down the circulation;
- physical trauma, which directly cause local stagnation.

Development

- Haemorrhages (of the intermittent and dark type, whereas those due to heat are more sudden and abundant), because stasis blocks blood, which accumulates and in the end is forced out of the vessels or, because stasis produces heat, which moves the blood in a disorderly fashion.
- Blood emptiness, since the stasis impedes the production of new blood.
- Heat in the blood, given that every accumulation that persists over time leads to constricted heat.
- *Qi* emptiness, since it lacks nourishment (blood is the mother of *qi*).

Clinical Manifestations

- Insomnia and poor memory, restlessness, mood swings, emotional frailty, continuous states of panic, up to and including *diankuang* syndromes.
- Palpitations, tightness of the chest and heart pain, which can rise to the throat or radiate to the upper back.
- Worsening of symptoms during the night (agitation, palpitations, headache, or typical restless legs syndrome).
- Dry mouth, dark complexion.
- Purple, red-violet (heat), or pale blue (deficient) tongue, spots, congested sublingual vessels.
- Rough pulse; depending on the accompanying features it can also be short or, in more serious cases, hurried or knotted.

The general signs of blood stasis are fixed, dull or stabbing pain, which generally worsens with pressure, painful menstruation with dark blood and clots or amenorrhea, fixed masses, numbness, haemorrhoids, varicose vessels, haemangioma, red spots or skin spots, dark complexion, cyanotic lips and nails, rough skin, purple tongue, with red spots, a pulse with 'complicated' qualities.

Clinical Notes

- Even if pain is a cardinal sign of blood stasis, the classics outline many different signs and precisely describe the relationship between illnesses of the psyche and blood stasis.
- A patient with blood stasis has symptoms that worsen at night (for example, palpitations), a diffuse restlessness, cannot find peace, cries often and sobs for apparently banal reasons; is emotionally unstable and has frequent mood swings; complains of a poor memory, 'forgets everything', but in general it is actually a question of lack of attention; finds himself in a sort of continuous state of panic as a result of which he is frightened and jumps at sudden sounds. In Chinese texts these symptoms of blood stasis are defined as: agitation and restlessness (*fanzao*), continuous crying, sudden crying, laughter and crying, amnesia, starting, easily frightened.
- Blood stasis easily produces heat, which increases the restlessness and impatience, gives origin to a sensation of internal heat, dries the liquids (dry mouth and thirst, dark urine, dry stool, yellow tongue coating), agitates the blood further facilitating bleeding (haematosis, blood in the sputum, faeces or urine, excessive menstruation or uterine bleeding, easy bruises or broken small vessels), often manifests on the skin (eczema or erythematic lesions) and confuses the *shen* (confusion, delirium, loss of consciousness).

- The illness called 'lantern sickness' in Chinese, *denglong bing*, is specific to the internal heat caused by blood stasis with a cool body on the outside, but with heat internally, diffuse impatience and irritability in people with a normally calm character.[7]

Therapeutic Principles

Move the blood, activate the *qi* and calm the *shen*.

Treatment Rationale

P-4 *Ximen* + BL-17 *Geshu*

This pair of points is indicated particularly when the compromising mostly involves the *shen* and the upper *jiao* or where there is acute heat in the blood.

P-4 *Ximen*

Xi point.

Principal actions

–Moves and cools the blood.
–Calms the *shen* and clears heat in acute fever.
–Regulates rebellious stomach and lung *qi* with diaphragmatic spasms.

Notes

Being a *xi* point it resolves acute pain and since it is on a *yin* channel it is specifically applicable in blood disorders. It removes blood stasis so the blood can adequately nourish the heart, and the *shen* has a place to reside.

Furthermore, its ability to cool the blood makes it particularly indicated in cases of agitation of the *shen* in acute febrile illnesses when the heat has penetrated to the level of the blood and nourishment (the *xi* point of the heart channel is instead more indicated in empty heat, to nourish the *yin* and liquids).

BL-17 *Geshu*

Shu point of the diaphragm, *hui*-meeting point of *xue*.

---

[7] Wang Qingren's description is cited and discussed in Chapter 5 on heat and fire.

Principal actions

–Moves and cools the blood.
–Nourishes and regulates the blood.
–Regulates the diaphragm and brings down counterflowing *qi* of the lung and stomach.

Notes

Given its wide range of actions on all types of blood pathologies (stasis, heat or deficiency), this point is indicated both when the blood stasis directly disturbs the *shen* and also when it agitates it through the production of heat.

SP-10 *Xuehi* + SP-6 *Sanyinjiao*

These two spleen points are a first choice when the signs manifest more on a somatic level with bleeding, gynaecological disorders, or dermatological pathologies.

SP-10 *Xuehai*

Principal actions

–Moves and cools blood.
–Regulates menstruation and benefits the skin.

Notes

Cools the blood and activates its circulation, dispersing stasis.

It is indicated in those very frequent conditions where the emotions produce a stasis of blood and an accumulation of heat with manifestations of a gynae-cological nature, haemorrhages of the gastrointestinal tract because the heat forces the blood out of its vessels or dermatological manifestations due to heat in the blood or stasis with blood emptiness.

The resolution of the stasis also permits the production of new blood; in order to nourish the blood it has to be moved.

SP-6 *Sanyinjiao*

Meeting point of the three *yin* channels of the leg.

Principal actions

–Nourishes *yin* and blood and tonifies *qi*.
–Calms the *shen* and regulates liver *qi*.
–Tonifies the middle *jiao* and resolves dampness.
–Moves and cools blood.

Notes

In combination with SP-10 it reinforces the action of cooling and moving the blood. For the other functions, see the discussion regarding deficiency syndromes in Chapter 11.

Other Points

- The points on *Renmai* and *Dumai* (see Chapter 13).

    It is important to treat the causes of blood stasis and prevent its pathological developments.
    To activate *qi*:

- LI-4 *Hegu*, LIV-3 *Taichong*, GB-34 *Yanglingquan*, P-6 *Neiguan*.

    To clear heat:

- P-7 *Daling*, LIV-2 *Xingjian*.

    To tonify *qi* and *yang* and eliminate internal cold:

- ST-36 *Zusanli*, BL-23 *Shenshu*.

    To nourish blood and *yin*:

- SP-6 *Sanyinjiao*, BL-17 *Geshu*, BL-18 *Ganshu*, BL-20 *Pishu*.

    To tonify *qi* and the heart:

- BL-15 *Xinshu*, BL-44 *Shentang*, HE-7 *Shenmen*.

Case Study 10.1

JAMS[8]

A 40-year-old female graphic artist turns to acupuncture for a fibromyoma that she would like to treat without repeating surgery, which she had 4 years previously.

The procession of symptoms consists of pelvic pain, a sensation of swelling and heaviness and frequent urination, sometimes followed by pain. The patient also complains of digestive troubles with light nausea, frequent diarrhoea or incompletely formed stools. She also suffers from a heavy sensation in the legs.

---

[8] In this respect, see also the discussion in Chapter 12 on stimulation methods and compare with cases 9.4 and 16.2.

Her premenstrual period is marked by extreme abdominal distension, tension in the breasts, irritability and sadness, but the menstrual flow resolves all sensations of swelling and brings a great sense of wellbeing. In the past the patient has also suffered from leucorrhoea.

She has been taking oestro-progesterones during the past few months; however, her period was regular even before that.

The tongue is slightly swollen and tooth marked with scalloped edges, the tongue coating is thin and yellow, the sublingual zone has notably shiny yellow mucus at the level of the frenula and in particular the carunculus. The pulse is deep and slippery.

Diagnosis
Stagnation of liver *qi*, damp-heat from emptiness of spleen *qi*.

Therapeutic principles
Activate liver *qi* and regulate *Daimai*, clear damp-heat and strengthen the spleen.

Treatment
Fifteen treatments, initially more frequently and then weekly, for a total of 4 months, including a break of 18 days.

The choice was mainly between the following points:

- Ren-4 *Guanyuan*: to regulate the uterus and reinforce *yuanqi*;
- P-6 *Neiguan*: to regulate the *qi* and calm the *shen*;
- LIV-3 *Taichong* and LI-4 *Hegu*, the 'four gates': to activate and regulate the *qi*. In particular, LI-4 *Hegu* activates the *qi* and has a specific action on the uterus, while LIV-3 *Taichong* moves *qi* and regulates the lower *jiao*;
- Ren-12 *Zhongwan*, SP-3 *Taibai*, SP-6 *Sanyinjiao*, SP-9 *Yinlingquan*, ST-25 *Tianshu*, BL-20 *Pishu* and BL-21 *Weishu*: to tonify the spleen and eliminate dampness;
- GB-41 *Zulinqi* and SJ-5 *Waiguan*: confluent points of the *Daimai* and points which activate *qi* strongly;
- GB-27 *Wushu* and GB-28 *Weidao*: points of the *Daimai* that act on localised stagnation;
- LIV-13 *Zhangmen*: the area from which *Daimai* originates and the *mu* point of the spleen, which reinforces the spleen, regulates liver *qi* and moves abdominal *qi*.

During the third appointment I also used electrostimulation (dense-disperse current at low intensity) on: Ren-4 *Guanyuan* and ST-29 *Guilai* on the left, ST-29 *Guilai* and GB-28 *Weidao* on the right.

During the first month the sensation of heaviness and pain after urination regresses and the pelvic pains are more moderate; bowels remains irregular with soft stools or at times yellow, liquid and 'hot' stools.

After 2 months, during the ninth treatment, the patient has me note that her fingernails are less tormented. She says that she feels definitely better, so much so that we decide on an overall decrease in the frequency of the treatments, also due to the fact that external causes dictate an interruption of 18 days in any case.

When treatments begin once more the patient is agitated, having again had abdominal pain, saying that 'things are not going well, I feel weak in my body and mind, I get dizzy, my vision gets blurred, I am depressed, I have a sensation of having no consistency, of losing myself, of not feeling myself', owing to which we return to weekly treatments for the last month before her summer holiday.

During this month the pelvic pains completely disappear while a swollen sensation sometimes remains, but no longer that of being 'soft in the belly', she is not excessively tired considering the extremely hot-damp climate and the size of the preholiday workload and the last menstruations were not preceded by important mood swings. The patient no longer chews her nails and says that she is less paralysed when faced with situations that previously created great agitation.

She takes into consideration the possibility of starting to practise *qigong*.

The gynaecologist delays her scheduled ultrasound test because his examination reveals that the situation has not changed.

The tongue, however, is still a little pale and tooth marked, the tongue coating is thin but still tends to yellowness and a certain slipperiness is still present in the pulse.

Comments

The stagnation of *qi* is quite evident in this case in the constraints and jams that are manifested at various levels. The symptomatology is characteristically correlated with the menstrual cycle and includes: the various sensations of swelling, distension and pain; the irritability and mood swings; the tension in the tongue due to which the edges are raised; the solid masses at a gynaecological level where the stagnation also produces stasis of blood.

Stagnation also produces depressive/internal heat which then agitates the *shen*, colours the tongue coating, warms the lower *jiao*, combining with the dampness and producing disorders in bowel movements and urination.

Dampness is an important part of the picture: it derives from the weakness of spleen *qi*, which does not carry out its transforming and transporting functions and manifests higher up with dizziness and blurry vision, in the central region with digestive difficulties, abdominal swelling, sensations of heaviness and fatigue in the four limbs and in the lower regions with heaviness in the legs.

The tongue is swollen and tooth marked because the excess of *yin* renders it too soft, while the pulse is slippery because it is full of heavy matter.

The treatment was also addressed to a regulation of the *Daimai* along its pathway given its influence on the waist area and the genital–urinary system, and its function of harmonising the liver and gall bladder in excess patterns and of clearing damp-heat in the lower part of the body and, finally, for its action on the circulation of stomach *qi* and of all the channels in the legs.

Given the particular sensitivity of the patient, it was important in this case to differentiate between the act of inserting the needle and that of stimulating the *qi*. Especially during the first two treatments, these two operations were kept distinctly separate: I first inserted all of the needles with extreme delicacy and only later did I seek to reach *qi* and finally only after receiving her permission did I manipulate it.

In this case, the signs and symptoms point to a disorder in which somatic and psychological elements intermingle. In a similar fashion to what happens in a Chinese clinic, I did not investigate in a particularly detailed way on how, when and why there were emotional alterations and confusion of the *shen*. The energetic diagnosis was sufficiently clear to define the therapeutic principles and to devise a treatment that would resolve the coarser symptomatology.

The initial request involved a problem of a physical order, whereas the therapeutic response had also later included psychic and emotional aspects. The patient, in fact, commented: 'When I come here I notice that I am calmer, things seem more possible to overcome, whereas generally I get agitated; it is stronger than me, even if they are things that I like to do, I always feel like there is not enough time and it immediately affects me physically'.

It is difficult to theorise on how long this new alignment will last; the hope is that the resources mobilised will also permit the patient to start on a path in which she assumes a more active role in her own health.

At times acupuncture makes only small changes in a pathogenic system, but this restructuring and rebalancing on a different level enables the patient to use her own resources in a better way. For example, relieving the symptoms also means breaking the vicious, self-feeding cycle of suffering, and realigning her energetic system implies the possibility that the patient perceives herself as different; this concrete experience favours her attempt to try and effect changes.

Follow-up

Six months later the ultrasound results can be added to the previous ones; the patient has had many family problems without, however, being overwhelmed. Physically things aren't going poorly, but she would like to begin acupuncture again because 'it made me feel good, relaxed and calm'.

Case Study 10.2

The Pink-Skinned Woman With Blue Hair

Two women enter the office together; one has an interesting, but tired and wrinkled face and the other has light coloured eyes, smooth, pink skin, and light blue-tinted hair. The latter is the mother of the former, sent to me by her regular doctor due to a severe migraine. She also suffers from a bipolar mood disorder, with alternating periods of depression and euphoria.

The woman is 85 years old and mentions that the headache has been with her from the age of 18 when she had her first pregnancy and that the first episode of depression coincided with her second pregnancy and the death of her mother. The headache had worsened over the past few months, with bilateral, continuous pain that generally started around dawn, was located in the supraorbital and temporal areas, with no symptoms or signs in the eyes, and was accompanied by light nausea that was relieved by eating.

The daughter describes her mother's depression as being characterised by agitation, crying and sudden fear; the patient complains mostly of the lack of desire to go out or read, a sensation of dulling of her intelligence, the lack of memory and concentration. The manic or hypomanic manifestations that determine the bipolarity are less clear. Both mother and daughter agree that the headache and periods of depression are related.

Appetite and digestion are good; bowel movements and urination are regular. The patient suffers from hypertension that is under medical control and takes both tranquillisers and antidepressants.

The patient's tongue does not present particular characteristics except for a slight paleness around the edges; her pulse is deep and with a decidedly wiry characteristic. Her attitude is very courteous, but she is nevertheless a determined and volatile character and unquestionably present are elements of inflexibility and a diffuse impatience that is ready to transform itself into anger. Together with sincere gratitude a contentious and coercive temperament are also well perceivable.

Diagnosis
Constraint of *qi* and converse rising of *qi* in the *Shao yang*, and phlegm that obscures the portals of the heart.

Therapeutic principles
Regulate liver *qi* and *qi* in the *Shao yang,* and, resolve phlegm.

Treatment
Twice a week for 1 month, weekly for another month and subsequently once every 2 weeks.

In general, the following points were maintained:
- GB-20 *Fengchi*, LI-4 *Hegu*, LIV-3 *Taichong*, GB-34 *Yanglingquan*;
- GB-20 *Fengchi* and GB-34 *Yanglingquan* to extinguish wind, move *qi* and bring down liver *qi*; LI-4 *Hegu* and LIV-3 *Taichong* ('the four gates') to move the *qi*.

Furthermore, the following points were alternated:
- GB-14 *Yangbai*
  and
- GB-13 *Benshen* (at times, using a light bleeding);
- GB-14 *Yangbai* and GB-13 *Benshen* to act upon the excess of *yang* above and on the phlegm in the portals of the heart.

In the summer the therapy is interrupted for almost 4 months and when the patient returns at the end of September she states that she felt fine until 2 weeks earlier. Treatment is restarted: during the first month the mood is depressed and agitated and the episodes of headache return, then the situation calms down and afterwards two treatments a month are basically sufficient to keep the mood stable and to reduce the headaches to sporadic episodes.

The pharmaceutical treatment remains unvaried, but it seems to have an increased effect, especially being more reliable in its therapeutic effect.

Comments

Even though the case is aimed essentially at the resolution of the symptomatology of the headaches rather than the mental disorder, it is cited here because it offers a number of points for reflection.

A first point refers specifically to the fact that the treatment appears to have had an influence on the course of the mental pathology, improving the efficacy of the drugs. The connection between the manifestations of pain and the psychological ones was in this case evident both to the patient and to her family: even if it is theoretically obvious that a regulation of *qi* has an influence on a variety of symptoms, in this case the response to therapy constitutes an interesting confirmation. The mood improved even though the therapy was aimed at curing the headaches, both because this was the request of the patient and also because a treatment designed for chronic bipolar depression would have required a totally different therapeutic approach.

A second consideration is that of the effect that an intervention of regulation of *qi* also has on more residual aspects like phlegm, which obscures the portals of the heart. In this case, one can reasonably trace the cause of the initial alteration to a stagnation of *qi*, while the present manifestations are attributable to a disordered movement of *qi* with sudden converse rising and a by now consistent accumulation of phlegm, which obscures the portals of the heart. In this patient, regulating the *qi* movement was considered a priority since the patient's constitutional tendency or old constraints were the origin of a disruption of normal circulation causing sudden disorder and violent explosions. Treatment was therefore not addressed directly to the phlegm, even though this was kept under consideration, for example, in the choice of points on the head. Furthermore, in order to resolve blocked phlegm you must start by moving *qi*.[9]

A third interesting aspect of this case is that there is not necessarily a correlation between advanced age and a pattern of emptiness of the kidney. Notwithstanding her 85 years and a few signs of emptiness such as the pale edges of her tongue, the main symptoms of this patient nevertheless suggested fullness, with constraint and fire.

In the aged there is a physiological consumption of *qi*, blood and *jing*, but this does not necessarily imply a priority to tonify the kidney. Cases in which it is necessary to move the blood in order to facilitate the production of new blood are frequent. Furthermore, it often happens that one must focus the treatment on modifying an underlying pathological situation that has accompanied the patient throughout life.

A number of cautions remain obvious: stimulation cannot be excessive, one should favour points that activate *qi* rather than disperse it, the actions taken to

---

[9] See also in this respect the discussion on constraint-*yu* and phlegm-*tan* in Chapter 4. Also compare with the therapeutic methods of Julian Scott, who in children recommends not addressing action initially to the phlegm, but first clearing heat, fullness and accumulation, or tonifying in cases of emptiness.

extinguish wind and drain fire should not be too violent, and an attempt to nourish should in any case begin.

Follow-up

After an interval of one and a half years, I call the patient to extend holiday wishes and hear how she is doing: she tells me that she is fine, although she does have a slight lack of memory, but that when one is 88 years old these things happen. She no longer has headaches, only a hint of one sometimes in the evening, but she does not have to take any medication for it. She asks me if she should come in for some treatments. Her mood also seems good; since our previous treatments one antidepressant pill in the morning has been sufficient to keep her stable. 'Great', I think, 'Age does not always worsen the situation'.

Case Study 10.3

The Very Restless Friend

I was already acquainted with this 50-year-old patient through mutual friends and also because I had already treated him for a recurring case of lumbar sciatica. He worked in a factory with duties and hours that were often physically onerous and over the last 4 years the reappearance of pain had required a number of treatments on several occasions.

The same *Shao yang* type of lumbago had been treated a month previously with a cycle of three treatments. On those occasions I had noted the restlessness that accompanied the patient, but without noting any signs that were different to previous occasions I had treated him.

Three weeks later the patient returns much thinner and in a state of excitation so strong that he appears not even to hear what I am saying. His manner of speech, which was normally quite intense and strong, this time is convulsed, his gaze is disturbed and his gestures excited. Everything he speaks about – regarding both his work and his family – has a decisively persecutory tone; he continuously draws small designs relating to events and his moods which he shows me and also leaves for his wife; he arrives at appointments in hours nowhere near the agreed times; he engages in building projects for which he continuously purchases expensive materials.

The patient is a very intelligent, cultured and active person; however, I am presently struck by his hurried speech, without pause, with no space for reply, with his mind desperately returning to the same subjects. He is mainly anguished about lack of recognition and respect in the job, but possibly even more so about lack of tenderness and warmth at home.

He sleeps very little, has absolutely no appetite, and the stomach pain which he suffered from in the past has returned, his stools are not well formed and yellowish, urination seems normal, with sporadic nocturia.

His face is signed, the tongue red and with a very scarlet tip, the tongue coating is yellow and fairly thin, the pulse is strong, fast and slippery.

First diagnosis
Heart, liver and stomach fire; phlegm and fire that obscure the portals of the heart, agitating and confusing the *shen*.

Therapeutic principles
Clear heart, liver and stomach fire and resolve phlegm.
Calm the *shen*.

Treatment
Four twice-weekly treatments.
First treatment:
- Du-14 *Dazhui*, Du-16-*Fengfu*, EX-HN-3 *Yintang*, HE-5 *Tongli*, KI-1 *Yongquan*.
Second treatment:
- EX-HN-1 *Sishencong*, Du-20 *Bahui*, HE-5 *Tongli*, KI-1 *Yongquan*.
Third and fourth treatments:
- EX-HN-1 *Sishencong*, Du-20 *Bahui*, ST-44 *Neiting*, LIV-2 *Xingjian*.

Du-14 *Dazhui*, Du-16 *Fengfu*, Du-20 *Bahui*, EX-HN-3 *Yintang*, EX-HN-1 *Sishencong* are used to eliminate the excess of *yang* above and transform phlegm that obscures the portals of the heart; HE-5 *Tongli*, KI-1 *Yongquan*: to calm the *shen*'s restlessness through the heart's *luo* point and the *jing* point of water; ST-44 *Neiting*, LIV-2 *Xingjian*: to clear stomach and liver fire.

During the first 10 days there seems to be no change in the situation. During the first three treatments, I am struck by the total lack of the slightest stillness, which is usually produced at least temporarily by the treatment; even though I remind the patient that it is better to remain silent during the treatment, as soon as I remove the needles the torrent of words starts anew without interruption.

During the fourth treatment, however, he falls asleep. The general situation is also more contained and the *shen* manages to find a sufficient stability so that the patient can put into action the plan that he had in mind, which is to return to his town of origin in the Marche region for a period of time. He remains there for more than a month and manages to gather enough forces to 'put the pieces back together again'.

When he returns, he tells me that initially he had a hard time, but after a while 'he breathed, ate and slept' and the acute crisis resolved itself. He is now sad, has no somatic symptoms other than stools that are not well formed; the tongue is pale, slightly swollen with red, raised and tooth marked edges; the pulse is still full and a little slippery, but no longer fast.

Second diagnosis
Stagnation of liver *qi*, emptiness of heart and spleen.

Therapeutic principles
Activate liver *qi*, and tonify the blood of the heart and the *qi* of the spleen.

Treatment

I see the patient four times, and not more than once a week, as he asks.

The following points are alternated:

- HE-7 *Shenmen*, KI-3 *Taixi*, ST-36 *Zusanli*

  and:

- LI-4 *Hegu*, LIV-3 *Taichong*.

EX-HN-3 *Yintang*, Du-24 *Shenting* are used to maintain the action on the excess of *yang* above and the phlegm which obscures the portals of the heart, but more delicately than the points on the top of the head; HE-7 *Shenmen* and KI-3 *Taixi*: to maintain the action of harmonising fire and water, but working mainly on *yuanqi* through the relative *yuan* points; LI-4 *Hegu* and LIV-3 *Taichong*: to promote the circulation of *qi* through the 'four gates'; ST-36 *Zusanli*: to tonify *qi* and blood through post-heaven.

At the end of the month the patient says that he is still sad and sometimes gloomy, but he knows that it will pass. He feels that he is improving, the relationship with his wife is definitely going better, he has started working again; sleep, appetite and bowels have normalised.

Comments

The treatment was essentially addressed towards the draining of fire and the moving down of excess *yang*, which had ascended and disturbed the *shen*. I chose to concentrate on draining the fire rather than resolving the phlegm directly, because I felt that the phlegm had not yet condensed and become too fixed. Considering the acuteness of the case, its insurgence could have corresponded with the manifestation of the substantial part of the fire and I hoped that resolution of the phlegm would follow directly from the calming of the fire.

I therefore used the points on the head that act upon the excess of *yang*, calm the *shen* and in any event clear the portals of the heart. Furthermore, in the first phase, the choice was made to act upon the fire–water axis through the *luo* point of the heart and the *jing* point of the kidney to move the *qi* and bring it down; then attention was shifted to the points of the stomach and liver channels that disperse fire.

The second part of the treatment was aimed at helping re-establish the balance which had been put to a hard test; tongue, pulse, attitude, and bowels suggested that action was needed to nourish the heart, to supplement the post-heaven and to regulate the *qi*.

The handling of this case was rather delicate. It did not seem possible to prescribe psychopharmaceuticals because the patent was totally against it and even a minimal hint of this hypothesis had risked breaking the bond of trust that he continued to declare he had in me, and which was fundamental for him in that moment.

When I started the treatment, friends and relatives were already mobilising around him, about which I had clear feedback both through a mutual friend–colleague and through the patient's own descriptions. His wife called, very worried, and requesting an appointment; however, I kept my relationship with her to a minimum because the main point is to keep all the space for my patient: I listen to her and express my understanding, but exclude the possibility of seeing her and refer her instead to a colleague for support.

Follow-up

After 4 months, I call the patient's home and his wife answers. She says that she is very relieved, 'I can't believe how things are going'. She adds that in the beginning her husband was embarrassed and his face would darken when he thought back to that period, and that now he is still sad at times, but has not been so desperate, restless and out of control as before. Later I find a message on my answering machine, he said goodbye and thanked me.

Principal Patterns of Emptiness-*Xu*

11

In patterns with stagnation, fire and phlegm – in other words, patterns of fullness – the *shen* 'fills up', and becomes agitated and the manifestations assume extreme characteristics, ranging from a disposition to inflammation – with symptoms such as irascibility and tongue ulceration – to the confusion of *diankuang*-madness. Empty patterns are, in contrast, characterised by a *shen* that cannot find rest and wanders without a home.

If *yin* and blood are deficient, they cannot nourish the heart sufficiently and the 'material' base in which the *shen* is stored and given root is absent. The *shen* therefore has no place to reside and becomes restless; this fundamental restlessness manifests at night in sleep disorders and during the day in a state of anxiety, apprehension and faulty memory. This restlessness is evident both in the patient's behaviour and in what he tells us: he cannot find peace, lives in a continuous state of alarm, or is upset by every event and emotion.

There are a number of apparently different ways in which it manifests: some patients tell us that they are in a state of continuous anguish over what might occur (up to the feeling of dying that is typical of panic attacks); others complain of a lack of memory or concentration (the inability to remember turns out to be due to lack of attention, an incapability of following conversations or events, given that the thoughts are unable to remain fixed on the subject and are always somewhere else); others still are at the mercy of emotional weakness such that every image, word or deed can upset them, stirring up uncontrollable agitation.

Categorising patterns of emptiness into specific syndromes is a particularly delicate task, because a deficiency always seems to involve a number of aspects.

This complexity is evident in clinical reality: the more the classification of patterns is detailed, the more often symptoms and therapeutic choices overlap. Therefore, we concentrate here on a structure of reference that reflects the fundamental changes from which illnesses develop, attributing the various possibilities to two main roots (emptiness of *qi* and blood, and emptiness of *yin*).

EMPTINESS OF HEART AND SPLEEN

Aetiology

The process of living consumes *qi*, and is simultaneously the precondition for generating *qi*.

A serious or persistent alteration of the balance of *yin* and *yang* tends to deplete *qi*, resulting in patterns of emptiness. Illness increases the consumption of *qi* and hinders its reconstitution.

In particular, we know that sadness, pain and suffering deplete *qi*, just as chronic illnesses, fatigue and excess of activity, accumulation of pathogens and blood deficiency consume *qi*.

Emptiness of *qi* also generates a state of emptiness of blood, owing to which the *shen* is not nourished and wanders without an abode.

In clinical cases of *shen* disorders, emptiness of spleen and heart, a synonym of 'emptiness of spleen *qi* and heart blood' is therefore an extremely frequent condition.

Clinical Manifestations

- Palpitations, restlessness, anxiety, insomnia, lack of memory.
- Asthenia, fatigability, pale face and lips.
- Pale, swollen or thin tongue, depending on whether there is a prevalence of *qi* or blood emptiness.
- Thin, weak pulse.

Clinical Notes

Post-heaven *qi* is generally consumed first, which leads to an emptiness of spleen *qi*. Later on, pre-heaven *qi* is drawn upon – from which ensues an increasingly serious kidney emptiness with insufficiency of *qi* and *yang*, but also of *yin* and *jing*.

The presence of heat, with its relative symptoms of a cracked tongue body or red tip and acceleration of the pulse, is frequent.

It is important to keep in mind the possible evolution of the pathology and to know the state of the other organs: later, the specific patterns of spleen or kidney *qi/yang* emptiness, emptiness of heart and gall bladder *qi*, and emptiness of liver blood are described.

In the pattern of heart blood emptiness and spleen *qi* emptiness, one of the two can dominate: we will therefore list separately the general signs and symptoms of emptiness of *qi* and those of emptiness of blood.

Blood emptiness

- Dizziness, unsteadiness.
- Paraesthesia, hypoaesthesia, itch *sine materia*.
- Dry eyes, vision disorders, muscle spasms.
- Dry skin, fragile nails, weak hair, dull complexion and pale lips.
- Decreased quantity of menstrual blood, late cycle, up to amenorrhoea.
- Pale, short, thin, tongue with possible superficial cracks, indented tip if serious.
- Thin, weak or minute pulse; choppy if there is also blood stasis; drenched or like drum skin if serious.

Qi emptiness

- Physical and mental tiredness, disposition to fatigue.
- Shortness of breath, sweating at minimal exertion, pale complexion.
- Weak voice or difficulty in speaking.
- Tendency to feel cold and to be invaded by external cold.
- Worsening of symptoms after effort.
- Pale, tooth marked, or soft tongues.
- Weak, minute, short or slackened pulse; scattered if serious.

Therapeutic Principles

- Tonify *qi*, nourish blood, and calm the *shen*.

Treatment Rationale

HE-7 *Sishencong* + ST-36 *Zusanli* + SP-6 *Sanyinjiao* (or SP-3 *Taibai*)

This combination is widely used as it calms the *shen*, tonifies the *qi* and nour-ishes the blood. It is an excellent basic choice for all those situations in which both the *shen* and the body are starting to show signs of instability or fatigue.

With timely additions it is also extremely useful in more serious condi-tions in which action on fire or phlegm is necessary, but the base also needs consolidation.

It acts directly on the heart through HE-7 *Shenmen*, whose action in calming *shen* is shared by SP-6 *Sanyinjiao* and ST-36 *Zusanli*, which amplify the effect. SP-6 *Sanyinjiao* furthermore nourishes *yin* and blood through the lower three *yin* and ST-36 *Zusanli* tonifies *qi*, and also blood.

If the stomach and spleen deficiency is more pertinent, SP-6 *Sanyinjiao* may be replaced by SP-3 *Taibai* in order to support substantially both the middle *jiao* and the production of post-heaven *qi*.

HE-7 Shenmen

Yuan and *shu* point, earth point, sedation point.

Principal actions

— Calms the *shen* and regulates *qi*.
— Tonifies the four emptinesses of the heart (*qi* and blood, *yin* and *yang*).
— Clears heat from the channels and opens the orifices.

Notes

The 'gate of *shen*' *shenmen* is probably the most used point in emotional disorders precisely because it is indicated both in patterns of emptiness and in those of stagnation. It in fact nourishes *yin* and blood, in this way providing a root and a home for the *shen*, but is also able to regulate *qi* and calm agitation.[1]

ST-36 Zusanli

He point of stomach, earth point, *Chong Mai* point

Principal actions

— Tonifies *qi* and nourishes blood.
— Reinforces the middle *jiao* and regulates stomach *qi*.
— Calms the *shen* and clears heat.
— Supports the spleen and resolves dampness.
— Regulates defensive and nutritive *qi* and nourishes *yuanqi*.
— Reinforces true *qi* and activates *qi* in the channels.

Notes

Called 'the point of the hundred illnesses', it is one of the most well-known points precisely because it has a wide range of applications and powerful effect.

---

[1] Classically it is localised medial to the ulnar flexor tendon of the carpus, but in contemporary clinic it is usually reached by inserting the needle on the ulnar side of the tendon. Moreover some practitioners direct the needle towards *Neiguan* P-6. The *Sishencong* point in the ear is also often used to calm the *shen*, and particularly to treat the emotional aspect of pain (see also Chapter 12 on stimulation methods).

Being a *he* point, it acts directly on the stomach, the root of the organs and the seas of *qi* and blood (the pulse must have stomach *qi*, *shen* and root – elements that are also prognostic indicators).

ST-36 *Zusanli's* tonifying action on *qi* derives from its ability to act on post-heaven *qi*, but also on *yuanqi*.[2]

It is of fundamental importance in disorders of the *shen*, which so often is agitated because of an insufficiency of heart blood; in fact, it promotes the transforming and transporting functions of earth and stimulates the spleen and stomach to produce *qi* and blood.

Its action in regulating stomach *qi* also permits it to resolve disorders due to conversely rising *qi*.

Its ability to clear heat in the *yangming* and to support the spleen's action of transforming dampness and phlegm renders it a fundamental point in *diankung*-type syndromes of the stomach channel in which fire and phlegm are preponderant.

SP-6 Sanyinjiao

Meeting point of the three *yin* channels of the leg.

Principal actions

— Nourishes *yin* and blood and tonifies *qi*.
— Calms the *shen* and regulates liver *qi*.
— Tonifies the middle *jiao* and transforms dampness.
— Invigorates and cools blood.

Notes

The range of its functions renders it one of the most useful and utilised points: it is, in fact, indicated in cases of *qi* deficiency, insufficiency of *yin*, emptiness, stasis or heat in the blood, accumulation of dampness, pathology of the lower *jiao* and obstruction of the channels.

It is a fundamental point for calming the *shen*, through various actions: it tonifies spleen and heart *qi* and nourishes the blood, and is therefore effective in cases of emptiness of heart and spleen, but at the same time is also important in emptiness of *yin* because it nourishes liver and kidney *yin*.

It furthermore cools blood if there is heat, transforms dampness and invigorates *qi*, also acting on liver stagnation.

---

[2] Hua Tuo recommends it for the five exhaustions-*lao* and for the seven damages-*sun*. The five exhaustions-*lao*, mentioned for the first time in the *Lingshu*, are: to use the eyes excessively harms the blood, to lie down harms the *qi*, to sit down harms the flesh, to stand up harms the bones, to walk harms the tendons; the seven damages-*sun* are: excess of food damages the spleen, rage damages the liver, cold damages the lung, suffering and preoccupation damage the heart, fear damages the will-*zhi*, and wind-cold and summer heat damage the body.

SP-3 Taibai

Yuan and *shu* point, earth point.

Principal actions

— Tonifies spleen *qi*
— Resolves dampness and damp-heat.
— Harmonises spleen and stomach and regulates *qi*.

Notes

Being a *yuan* point, it reinforces and regulates stomach and spleen *qi*: it is remarkably effective in cases in which the transforming and transporting functions are deficient, and thoughts and body become too ponderous or heavy.

Together with ST-36 *Zusanli*, it acts on abdominal swelling and pain, and oppression in the lateral costal region or chest when they are caused by a difficulty in the circulation of *qi* due to an emptiness of *qi* or dampness, which obstructs its movement.

Its action on dampness is also important with regard to the possibility that dampness condenses into phlegm (with easy obstruction of the heart's portals), combines with heat (with agitation, and 'hot' diarrhoea), and joins with wind (pain in the neck and shoulders, painful obstruction and *bi* syndromes).

KI-4 *Dazhong* + HE-5 *Tongli* (or LU-7 *Lieque*)

This combination makes sense particularly in those patterns where there are signs of *qi* that goes upward instead of entering into the *yin* – in other words, in which the emptiness is mainly related to disordered movement of *qi*.

The classics gave extreme relevance to the concept of *qi* disorder, which includes counterflow *qi*, *qi* that attacks above, *yang* that is liberated above due to *yin* emptiness, but also *yang* that, being deficient, does not enter into the *yin* below and floats upward to disturb the *shen*.

In clinical cases of emotional disorder this pathology of *qi* is seen daily, and these points, which not by chance are cited often in the classics in relation to psychic disturbances, represent a good therapeutic rationale. [3]

---

[3] Some examples of classical indications of these points are the following: 'Desire to speak but no sound comes out, agitation and irritability, palpitations from fear, fullness which induces heaviness in the four limbs, reddening of the head, cheek and face, emptiness which prevents from eating, sudden muteness, inexpressive face. Prick *Tongli* HE-5 lightly with a thin needle and its miraculous effect will be evident.' In: Wang Guorui *Ma danyang tianxing shierxue bingzhi zabing ge* ('Chant by Ma Danyang of the 12 star points for the treatment of various illnesses'). In relation to *Dazhong* KI-4 is suggested for 'fear of people, emptiness of the *shen*', in: Sun Simiao, *Qianjin yaofang* ('Remedies worth a thousands golden pieces for urgencies') and for 'the ill wants to close the doors and stay home', in: Wang Weiyi, *Tongren shuxue zhenjiu tujing* ('Illustrated classic of the points of the bronze statue'), a condition appearing also in the work of the imperial medical staff *Shengji zonglu* ('Compendium of sacred remedies'). Mei Jianhan suggests it for 'the alternation of clear and confused mind'

Being *luo* points, they move *qi* well: the KI-4 *Dazhong* + HE-5 *Tongli* couple acts on the water–fire axis and is very efficient if there are direct signs of agitation of the heart (palpitations, insomnia), while the pairing of KI-4 *Dazhong* and LU-7 *Lieque* directs action more towards the regulation of the containing/spreading functions of the *qi* of the kidney and lung system.

KI-4 Dazhong

Luo point.

Principal actions

— Moves down excess *qi* from above.
— Reinforces the kidney.

Notes

Rarely used in modern clinical TCM, it is often cited in the classics in relation to psychic symptomatology.

Situations in which there is an excess of *qi* above with an emptiness below (*shangshi xiaxu*) are, in fact, very frequent: being a *luo* point KI-4 *Dazhong* has the ability to invigorate *qi* strongly and, more importantly, to move it down, in this way nourishing the kidney. For this reason, even if it tonifies and nourishes less than KI-3 *Taixi*, it is indicated in those *shen* disorders in which there is an emptiness of kidney *qi*.

HE-5 Tongli

Luo point.

Principal actions

— Regulates heart *qi* and calms the *shen*.
— Clears heat and activates the *qi* of the channels.

Notes

As well as cases in which it is necessary to regulate fullness, it is also indicated in conditions of emptiness.

It is particularly effective in cases of palpitations, sensations of an overly strong or disorderly heartbeat, and alterations of rhythm; it in fact regulates heart *qi*, which in turn governs blood circulation, of which the heartbeat is an expression.

(MediCina seminar September 1996). Notice that the point *luo* coupled by *Feiyang* BL-58 in the classics is suggested for signs of high *qi* and emptiness of the kidney. For example Mei Jianhan recommends it in hypertensive crises, when *Quchi* LI-11 does not produce any result. *Lieque* LU-7 is mentioned in Huangfu Mi, *Jiayijing* ('The systematic classic of acupuncture and moxibustion'), both in the case of heart restlessness and in that of disturbed sleep.

It is a fundamental point in those certainly not infrequent cases in which a person tends to suffer from recurring urinary disturbances that are often related to difficult emotional periods; it has, indeed, a strong ability to clear heat that travels from the heart to its associated small intestine channel and through the *Tai Yang* to the bladder.

It is just as important in those conditions in which heat from the heart agitates the uterus through the *Bao Mai*, with excessive menstrual flow and prolonged spotting.

LU-7 Lieque

Luo point, confluent point of the *Renmai*.

Principal actions

–Regulates defensive *qi* and frees the surface from invasions of external pathogens.
–Stimulates the lung's functions of descending and diffusing *qi*.
–Resolves phlegm, both substantial and insubstantial, and opens the water passages.

Notes

Just as with the other *luo* points of the *yin* channels, it has the ability to invigorate *qi* and to treat emotional disorders, but in a particularly effective way. It is often cited in the classics in cases of headaches and with regard to manifestations such as lack of memory, palpitations, propensity to laughter, and frequent yawning or stretching (heart and kidney signs).

When one has the sensation that the condition is 'delicate', when the *qi* lacks root below, when there is obstructing phlegm, LU-7 *Lieque* is a point to take into consideration as an alternative to LIV-3 *Taichong*, as it also has the ability to nourish blood.

The kidney is the root of *qi*, receiving and storing it. The lung spreads *qi* in the whole body, and governs *qi* and the movements of all the organs, putting them in condition to carry out their functions; therefore, all *qi* is 'based' on the lung.

The grand circulation of *qi* begins in the lung channel, which originates in the middle *jiao*.

The lung governs central qi-*zhongqi* – in other words, breathing and the circulation of blood; *qi* and blood are used daily for living, while the kidney is at the root of the longer rhythms, both monthly and those of the entire life.

The kidney controls opening and closing; the lung is called *huagai*, or 'lid' – a term which refers to its function of gathering and condensing vapour-*qi*, which then rises to be spread in the whole body.[4]

---

[4] *Huagai* is often translated as 'canopy' in the sense of precious covering.

BL-15 *Xinshu* + BL-44 *Shentang* + Du-11 *Shendao*

Principal actions

For the functions of the individual points see Chapter 13.

Notes

The association of the *shu* point of heart with the corresponding point on the external branch of the bladder and on the *Du Mai* is used a great deal to calm the *shen* since it has a tonifying action on the organ and clears heat. The *huatu-ojiaji* may also be taken into consideration.

Combinations that include the dorsal points located at the same level have the quality of reinforcing the action of the *shu* point.

In the case of dorsal points, palpation is particularly important for determining their selection. Differences in the consistency of the tissues, reactivity to pressure, temperature, colour, and eventual skin alterations guide the diagnosis and treatment.

Du-24 *Shenting* (or EX-HN-3 *Yintang*) + Ren-17 *Shanzhong* (or Ren-14 *Juque* or Ren-12 *Zhongwan*)+ Ren-6 *Qihai* (or Ren-4 *Guanyuan*)

Principal actions

For the functions of the individual points see Chapter 13.

Notes

The combination of *Du* and *Renmai* points is particularly useful when the deficiency is in relation to disordered movements of *qi*.

Du-24 *Shenting* and EX-HN-3 *Yintang* possess a similar action in calming the *shen*: the first acts more on internal wind, and the second on phlegm that obstructs the orifices.

Ren-17 *Shanzhong*, Ren-14 *Juque* and Ren-12 *Zhongwan* tonify and regulate *qi* at their respective levels: the first acts on constraints at the level of the chest and throat, the second dissolves the knotting of *qi* of an emotional origin which manifests at the level of the lateral costal region, the third regulates the middle *jiao*, possibly in association with Ren-13 *Shangwan* and Ren-10 *Xiawan*.

Ren-4 *Guanyuan* is more indicated for nourishing *yin* and blood, reinforcing *yuanqi* and blood, whereas the action of Ren-6 *Qihai* is directed more at the *qi*, tonifying, invigorating and moving it downwards.

Emptiness of spleen *qi*

- A feeling of fatigue and heaviness that increases after meals.
- Decreased appetite, abdominal swelling, stools that are not well formed or diarrhoea.
- Dizziness from orthostatic hypotension, 'coldness in the four limbs'.
- Haemorrhoids, a feeling of heaviness in the lower abdomen or leaking of urine under pressure.
- Tendency to bleeding (red spots, haematomas, haematuria, melaena, menometrorrhagia).
- Soft and tooth-marked tongue.
- Empty, weak, pulse.

Notes

One of the most frequent patterns is a disharmony between liver and spleen: if the spleen is weak even a moderate stagnation of liver–wood is sufficient to invade earth, with symptoms of *qi* constraint and a tight pulse.

Bowels may be constipated if the *qi* deficiency does not move the intestine.

The deficiency of spleen *qi* easily leads to an accumulation of cold-damp, with symptoms and signs such as nausea and vomiting, a heavy headed feeling, a yellowish complexion, a swollen and damp tongue, and a scattered or slippery pulse.

Dampness may transform into damp-heat that attacks the intestines, with diarrhoeic, yellow and foul-smelling stools.

Dampness may condense into phlegm.

Stomach heat may also be present together with spleen emptiness.

Useful points

To tonify spleen *qi* and clear heat:

- SP-3 *Taibai*.

  To reinforce and regulate the middle *jiao*:

- Ren-12 *Zhongwan* (possibly with moxa).

  To tonify spleen and stomach:

- Bl-20 *Pishu* and BL-21 *Weishu* (possibly with moxa).

  To lead *qi* upward:

- Du-20 *Baihui* (possibly with moxa).

To support earth that is attacked by wood:

- LIV-3 *Taichong* and LIV-13 *Zhangmen*.

To regulate the relationship between spleen and intestines:

- SP-15 *Daheng*, ST-25 *Tianshu*, Ren-6 *Qihai*.

To resolve dampness:

- SP-9 *Yinlingquan*.

To resolve damp-heat in the intestines:

- ST-37 *Shangjuxu* and ST-39 *Xiajuxu*.
- P-5 *Jianshu*, ST-40 *Fenglong* to resolve phlegm.

Emptiness of *yang*

- Greater severity of all the symptoms present in cases of emptiness of *qi*.
- Cold sensation, cold limbs, spontaneous sweating.
- Aching, pain or coldness in the lumbar area or in the knees: emptiness of kidney *yang*.
- Decrease of libido or disturbance in sexual activity: emptiness of kidney *yang*.
- Poliurea, bed wetting, or incontinence, diarrhoea at dawn: emptiness of kidney *yang*.
- Severe diarrhoea with undigested food: emptiness of spleen *yang*.
- Oedemas: emptiness of spleen or kidney (declivous oedema) *yang*.
- Arrhythmia: emptiness of heart *yang*.
- Cold sweats, gelid limbs, dyspnoea, cyanosis, loss of consciousness: collapse of *yang*.
- Sudden and severe cardiac pain: collapse of heart *yang*.
- Very soft tongue, pale at the tip.
- Weak, deep, slowed-down, floating or hollow pulse.
- Intermittent, knotted, or hidden pulse: collapse of *yang*.

Notes

Emptiness of *yang* corresponds to a lack of the warm and dry aspect of *qi*, to a deficiency in movement with respect to stillness, and the upwards and outwards motion is missing in the movement; symptoms and signs reflect the falling of this fire that supports the functions of the organs and the circulation of *qi* and blood.

From a psychic viewpoint if *yang* is lacking it does not furnish the warmth necessary for mental and emotional movement and there can be depression or cognitive deficits.

Useful points

To tonify *yang*:

- BL-23 *Shenshu*, BL-52 *Zhishi*, Du-4 *Mingmen* (possibly with moxa).

  To tonify kidney *yang* and nourish kidney *yin*:

- KI-3 *Taixi*.

  To regulate kidney *qi* and reinforce the action on the water passages:

- KI-7 *Fuliu*.

Emptiness of heart and gall bladder *qi*

- Uncertainty, indecision, lack of courage, determination and timidity.
- A state of apprehension or of alarm ('easily frightened', 'easily startled').
- Dreams that awaken the patient in terror, palpitations.

Notes

In daily practice, this image of an apprehensive, easily startled patient, as though there were always someone or something to be afraid of, is commonly found. The same condition is described a number of times in classic texts, where a close relationship between fright, heart and gall bladder *qi* is posited.

A number of modern texts also underline the role of the gall bladder in the response to anxiety-producing events. 'If gall bladder *qi* is sufficiently strong it can face up to the stress deriving from external pressure, from the continuous changes that occur around us, and one can easily overcome the emotional changes that are a consequence.'[5]

Useful points

To reinforce gall bladder *qi*:

- GB-40 *Qiuxu*, GB-24 *Riyue* and BL-19 *Danshu*.

  To regulate gall bladder *qi*:

- GB-34 *Yanglinquan*.

Emptiness of liver blood

- Sleep disturbed by dreams, eyesight disturbances that are more evident at night, paraesthesia: emptiness of liver blood.

---

[5] Qiao Wenlei, Chapter 18. For a discussion on the aspects of determination or cowardice of the gall bladder see Chapter 2. According to Bob Flaws the emptiness of the heart and gall bladder *qi* is actually a complex syndrome in which there is a spleen emptiness resulting in a heart and blood emptiness, and also constraint of liver and stagnation of *qi*, accumulation of phlegm-dampness and frequent constricted fire due to liver stagnation (MediCina seminar, 14–15 October 2001).

- Dizziness, ringing in the ears, headaches, tremors, cramps, convulsions, and loss of consciousness: *yang* above and wind.
- Red and sore eyes, *Shao yang* type headaches, bitter mouth, yellow tongue coating: liver fire.
- Tongue body with pale edges.
- Thin, weak or minute pulse; scattered or leather pulse if serious; choppy if there is also stasis of blood.

Notes

This pattern overlaps with the 'heart and liver disharmony' syndrome.

The liver stores blood and the heart governs it: an emptiness of liver blood manifests as general signs of insufficient blood accompanied by a rising of *yang*, production of wind, transformation into fire or a wandering *hun* due to a lack of an abode.

Liver and kidney have the same source and influence each other, so emptiness of liver blood often magnifies into an emptiness of liver and kidney *yin*, with its relative signs and symptoms.

Useful points

To nourish liver blood:

- BL-17 *Geshu*, BL-18 *Ganshu*, LIV-8 *Ququan*, LIV-3 *Taichong*.

  To calm *yang* and extinguish wind:

- GB-20 *Fengchi*, GB-21 *Jianjing*, GB-7 *Qubin*, GB-12 *Wangu*, GB-43 *Xiaxi*.

  To drain fire of the *shaoyang*:

- GB-13 *Benshen* or EX-HN-9 *Taiyang* (possibly with bleeding).

  To nourish *yin* and liquids:

- HE-6 *Yinxi*, SP-6 *Sanyinjiao*, KI-6 *Zhaohai*.

EMPTINESS OF HEART *YIN* WITH EMPTY FIRE

Aetiology

As in the case of emptiness of *qi* and blood, emptiness of *yin* is also a result of pathology that persists over time, whether emotional, chronic illness or lifestyle habits such as an excess of sexual activity or overwork, especially mental.

An excess of mental labour tends to injure the *yin* more than physical work, and emotions directly attack the *yin*. That which is least substantial acts on its opposite: the dense substance of *yin*.

If kidney *yin* is deficient it cannot nourish the heart; the *shen* has its root in *jing*, and if *jing* is insufficient the *shen* is injured.

Water and fire must communicate and interchange in order to assist each other mutually, while if kidney water does not control heart fire an imbalance between *yin* and *yang* follows, with accompanying agitation by fire and restlessness of the *shen*.

See the chapters on heat (Chapter 5), *fanzao* (Chapter 6), and classic patterns (Chapter 9) for an analysis of the relationship between fire, emotions and compromising of *yin*.

Clinical Manifestations

- Red (or with a redder tip), dry, cracked tongue (the cracks are related to empty kidney *yin* if they are all over, to the stomach if central, to the lung if at the tip, and to the heart if the longitudinal crack reaches the tip); absence of coating or with a dark root if fire has consumed the *yin*.
- Thin, rapid pulse; hurried if serious.
- Signs of empty heart *yin* with empty fire:
  — palpitations, restlessness, lack of memory;
  — state of alarm, apprehension, anxiety;
  — interrupted sleep disturbed by dreams and not very restoring.
- Signs of empty kidney *yin* with empty heat:
  — ringing in the ears, dizziness, weakness or soreness in the lumbar or knee areas;
  — malar flush, feverish sensation in the evening, nocturnal sweating, dry mouth;
  — heat in the 'five hearts', frequent urination with dark urine, dry stools.

Clinical notes

Yin deficiency is often accompanied by empty fire, from which a vague uneasiness originates.

The presence of fire disperses the *shen*, as though a part of it were always elsewhere in time, in space and in thought: the classics speak of keeping the *shen* united as a precondition for adhering to the *dao*.

Internal agitation can have very specific manifestations such as anxiety when facing everyday activities (think of how often the hot flashes of menopause accompany this fear of 'not being able to do things in time'), or deeply affect the relationship between the self and the external world, rendering, for example, making it impossible to live simply in the present moment.

Heat in turn consumes *yin*, in a vicious cycle in which tranquillity, rest, and liquids are exhausted.

This pattern in which fire does not descend to warm the kidney and water does not rise to cool the heart overlaps with the 'heart and kidney do not communicate' (*xinshen bujiao*) and 'kidney and heart not harmonised' (*xinshen buhe*) patterns, which, however, may present with a greater measure of kidney symptoms.

The pathogenic mechanism and clinical manifestations of agitation of *shen* remind us of a number of aspects of the full heart fire pattern, but the fire that derives from a *yin* deficiency manifests through specific signs of empty heat.

If full fire persists over time, it consumes the *yin* in any event and the patterns of fullness are then complicated by elements of emptiness.

If *yin* is truly compromised this means that the damage to the energetic balance is at a deeper level, and these are the situations in which internal practice and a change in attitudes seem to be fundamental.

Therapeutic Principles

Nourish heart and kidney *yin*, clear empty heat, and calm the *shen*.

Treatment Rationale

HE-6 *Yinxi* + KI- 6 *Zhaohai*

This is a combination of two points that nourish *yin* and liquids and have a fortifying effect in emptiness of *yin*, especially when the consumption of substances has produced widespread dryness.

In these cases, in fact, a number of organs may be injured: the heart, with agitation of the *shen*; the lung, with dry and persistent coughing; the kidney, with a decrease in urination; the liver, with disturbances of the eyes; the stomach, with pain and languor; and the intestines, with constipation.

HE-6 *Yinxi*

Xi point.

Principal actions

— Nourishes heart *yin* and liquids.
— Drains empty fire and calms the *shen*.

Notes

This is the main heart point for nourishing *yin* and liquids, and is very effective for symptoms arising from empty heat such as nocturnal sweating, 'boiling bones',[6] disturbed sleep and restlessness.

Being a *xi* point of a *yin* channel it is also indicated for blood stasis and haemorrhage due to heat agitating the blood, even if in these cases the first choice of point is *Ximen* P-4.

KI-6 Zhaohai

Confluent point of the *Yin Qiao Mai*.

Principal actions

— Nourishes *yin* and liquids.
— Clears empty heat.

Notes

A fundamental point in empty *yin* pathologies with drying up of body fluids, it is extremely useful in pathologies of the elderly when *yin* deficiency results in dryness, of both a more 'material' type (throat, eyes, skin, stools) and a more 'immaterial' type (such as restlessness, anxiety or insomnia).

Ren-4 Guanyuan + HE-7 Shenmen + SP-6 Sanyinjiao

This combination recalls the HE-7 *Shenman* + SP-6 *Sanyinjiao* point combination already detailed in heart and spleen emptiness. The substitution of Ren-4 *Guanyuan* for ST-36 *Zusanli*, however, directs its actions towards the *yin*. In fact, Ren-4 *Guanyuan* is one of the most important points for nourishing blood and *yin*, reinforcing *yuanqi* and benefiting *jing*.

Specific patterns

Empty *jing*

• The tongue loses substance at the root, retreats and forms a depression.
• The pulse may be weak, scattered, leather or choppy if there is stasis.

---

[6] Qiao Wenlei, Chapter 18. For a discussion on the aspects of determination or cowardice of the gall bladder see Chapter 2. According to Bob Flaws the emptiness of the heart and gall bladder *qi* is actually a complex syndrome in which there is a spleen emptiness resulting in a heart and blood emptiness, and also constraint of liver and stagnation of *qi*, accumulation of humidity-phlegm and frequent constricted fire due to liver stagnation (MediCina seminar, 14–15 October 2001).

Notes

Empty *jing* derives from excessive consumption or from a congenital deficiency.

Jing deficiency pathologies in relation to the *shen* essentially involve the cognitive system – for example, various types of dementia, memory disorders and mental retardation.

In *jing* deficiencies phlegm accumulates easily, obstructing the heart's portals and dimming the *shen*.

Useful points

To tonify the kidney:

- BL-23 *Shenshu*, BL-52 *Zhishi*, Du-4 *Mingmen*, Ren-4 *Guanyuan*, KI-3 *Taixi*.
  To ascend *qi* and resolve phlegm:
- Du-20 *Baihui*, EX-HN-1 *Sishencong*, Du-24 *Shenting*, EX-HN-3 *Yintang*.

Lung *yin* emptiness

- Distraction and agitation, sadness and a continuous desire to weep, emotional frailness.
- Difficulty in falling asleep, many dreams, desire for tranquillity, hallucinations.
- Feeling of hunger with no desire to eat, frequent yawning.
- Malar flush, feverish feeling in the evening, nocturnal sweating, heat in the 'five hearts'.
- Bitter taste, dry cough, dry mouth or throat, dry stools, dark urine.
- Red, dry, tongue with a crack in the tip; scanty or absent coating.
- Rapid, thin, minute pulse.

Notes

The lung is a 'delicate' organ; it detests dryness, and its *yin* is fragile and easily consumed by heat.

The description of the empty *yin* pattern of the lung repeats a number of signs and symptoms seen in classic syndromes, especially *zanzao* and *baihebing* (see Chapter 9) – in other words, those illnesses with prevalently psychic expressions that are related most closely to the organs and *yin*.

A specific characteristic of empty lung *yin* and its relative dryness is a pervasive uneasiness.

Emptiness of lung *yin* is seen frequently in the clinic: the somatic symptoms often remain hidden, but the empty fire can be deduced from the underlying uneasiness, which has similar characteristics to those of the dryness of metal. With the depletion of *yin*, moisture and stillness are lacking and there is no rest.

Useful points

To tonify the lung:

- LU-1 *Zhongfu*, LU-9 *Taiyuan*, BL-13 *Feishu*, BL-42 *Pohu*.

  To nourish *yin*, clear heat and tonify *yuanqi*:

- BL-43 *Gaohuangshu* (possibly with moxa).

  To harmonise the movement of *qi* between body and head:

- LU-3 *Tianfu*.

Notes

BL-42 *Pohu* nourishes and tonifies the lung and clears it of empty heat. It is indicated for cases of 'possession of the three corpses'. According to popular Beidi Daoism, in the 57th day of the *jiazi* 60-day cycle the Northern Emperor opens the door, sees all our deficiencies and gathers the requests of all the spirits. Every deed is evaluated in days of life and registered in the great ledger of destiny: the earlier one dies, the earlier the corpses leave the prison of the body and again become demons of darkness. If a person dies a violent death his soul may have the power to enter and possess another body. Certain stretches of road or mountain paths or areas of navigation concentrate this anger for having left life too early and thus the desire to provoke accidents.

The corpse of above is called *pengju*; it resides in the centre of the head and consumes the higher parts of the body, causing dimming of the eyes, loss of hair, a bad taste in the mouth, a stiff face and loss of teeth. It is also called *qinggu* (blue worm), which resides in the *niwan* (the mud pill), at the top of the head. The corpse of the centre is called *pengzhi*: it erodes the five *zang* organs, weakens memory, causes a love of bad things, and produces dreams, sleep, perversions and confusion. It corresponds to *baigu* (white worm), which resides in the *xianggong* (scarlet palace) in the chest. The corpse below is called *pengqiao*: it resides in the centre of man's feet, it upsets and convulses the *mingmen*, and causes the five emotions to be agitated and displaced, and the pathogens to overflow without stop. It corresponds to *xueshi* (corpse of blood), which resides in the lower *dantian*.[7]

BL-43 *Gaohuangshu* has properties that are similar to BL-42 *Pohu*, but with a more profound action on serious emptiness of *yin* and on *yuanqi*.

Gaohuang is the vital area between the heart and the diaphragm, and has already been discussed in works that predate the *Neijing*, such as *Lushi Chunqiu* (Annals of the Spring and Summer by Master Lu) on incurable diseases, and

---

[7] From J.M. Eyssalet, *Le Secret de la Maison des Ancetres*, 1990, p. 214 and following, who quotes the Daoist text *Yuhan Bidian*. See also the annotations on *niwan* and on the *dantian* in Chapter 13 on points.

in the classic medical texts this point was recommended – often with moxa granules – for serious consumptive diseases.

LU-3 *Tianfu*, which is rarely used in the modern clinic, is one of the so-called 'window of heaven' points cited in the *Lingshu*.[8]

In the *Neijing* it is suggested for bleeding of the nose and mouth due to fire that attacks the lungs. In a more general sense it shares with the other heaven-*tan* points the ability to act on disordered movements of *qi* between the body and the head with counterflow *qi* or blood.

In a number of classic passages it appears in relation to emotional disorders, especially those in which ghosts are seen, since it calms the *po*. It is suggested in patterns with insomnia, sadness, weeping, melancholy, speaking with/of ghosts – disorders that are probably associated with the emptiness of *yin* with a fluctuating *shen* found in advanced stages of tuberculosis (once called 'flying corpses'-*feishi* owing to the delirium that Sun Simiao had already recognised as being related to the lung rather than possession by ghosts-*gui*).[9]

Case Study 11.1

Pain and Phantoms

I already knew this 40-year-old businessman, as I had treated him some months previously. I had also treated his son, who presented with many similar features to the father: they both had pale complexions, a complaining attitude and spontane-ous sweating at the smallest exertion.[10]

The father had come for allergic asthma that had resolved fairly well, although it had been decidedly more difficult to cope with the emptiness of spleen and kidney *qi* and *yang*, which manifested with sudden drops in energy, especially after meals, and stools that were not well formed.

The deficiency also involved the heart *qi*: the episodes of sudden loss of strength were, in fact, accompanied by a feeling of 'fogginess in thinking', as well as insom-nia, agitation, anxiety and palpitations. He gave the impression of not being able

---

[8] *Lingshu*, Chapters 2 and 21. See also the article by Mazin Al-Khafaji and Peter Deadman, 'The Points of the Window of Heaven', 1993.

[9] For example: 'Sadness and tears, *gui*-words, 50 cones of moxa on *tianfu*', in: *Qianjin yaofang* ('Remedies worth a thousand golden pieces for urgencies'); 'Sudden and strong thirst, reverse qi rising on the inside, liver and lung fight, blood coming out from the mouth and nose, use *tianfu*.' in: *Lingshu*, Chapter 21; 'Excessive desire to sleep' in: *Jiayijing* ('The systematic classic of acupuncture and moxibustion').

[10] The 8-year-old child sweated mostly from the head (as happens with children) and easily got an infection in the upper respiratory tract during winter: it was a clear framework of *qi* deficit (in particu-lar of *weiqi*), which instantly responded to the preventive treatment with moxa and *Yupingfeng san*, a formula that strengthens the exterior and tonifies the lung.

to make decisions or identify a strategy at a moment that was certainly not easy financially. The previous year he had suffered a myocardial attack.

His wife had died suddenly during the summer in a car accident, for which he feels in part indirectly responsible. His wife was a great support in his work, besides being his companion in life.

When I see him again in November, the situation has worsened once more and all the previous symptoms (except the asthma) have reappeared. Every demand that everyday life makes on him assumes gigantic proportions, anxiety and agitation are continuous, his mind is not very clear, he has nocturnal episodes of panic with feelings of depersonalisation, sweating, laboured breathing and tachycardia. He has turned to the emergency department a number of times for attacks of lateral costal pain, nausea and heaviness in the chest, but examinations excluded any cardiac involvement.

He is exhausted even if work is scarce, he needs to sleep every 3 to 4 hours, he always feels cold, so much so that he sleeps with a vest and sweater at night, he is losing weight, is pale and has deep circles around the eyes, his stools are soft, and often there is an urgent need to empty the bowels upon awakening.

In a short time, the pain and desperation take a psychic form, and the engineer starts to be attracted by the world of the paranormal.

Signs of a serious depression also appear: loss of interest in life with feelings of guilt, lack of willpower in behaviour and inhibition of thought, loss of initiative, scarcity of ideation, monotonous and repetitive thought patterns and a desire to die.

His tongue is pale, tooth marked and swollen, and the pulse is rapid and weak.

Diagnosis
The emptiness of kidney and spleen *qi* of the initial diagnosis has now become an emptiness of *yang*. The deficiency of heart *qi* has worsened and an emptiness of blood has also developed, so that the *hun* wanders with no abode.

Therapeutic principles
Tonify spleen, heart and kidney *qi* and blood; stabilise the *zhi*, root the *hun* and calm the *shen*.

Treatment
Weekly treatments for more than 1 year, then more sporadically for another 3 years.
Principally, the following are stimulated:

- Du-20 *Baihui*, Du-24 *Shenting* and GB-18 *Chengling* to calm the *shen*;
- SP-6 *Sanyinjiao*, KI-3 *Taixi* and HE-7 *Shenman* to nourish *yin* and blood;
- Ren-12 *Zhongwan*, ST-36 *Zusanli* and SP-3 *Taibai* to tonify spleen and stomach;
- BL-15 *Xinshu*, BL-44 *Shentang* and Du-11 *Shendao*, BL-18 *Ganshu*, and BL-47 *Hunmen* to nourish the heart and pacify the liver;
- BL-20 *Pishu*, BL-23 *Shenshu* and Du-4 *Mingmen* to tonify spleen and kidney.

Comments

The diagnosis of empty *yang* is deduced from signs such as diarrhoea at dawn, the facial appearance, and extreme disposition to fatigue. A fundamental difference between empty *qi* and empty *yang* is the 'cold' symptom, about which we read in the Chinese texts: it is a deep and unassailable cold that no sweater can eliminate.

The tendency to coldness that we find, for example, in the decrease of *yang* possibly occurring during menopause manifests only as a corresponding tendency towards a *yang* deficiency (not to be confused with the much more frequent pattern in which cold derives from constraint of *qi*, which no longer circulates well and therefore does not warm the extremities).

Yang warms and transforms; if this energy that drives life becomes too depleted the organs no longer perform their functions, physical and mental strength become depleted, and there is true psychological depression.

The fact that the tongue tip is not red in this case seems to be an indication of the severity: the emptiness of *yang* is such that it is not able to warm the heart (we recall that the presence of fire from empty *yin* or patterns with relative excess *yang* manifestations is generally less serious than a situation in which the degree of consumption and exhaustion have led to an emptiness both of *yin* and of *qi/yang*).

The pulse may be rapid owing to false heat – in other words, to a condition of floating of the residual *yang*, but originating from an emptiness of *yang* (the pulse should, however, be bigger, whereas in this case it was weak, that is, soft, deep and thin).

In this situation a weak-*rou* pulse may appear and, in fact, I noticed a 'strange' quality in the pulse of this patient, but I was not able to define it exactly.[11]

Follow-up

The results of this treatment were not encouraging: agitation, restlessness and propensity to fatigue all remained, although more contained; however, the more alarming features had retreated sufficiently for him to be able to take care of both his son and his business.

His experience of tragedy does not seem to have modified his internal attitudes and behaviour modes, nor has he allowed himself a space for mourning; the absence of an internal period of withdrawal probably interfered with the restitution of his *qi*.

His recovery was later also impeded by his lifestyle – for example, just when a more stable base of *qi* had been restored the patient started a personal relationship, resulting in excessively intense sexual activity given his condition (three times a week, twice per night).

---

[11] In relation to these comments see also the 'exhaustion' phase in the discussion by Qiao Wenlei on stress syndromes (Chapter 18), the annotations by Barbara Kirschbaum on the semeiotic of the tongue (Chapter 17) and Appendix A on pulse.

Case Study 11.2

If Eating Is Too Difficult

A 45-year-old MD, who has never been particularly interested in Chinese medicine, was treated at the MediCina clinic during the period when Dr Qiao was present and afterwards by me.

The main motive for her first visit to the school was migraine, which she has been subject to since adolescence. The migraine attacks, which initially were linked to her menstrual period (which is scanty, with red blood and a cycle of 22–24 days) and to ovulation, had worsened over the past few years, in both frequency and intensity. The pain, which generally was intense enough to prevent her from working, is localised on the right side in the temporal–parietal zone, radiating to the nose, eyes and temple, with nasal obstruction and tears.

At the initial consultation she was decidedly underweight and very tired, with a meagre appetite, interrupted and non-restoring sleep, an often-early awakening immediately followed by a state of anxiety. She tended to feel cold, with cold extremities and frequent lumbar soreness.

Her tongue was soft, tooth marked, slightly pale but with a blue tinge and a redder tip, and the coating was yellow, slightly dry and not very thick. The pulse was wiry, thin especially in the *cun* position, and slightly choppy.

Dr Qiao's diagnosis was liver *qi* stagnation and emptiness of kidney.

The therapeutic principles were: tonify the kidney, invigorate *qi*, regulate the *Ren* and *Chong mai*, and tonify the emptiness of blood following the menstrual period.

Treatment consisted of four visits with weekly frequency where she needled a number of sore points on one side: TB-23 *Sizhukong*, GB-12 *Wangu* and EX-HN-9 *Taiyang* (in acute cases you first needle the point on the opposite side) and a number of points related to *Shao Yang*: GB-20 *Fengchi*, GB-21 *Jianjing*, GB-34 *Yanglingquan*, BL-18 *Ganshu* and BL-19 *Danshu*.

After the first treatment, with an immediate positive effect on the pain, Dr Qiao retained a few local points with light stimulation and added others to tonify the kidney, nourish the blood and regulate the *Chong mai*: Ren-4 *Guanyuan* and BL-23 *Shenshu*; SP-6 *Sanyinjiao* and HE-7 *Shenmen*; KI-12 *Dahe* and SP-4 *Gongsun*.

A number of ear acupuncture therapy points were also used with 'permanent' seeds (Liver, Gall bladder, *Shenmen*, Endocrine, Ovaries, Subcortex, Occipital, Temporal, Shoulder, Eye, Cheek, Heart and Kidney) and the wrist–ankle technique, leaving the needle in residence for 24 hours at the Upper-2 point.

The improvement was immediate on the migraine symptoms, which manifested with only mild paraesthesia, disturbance or precursors that did not develop into true pain.

When, 2 months later, her treatment is handed over to me, her marital relationship has broken down into a quite painful separation and her general situation is seriously compromised. She fears developing anorexia, which she suffered from in the past, and has recently started taking antidepressive medication.

Work has become very difficult, she sleeps little even when taking a tranquilliser, eating even minimal quantities of food causes nausea and vomiting, so she eats very little and in any case feels as though she has a 'closed' stomach.

Her migraine has reappeared only recently, but she is subject to dizziness, sporadic hot flushes and nocturnal sweating. Her bowel movements are diarrhoeic and her menstrual cycle is shortened, with a very scanty flow.

Her low voice, her withdrawn manner and her constantly composed manner of speech give the impression that the patient has to be careful in order to not lose the small amount of remaining *qi*.

She is pale, with a dull and lifeless complexion; already underweight (petite, she is 1.50 metres tall and in general weighs about 41 kilos), she has lost 6 kilos, her tongue is small, very pale, with a reddened tip, and the pulse is weak and thin.

Diagnosis
Constraint of liver *qi*, emptiness of *qi*, blood and *yin*.

Therapeutic Principles
Regulate and tonify *qi*, and nourish blood and *yin*.

Treatment
The treatment lasts for 1 year, with weekly visits during the first 2 months and then twice a month. Essentially, a number of avenues are pursued:

- GB-14 *Yangbai*, GB-41 *Zulinqi*, GB-20 *Fengchi*, EX-HN-9 *Taiyang* to invigorate *qi*, especially in the *Shao Yang* area of the head;
- Ren-4 *Guanyuan*, ST-29 *Guilai* (or KI-12 *Dahe*), HE-7 *Shenmen* and SP-6 *Sanyinjiao* (or SP-4 *Gongsun* and P-6 *Neiguan*) + ear *Sishencong* with a 'permanent' seed to nourish the *yin*, regulate the *Chong Mai* and calm the *shen*;
- Ren-15 *Jiuwei*, Ren-12 *Zhongwan*, ST-36 *Zusanli*, SP-3 *Taibai* to regulate *qi* that rises conversely and support the middle *jiao* in order to tonify spleen *qi*;
- LI-4 *Hegu* and LIV-3 *Taichong* to aid the circulation of *qi* (starting from the point that there is sufficient *qi* to work on).

As had previously happened – and as happens in general – the migraine attacks diminish starting from the first treatment.

The reappearance of her appetite is much slower. In the beginning, the nausea diminishes and the vomiting becomes more sporadic, thanks to which she manages to eat a little, but only in the third month does she manage to cook, and to find pleasure in certain foods and situations and she manages to regain three kilos.

At the end of the fifth month she has returned to her normal weight, her appetite has stabilised, her bowels have become regular, sleep and mood are much improved, she has rediscovered the enjoyment of thinking about a holiday and the pleasure of taking it.

The episodes of migraine are now rare and her menstrual cycle has stabilised at 26–27 days with a more abundant flow.

After an interval of 1 year she decreases and then completely stops taking medication and starts to talk about ending the therapy. After the Christmas holidays she spontaneously decides that it is time to try and make it on her own.

Comments

The emotional upsets had violently disturbed the *shen*, which had difficulty in remaining united and showed its restlessness through the pulse and tongue signs and the classic symptoms. The relationship changes inserted themselves into a system that was already in precarious balance and they immediately exhausted the *qi* and consumed the *yin*.

The scanty menstruation, the dull complexion, the blue-violet shading of the tongue and the roughness of the pulse show that the stagnation of liver *qi* has led to stasis and deficiency of blood. A disorder of the middle *jiao* is also detectable, with stomach *qi* rising conversely (the nausea, vomiting and stomach knotting) and not cooperating with the spleen in its function of transforming and transporting *qi* (diarrhoea and tiredness from *qi* deficiency).

The dominant feature, however, is the deficiency of *yin*, already detectable in the ascending *yang* that is barely anchored by an insufficient *yin* and now also evident in the manifestations of empty fire (hot flushes, sweating, and a small tongue with a redder tip). In this case the empty *yin* does not manifest so much in the more frequent signs and symptoms, but mainly in the lack of material – there is no meat; thought has consumed all the substance.

In Chinese texts, anorexia is considered as a symptom and corresponds to lack of appetite, but it is not considered an autonomous illness. In TCM, therefore, there is no specific pattern of anorexia; in order to classify it we follow the normal diagnostic methods and consider its primary symptoms (amenorrhea, weight loss and possibly, vomiting).

The TCM interpretation of the aetiological mechanism is that emptiness of *yin* is the central element, which in turn can derive from a depletion of *qi*, from heat produced by a constraint of *qi*/emotions, etc. In the dynamic relationship of *yin* and *yang* the mutual interaction in which *yin* nourishes *yang* and *yang* invigorates *yin* is broken, and all that remains is the counterpoint of movement-*yang* to substance-*yin*. This opposition without reciprocation manifests in anorexia as a spirit-*yang* that denies the needs of the body-*yin*, like a flame that burns matter.

In this case it was a matter of accompanying the patient through this great suffering, so that it could be lived without ever pushing away or denying the pain, and respecting her reserve, which may be a choice of dignity, a personal characteristic or a necessity in confronting the high risk of destabilisation. We repeat that, at times when there has been a major depletion of *qi*, such reserve can be a necessary self-defence and even speaking of one's emotions also becomes too much to bear.

Follow-up

After an interval of 20 months I see her again for a twisted ankle: the episodes of headache are sporadic and contained, she eats regularly, weighs 46 kilos, her menstruation is regular, she has an intense work life and has a number of activities that interest her very much.

Case Study 11.3

The Man Who Could No Longer Work

A 46-year-old man mentions that he went to the emergency department 20 days previously for a sudden and violent stomach pain, accompanied by paroxysmal tachycardia and shortness of breath. Examinations revealed a hiatus hernia, but no cardiac pathology.

A number of episodes of minor intensity had occurred since then, but with similar characteristics: sudden onset without any obvious cause, a feeling of notable instability and immense tiredness, laboured breathing, sweating, feelings of oppression in the lateral costal region and tachycardia. He furthermore mentions a vague unwell feeling that is more non-localised but continuous and extenuating, and, above all, he lives in anguish that these attacks may be repeated. The first episode, so unexpected and violent, made him feel as though close to death.

He is a tall man, with a solid physique, relaxed deportment and a pleasant way of speaking: he gives the impression of being used to feeling confident and at ease. However at this moment he is profoundly shaken and frightened owing to the sudden collapse of his normal sense of being in the world. More than anything, he is struck by the impossibility of continuing to work as he was used to doing, which was a great deal and without apparent fatigue, and his decreased efficiency in responding to the demands of a position in which he needs to evaluate complex situations and take decisions of responsibility.

In reality, moments of lateral costal oppression and slight tachycardia had already occurred over the past year. The birth of a son affected by a serious congenital defect three years earlier had induced him to 'realise that an equilibrium had been shattered'. He has trouble falling asleep notwithstanding the fact that he takes tranquillisers. He tends to be constipated. His blood pressure is 140/100 mmHg.

His tongue is slightly swollen and bright red, without major signs of blood stasis except for a light turgidity in the sublingual veins. The coating is sparse and totally absent in a number of areas. The pulse is wiry and deep.

Diagnosis
Qi constraint, *yin* deficiency and agitation of the *shen*.

Therapeutic principles
Free constraint and knotting of *qi*, tonify *qi* and blood, nourish *yin* and calm the *shen*.

Treatment

Seven treatments, with biweekly frequency (until the summer holiday).

The following are maintained:

- EX-HN-3 *Yintang*, Ren-17 *Shanzhong*, Ren-6 *Qihai* to regulate *qi* at the level of the three *dantian*.

Furthermore, the following are alternated:

- Ren-14 *Juque*, P-6 *Neiguan*, SP-4 *Gongsun*

and

- Ren-15 *Jiuwei*, HE-7 *Shenmen*, SP-6 *Sanyinjiao* or KI-3 *Taixi*.

The *Yin Wei Mai* is paired with *Chong Mai*, the *Du* points of the heart and *luo* points of the *Ren Mai* activate *qi*, move it down and open the chest.

The *yuan* points of heart and kidney and the meeting points of the *yin* of the leg tonify *qi*, blood and *yin*.

During the first treatments the patient mentions that he already has much more energy and feels generally well, even though an underlying anxiety remains. The *shen* of his eyes seems steadier.

After the third treatment he stops taking tranquillisers even if a certain difficulty in falling asleep remains.

During the fifth treatment he mentions that he managed to play golf well: a pain in his right shoulder that he had not told me about because it was of marginal importance at the time seems to have disappeared.

When, after less than 1 month, the therapy is concluded due to the summer break, the situation has lost its quality of urgency: at times, he 'feels his breath' – a sensation that he recognises as a precursor of the chest constraint, tachycardia and panic crisis, but only once, on an aeroplane, did it actually develop into an attack of medium proportions, with dyspnoea, palpitations and sweating.

His blood pressure has normalised and he manages to maintain good eating habits.

Tongue and pulse are unchanged except for a slight increase in the coating of the tongue (the turbidity of the coating is a *yin* quality; its absence indicates a great emptiness).

Comments

This case brings to mind the words of the *Neijing*: thoughts and worries, anguish and sorrow had knotted and depleted the *qi*.

The pain and apprehension linked to the birth of his son could only have affected him deeply. His lifestyle in the following years and in particular the work overload, contributed to the consuming of *yin*.

While recognising at the start a more profound emptiness of *yin* than the pathological pattern, given the limited number of treatments available the intervention was directed predominantly towards activating and regularising the movements of *qi*, the constraint of which was indicated by symptomatic manifestations and pulse signs, among other things. The hope was that this would lead to a greater balance and furnish the possibility of reconstituting the consumed *yin*.

What really influenced the course and allowed an improvement were the changes made in lifestyle. The modification of behaviour and attitudes make up a precondition for maintaining a state of health, and the need for these changes is even more evident in those cases in which *qi* and *yin* are injured by emotions and lifestyle habits.

EX-HN-3 *Yintang* was chosen to calm *qi* which becomes agitated and confused above, Ren- 17 *Shanzhong* to loosen its knotting in the centre, and Ren-6 *Qihai* to move it down and give it root.

These two combinations take into account both the constraint and the emptiness, with points that balance each other internally: in the first, the *mu* point of heart, which nourishes *qi*, was paired with the two *luo* points that activate it; in the second, the *luo* point of the *Ren Mai,* which activates strongly, was used together with two points that have a tonifying effect.

Within this last combination, SP-6 *Sanyinjiao* directs the action of HE-7 *Sishencong* towards a tonification of *yin* and blood, the residence of *shen*, while the *yuan* point of kidney KI-3 *Taixi*, directs its attention to *yin* in relation to the water–fire dynamics.

Signs and symptoms also show heat; in the absence of excessively violent fire, however, I preferred to orientate action towards the *qi* constraint and the consumption of *yin*, which were the cause of it at that moment, rather than treating the heat directly.

The regression of the shoulder pain demonstrates how a treatment based on prevalently psychic manifestations can influence channel pathology, just as, vice versa, in other cases the resolution of a somatic symptomatology implies an improvement in mood and sleep.

Follow-up

After an interval of one and a half years I speak with him by telephone and he tells me that he no longer suffers from panic attacks and that he feels fairly well. In the evening he takes a low dosage tranquilliser. He has distinctly diminished his workload and pays careful attention to his diet and physical exercise.

Case Study 11.4

The Frightened Woman

A 37-year-old woman tells me that she has suffered from anxiety attacks for the past 2 years that leave her worn out, and she feels that she can no longer bear it. More than anything, she is frightened by the idea that this situation could continue indefinitely and that she will no longer be able to return to her old self.

She has a lively appearance, her hairstyle and way of dressing are those of a young girl, but she is instead, a woman who has two children and has worked since she finished high school. She tells me that she has always been a very active person, that she loves to travel, and is happy with her husband, who has stayed close to her in this situation.

She has a vivacious expression and the *shen* of her eyes is good, but she is truly very frightened. She attributes her first panic attack to the period in which she had received the news of the death of a friend, during a time in which she was very worn out by her small children and a difficult home move.

Her distress, which in the past seized her mainly in the throat, lately manifests with episodes that last approximately an hour, starting with: 'my legs pull all over and at the same time give out'. Difficulty in breathing, palpitations, internal trembling, and extreme weakness, follow together with 'ugly thoughts' regarding the future of her children in the case of her death, a paralysing fear and an uncontrollable weeping. During the worst attacks, she also has the feeling that her fingertips harden.

Whereas at first the situation seemed to be improving, it has instead precipitated in the last six months, after the woman had left her job due to incompatibility with her superiors.

Sleep remains fairly good, except that at times she awakens early; her appetite and digestion are regular, but her bowels are constipated. Her menstrual cycle has always been a little short (23–25 days) with an abundant, red flow and sporadic clots.

Her tongue is slightly swollen and tooth marked, rather pale, but with a very red tip. The pulse is rapid and thin.

Diagnosis

Disharmony between heart and kidney, with water that does not control fire.

Therapeutic principles

Induce communication between heart and kidney, nourish water and calm fire.

Treatment

Seven treatments, approximately every 5 days.

I speak to her about the practice of *qigong* and also the possibility of a psychological type of approach, but I prefer to start with a Chinese energetic one in order to attempt to alleviate the symptoms.

First treatment:

- EX-HN-3 *Yintang*, Ren-6 *Qihai*, HE-5 *Tongli*, KI-4 *Dazhong*
- + ear point *Shenmen* with a 'permanent' seed.

This group of points is chosen to activate kidney and heart *qi* through their *luo* points in order to re-establish communication between water and fire, and to act on the central *Ren–Du Mai* axis so as to move *qi* down and stabilise it.

Second treatment, after an interval of 5 days: she shows up very frightened, tells of having been at the mercy of a devastating anxiety, totally out of control, 'like never before', due to which she could not stop weeping and had slept very poorly, with continuous palpitations. The following days had gone better, but she was really frightened; she fears that she will not be able to bear it and weeps.

A combination of points which maintains the same basis as before is chosen, but now more directed at calming the *shen* by tonifying heart blood and spleen *qi*.

- EX-HN3 *Yintang*, Ren-17 *Shanzhong*, Ren-4 *Guanyuan*, HE-7 *Shenmen*, SP-6 *Sanyinjiao*
- + ear point *Sishencong* with a 'permanent' seed.

Third treatment, 2 days later, during the first day of her menstrual flow: she had still felt 'turmoil, agitation, nervousness, tiredness, internal trembling as though there was a fever', but there were no panic attacks.

- EX-HN3 *Yintang*, Ren-17 *Shanzhong*, Ren-4 *Guanyuan*, HE-7 *Shenmen*, SP-6 *Sanyinjiao*, ST-36 *Zusanli*
- + ear point *Sishencong* with a 'permanent' seed.

The prescription is repeated with the addition of ST-36 *Zusanli* to reinforce the action on *qi* and blood.

Fourth–seventh treatments, after an interval of approximately 5 days: during the fourth treatment she tells me she caught a sort of stomach bug that has already been resolved and that she feels less agitated, and no longer feels the internal trembling or the sudden weakness and fear. Sporadic palpitations remain, but she has only wept twice and in a more contained manner. Bowel movements are now regular.

She spontaneously returns to the conversation about the idea of a more profound type of intervention, because 'otherwise it would seem to me to leave something up in the air, I would like to understand better what is happening to me and what it means'. Because it is not possible for me to find a space for her immediately, we will continue another few acupuncture treatments, which are necessary in any case to consolidate the results.

The following points are maintained:

- EX-HN3 *Yintang*, Ren-17 *Shanzhong*, Ren-4 *Guanyuan*, ST-36 *Zusanli*
- + ear point *Shenmen* with a 'permanent' seed;
  while these points are alternated:
- HE-5 *Tongli* and LIV-3 *Taichong*
  and
- HE-7 *Shenmen*, SP-6 *Sanyinjiao*.

The *luo* point of heart regulates its *qi* and the *yuan* point nourishes it, the meeting point of the three *yin* of the leg tonifies *yin*, and LIV-3 *Taichong* activates and nourishes liver *qi*.

Even if a few moments of anxiety with palpitations still appear, these events are sporadic and of moderate intensity, while the episodes of distress and desperate weeping have no longer been repeated. She feels well, is calm, sleeps well, and her bowel movements have become regular.

A number of conversations with a psychodynamic basis follow. After five appointments in which a generic exploration is performed, the patient feels that the work done is sufficient.

Comments

The physical and emotional overload in this patient had probably weakened kidney *qi*, whose emptiness manifested with trembling, fear and knees that felt like they were giving out.

The agitation by fire was evident at the moment in the pulse and tongue and in the symptoms of anxiety and panic, but the heat was already detectable in a number of elements in her medical history (attitudes, menstruation and bowel movements).

In this case, the consumption of kidney *qi* had not yet deeply injured the *yin* and the disorder derived mainly from a deficiency of *qi* and blood with an interruption in communication between water and fire.

A doubt remains about the accuracy of the evaluation made on the first visit, at which time I focused the action purposefully on moving *qi* between the heart and kidney through the *luo* points; it is difficult to say whether this was nevertheless an intervention that helped in the resolution or whether I had underestimated the fragility of the underlying condition and the deficiency of *qi*. If *qi* is deficient it is difficult to change its incorrect movement. The aggravation of the symptoms after the treatment may have also depended on my having overlooked the fact that the patient was premenstrual.

Follow-up

After an interval of 1 year there have been no relapses.

Stimulation Methods

12

'*Qi* arrives like a flock of birds, expands as though in a field of millet, its movements are like flights of birds whose origin you do not know; in the same way the physician must be ready to shoot his arrow like an archer in an ambush when the moment comes.'[1]

Practising acupuncture therefore requires ability.

When beginning the art of calligraphy, one passes months just tracing the vertical stroke: in this simple movement of the brush there is *yin* in *yang* and *yang* in *yin*, or at least there should be, while poor results are evidence of their absence.

The learning of any practice whose final act has roots in the body, in its sensitivities and in its deep movements shares similar characteristics. The art of acupuncture is one of these disciplines: when using needles one needs to be able to achieve *qi*, to perceive its presence, quality, and movement, and finally to move and direct it.

All this does not come immediately, it is necessary to have someone teach you the technique; learning requires time and attention and there is no limit to the refining of sensitivity and precision in this act.

The therapeutic results are deeply influenced by the clearness of diagnosis and the accuracy in the choice of points, but also by the ability of the acupuncturist when stimulating the needle and therefore guiding the *qi*. It is this ability that underlies differences in the presence of the needle in the body, in its interaction with the points and in its effects on *qi*.

In the classics we find various descriptions of the attainment of *qi*, *deqi*, such as: '[If one feels the needle] light, slippery, slow, the *qi* has not arrived; if heavy, rough, tight, the *qi* has arrived. The arrival of *qi* is like a floating and sinking, like a fish that goes for the bait; when, instead, *qi* does not arrive it is like finding oneself in the stillness of an empty hall'.[2]

---

[1] *Suwen*, Chapter 25. The *Jiayijing* dedicates a long chapter to acupuncture techniques (Book 5, Chapter 4). For a discussion on the tool-needle see also the discussion on the act of acupuncture in Chapter 15. For the description of simple and complex stimulating techniques see general acupuncture texts.

[2] Dou Hanqin, *Biaoyoufu* ('Ode to reveal the mysteries' 1295).

As we also find evident in the modern clinic, the specific modalities of stimulation are quite varied and their effectiveness is comparable, but in any event the technique of needling in its widest sense has a notable effect on the results of the treatment.

The written word is nevertheless an inadequate instrument for conveying these aspects that require direct transmission; in this text we have chosen to not indicate the type of stimulation of the needles, given that the concept of tonification or dispersion (reduction, draining) is implicit in the therapeutic principles, whereas their material application pertains to the experiential sphere and depends on the teachers with whom one has worked.

I would like to remind the reader only that in emotional disorders there is often fullness to eliminate and emptiness to tonify, but possibly even more frequently, at least in the initial phase, disorders with a strong emotional component correspond to a disruption in the movements of *qi*.

In the *Neijing* it is also quite clear that it is not always a question of empty and full, tonifying and dispersing, but it is often a case of disorderly movements for which it is necessary to guide the *qi* properly or consolidate the *jing*.

When Huang Di asks about the five disorders, after having learned the various points in response to his questions about the method and the *dao* of acupuncture, he continues: 'And tonifying and dispersing?' 'Inserting slowly and withdrawing slowly is called guiding *qi*, tonifying and dispersing without form is called unifying the *jing*, it is not excess or deficiency, but a counterflow of disordered *qi*.'[3]

To recognise, feel and know how to manage *qi* is also important in the relationship with the patient, in particular when he/she is in a state of emotional frailty and psychic disarray. In this sense a number of small tactics can be of help:

–Differentiate in time between the insertion of the needle and acting on the *qi*, in order to distinguish the moment of penetration, which should be painless, from the sensation of the work on *qi*, which will then be recognised as a specific experience.

–Mention specifically the possibility of modulating this action on *qi* and make sure that the patient can serenely ask to moderate its intensity.

–Ask about the patient's sensations, but at the same time make it clear that you are aware of what is happening, that you are perceiving it directly.

–Communicate to the patient when you intend to stimulate with more energy and ask more or less explicitly for permission.[4]

---

[3] *Lingshu*, Chapter 34. The terms used are: *wu luan* 无 乱 'five disorders', *bu* 补 'tonifying', *xie* 泄 'dispersing', *dao* 导 ¼ 'conducting', *wuxing* 五行 'shapeless', *'zhuangyi* 专一 unify', *youyu* 有 余 'excess', *buzu* 不 足 'insufficiency', *ni* 逆 'inversion', *luanqi* 乱 'disordered qi'.
[4] As example consider cases 7.2, 9.4, 10.1, 15.1 and 15.2.

COMPLEMENTARY TECHNIQUES[5]

The so-called complementary techniques are substantially significant in many patterns of illness, some in acute cases, other in chronic cases.

In the treatment of pathologies with strong psychic components, they complement the primary therapy well and at times turn out to be decisive in unblocking a situation.

In some cases they perform a supporting function in the intervals between treatments (for example, in the various instances in which a needle is left embedded), or they solicit aspects of active cooperation from patients (for example, when it is necessary for them to press on ear acupuncture seeds or use a moxa stick).

Moxibustion-*Jiufa* (灸法)

A discussion on moxibustion outside the context of acupuncture often turns out to be artificial, because the two techniques are tightly interwoven – so much so that the Chinese term normally used is *zhenjiu* (针 灸), 'needle-moxa'.

In the treatment of patients with significant psychic aspects to their illness, moxibustion is used to nourish the *yin*, tonify and warm the *yang*, but also to invigorate *qi*.

Depending on the clinical pattern, a needle warmed with moxa, a moxa stick, direct cones or moxa interposed with ginger, etc. is used. The technique which is most used in clinical cases of emotions is direct moxa with small cones the size of grains of rice (generally five to seven grains).

The stimulation of points through 'rice grain' direct moxa, suggested in many classic texts, is an important method in those conditions with important psychic and emotional components, because emotions tend to produce heat and consume *yin* and liquids, while the grain of moxa has the ability to move *qi* and, at the same time, to tonify deeply without drying or heating.

The points that are most often used in clinical practice for *shen* disorders are the following.

- The *shu* points of the back to act on the relative *yin* organs through the *yang*, such as:
  BL-13 *Feishu*, BL-15 *Xinshu*, BL-18 *Ganshu*, BL-20 *Pishu*, BL-23 *Shenshu*.
- BL-43 *Gaohuangshu* to tonify *qi* and *jing* in chronic emptiness disorders.
- Points on the *Renmai* such as:
  — Ren-12 *Zhongwan* to tonify the middle *jiao*;

---

[5] Denomination and localisation of all points and areas according to standard WHO (World Health Organization) classification, 1991.

— Ren-8 *Shenque* for the collapse of *yang* (with interposing of salt);

— Ren-6 *Qihai* and Ren-4 *Guanyuan* to nourish original *qi-yuanqi* and give residence to the *shen*.

- Points on the *Du Mai* such as:

— Du-20 *Baihui* to guide *qi* upward;

— Du-14 *Dazhui* to tonify *yang*;

— Du-4 *Mingmen* to act on the *mingmen*.

- The ST-36 *Zusanli* point to reinforce the post-heaven, *qi*, blood and *yin*.

Moxa may also be used to treat heat directly, but these are decidedly more delicate situations in which it is fundamental to have good clinical experience.[6]

For example, in cases of heat above, this can be guided downward through the classic method of 'small fire calls the big fire', which comprises the stimulation of KI-1 *Yongquan* or other points located below through a very limited number of cones.

It is also possible to free constrained fire through moxa on Du-20 *Baihui*.[7]

Cupping-*Baguan Liaofa* (把 罐疗发)

This is used in accordance with the usual diagnostic methods and principles of treatment.

Light cupping is used in cases of emptiness, whereas a more decisive action is indicated in cases of fullness (with the formation of a mark, due to which the patient's agreement should be asked). It can be used together with the needle to reinforce its action, especially in conditions of emptiness or cold.

When, instead, the technique of bleeding is used in cases of heat, the successive and immediate application of a cup facilitates the microhaemorrhaging.

In clinical cases of *shen* disorders, cupping is particularly good when stagnation produces contraction and hardness on the back.

The technique of 'moving' cups, or *zuoguan*, is preferred in cases of depressive disorders due to stagnation: a thin layer of a neutral oil may be applied and the cups are then slid down the back with medium force, along the *Du Mai*, the two branches of the bladder channel and horizontally between the two BL-15 *Xinshu* points, Bl-18 *Ganshu* points, etc. This method moves *qi* and blood vigorously and generally is not used initially, but it can be of great help in cases of stagnation of *qi* and the emotions. It calms the *shen* because it brings *qi* downward.

---

[6] See for example the discussion by E. Wagner of the Walden House community on the use of moxa in HIV+ patients with fever: 'Moxibustion: its use in the HIV Clinic', 1996 (Original: 1995)

[7] Mei Jianhan said that 'liberating the constrained fire', *yuhuo fazhi* 郁 火发之 unlike 'purifying the fire', means leaving a way out for it, 'as in the use of *sangye* (Folium Mori Albae) in the hypertension from liver fire'. MediCina seminar, June 1995.

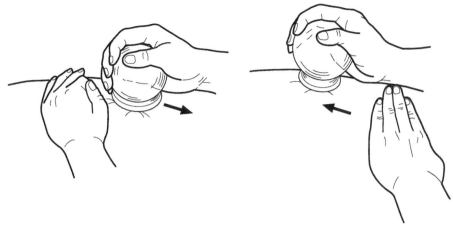

Figure 12.1 Cupping

'Plum-Blossom Needle'-*Meihuazhen* (梅花针)

Also known as 'cutaneous needling', this method can be of support in a wide variety of disorders, it does not penetrate into the tissues, and is extremely useful in children and in patients who are reluctant to have treatment with needles.

We recall that the 'plum-blossom' needle hammer has five needles, that of 'seven stars' has seven and the *luohan* type has eighteen. The hammer must be single use or sterilised after each treatment. The movement is one of percussion, rhythmic and flexible, coming from the wrist, and the head of the hammer moves perpendicularly to the skin without damaging it.

In cases of emptiness one tonifies with a light stimulation that slightly reddens the skin without causing pain. In cases of fullness, one disperses with a stronger stimulation, owing to which spots appear on the skin, or light bleeding may be produced, if one wishes to clear heat.

The 'plum-blossom' needle technique may precede 'moving' cupping in order to increase its specific effect.

In disorders with important psychic components, it is used mainly to move stagnation, which can manifest, for example, with asthma or breast pathologies. Stimulation of the upper back with the hammer can be of great help for freeing *qi* and circulating it.[8]

---

[8] See also the use of the plum-blossom needle in the treatment of insomnia according to Zhong Meiquan (Chapter 7).

Bleeding-*Sanlengzhen Liaofa* (Three-Edged Needle Method) (三 棱 针 疗法)

Bleeding clears heat and invigorates the blood. It is very effective in cases of heat above and in blood stasis. Its use should be kept in mind in cases with important emotional components when the restlessness of the *shen* is accompanied by signs of fire above, or when the pain related to blood stasis becomes chronic.

The points in which bleeding is most often used to calm the agitation or restlessness of the *shen* are as follows:

- EX-HN-10 *Erjian*, called the Apex of the ear in ear acupuncture: this is the primary point for clearing heat above that is of a full type; it is indicated in case of serious insomnia or chronic headaches and reduces systolic blood pressure. At least 8 to 10 drops of blood must be produced.
- EX-HN-5 *Taiyang*, GB-7 *Qubin*, Du-24 *Shenting*, Du-20 *Baihui*: these are used in cases of temporal, temporal–parietal, frontal and vertex symptoms respectively.
- GB-21 *Jianjing* or other points along the upper part of the gall bladder channel: these are used in cases of burning pain or contraction along the course of the main channel or the sinew-*jinjing* channel.
- Du-14 *Dazhui*: this point clears heat from the *yang* channels and regulates the immune system, especially in cases of itching or heat with skin signs.
- The back *shu* points: these are used in cases of heat in the *zangfu*, generally in the liver, gall bladder, and stomach.
- The *jing*-well points: these are used to clear heat and extinguish wind, especially in acute conditions, for example P-9 *Zhongchong*, HE-9 *Shaochong* or ST-45 *Lidui*.

The technique of pinching-*taici* – in which tissues of points in the *Tai Yang* area of the back are 'hooked' by the needle, shaken and possibly made to bleed– is utilised for clearing heat and stabilising emotions.[9]

Ear Acupuncture-*Erzhen* (耳 针)

The most widespread method involves the use of soapwort seeds, which in general are pressed by the patient three times a day or as needed (for example, in the evening in cases of insomnia), using 30 compressions each time or maintaining steady pressure for 1 minute.

The seeds may be substituted with magnetic plaques or metal spheres, which are, however, considered by many as being too hard and of too standard a size and surface quality.

---

[9] Mei Jianhan often uses this methodology. MediCina seminar, October 1997.

Needles are also used (generally 1 *cun* size, and rather thin), with the possibility of electrostimulation, or 2 mm intradermal needles may be applied leaving them in place for 4–5 days.

In any case, the correct localisation of the points is fundamental, and they should be searched for in the corresponding areas and defined according to their sensitivity in response to pressure (the patient should feel a sort of 'pain in the heart').

Five points are generally chosen (it is also possible to use a subcutaneous needle in order to reach more than one point) according to the following principles:

- somatotopic correspondence with the symptom;
- the *zangfu* are involved according to the theory of traditional Chinese medicine;
- the injured system according to conventional medicine;
- clinical experience.

The primary points for *shen* disorders are:

- Ear *Shenmen*: this is the most used point, whose action in calming the *shen* is fundamental in both agitation from fullness and in restlessness from empty heat; it is indicated in cases of anxiety or insomnia, but also in painful or dermatological pathologies, in order to calm down the emotions. It is used in all cases of dependency.
- Brain/Subcortex: this has a regulating action on the central nervous system (whereas *Shenmen* is more indicated for sedating). It treats disorders of the vegetative nervous system, pathologies of the digestive tract; cardiovascular, dermatological, allergic and inflammatory diseases. It has a pain reducing action and is one of the primary points for analgesia with ear acupuncture.
- Occiput: this calms the *shen* and extinguishes internal wind.
- Heart: this treats cardiac diseases and *shen* disorders.
- Mouth: this calms the *shen*, and is useful in all dependencies due to its calming effect on the mind.
- Ear apex: this clears heat. In general, bleeding is performed in mental disorders if there is fire present, in inflammatory diseases, fever, hypertension, itching, and burning pain in the lower limbs. In patterns with acute heat, in which the treatment must be repeated daily, Liver-*yang* and the six Helix points 1–6 are alternated with bleeding.

According to the clinical pattern, other points are added, for example:

- *qi* stagnation: Liver, Gall bladder, Triple Burner;
- emptiness of *qi*: Kidney, Spleen, + Diaphragm (in cases of blood emptiness);
- *yin* emptiness: Kidney, Liver + Heart (in cases of palpitations) or + Endocrine, Uterus, Ovaries (in cases of gynaecological disorders or menopause);
- autonomic nervous system disorders: Sympathetic.

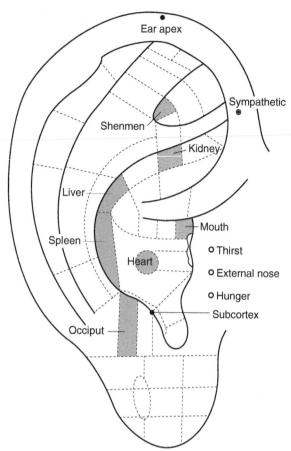

Figure 12.2 Primary points that are related to psychic disorders in ear acupuncture

For dependency, the primary points are:

- Smoking: Mouth, Ear *Shenmen*, Lung (in the point where there is pain under pressure, if both respond, needle both). In accordance with the various protocols, Brain/Subcortex, Sympathetic, Trachea are added, or points according to the specific pattern (for example, Liver, Spleen, Kidney or points which correspond to the location of a possible headache, etc.).
- Alcohol: Mouth, Ear *Shenmen*; Stomach.
- Food: Mouth, Ear *Shenmen*; Stomach, Triple Burner, the two Hunger and Thirst points (points classified in the charts which preceded the WHO standardisation, located on the tragus, above and below the External nose point).

Wrist–Ankle-*Wanhuaizhen* (腕踝 针) Technique

This reflexology-type technique elaborated in the early seventies, comprises the subcutaneous insertion of a needle, which should produce neither pain nor a sensation of *deqi*.[10]

The needle is then fixed with a plaster and generally left in place for a variable amount of time from 1 to 24–48 hours.

The two most used points in emotional disorders are:

- Upper-1: on the ulnar edge of the ulnar flexor tendon of the carpal, 2 fingers from the wrist crease. It is used for disorders that do not have a specific location; in particular for calming the mind.
- Upper-5: on the median line of the dorsal side of the forearm, at two fingers-width from the wrist crease. It is specifically indicated in those pathologies in which there is pain and contraction in the relevant area – the dorsal side of the upper extremity, shoulder, trapezoid, neck, or lateral area of the head.

Scalp Acupuncture-*Touzhen* (头针)

Scalp acupuncture was developed at the beginning of the seventies by physicians with Western medical training, who started from the study of acupuncture and combined with modern anatomical/physiological knowledge.[11]

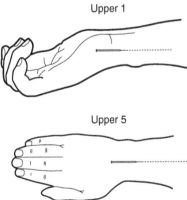

Upper 1

Upper 5

Figure 12.3 The two primary points for emotional disorders in the wrist–ankle technique

[10] The technique was created by Zhang Xinshu, a neurologist with a western background working at the Second Military Medical University in Shanghai. Liu Gongwang, 1998, ascribes its birth to the Neurology Department of the First Teaching Hospital affiliated to the Second Military Medical University of Xi'an, possibly because this university was moved to Xi'an for some years during the Cultural Revolution. See also the contribution by Qiao Wenlei on stress disorders (Chapter 18).
[11] See also: Jiao Shunfa, *Scalp Acupuncture and Clinical Cases*, 1997; 'Standard Acupuncture Nomenclature', WHO, 1991; the seminar on scalp acupuncture by Gu Yuehua, professor at the University of Nanjing, MediCina, October 2000. The classification follows the so-called 'standard' or 'new' style (WHO, Tokyo 1984), where lines are defined as MS (micro-systems).

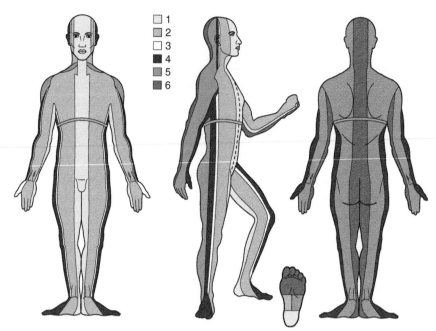

Figure 12.4 The six zones treated by points 1–6 of the wrist–ankle technique

Cutaneous zones that correspond to superficial projections of cortical areas are stimulated.

Scalp acupuncture is very effective in many pathologies of the central nervous system.

In 'emotional disorders' it is a secondary choice compared with somatic acupuncture, but is nevertheless suitable as a complementary method, or it may already be used from the start in cases in which the patient does not well tolerate somatic acupuncture and the sensation of *deqi*.

It can assume a decidedly important role in more serious pathologies, such as during psychotic crises and in *diankuang* patterns.

The most used points are:

- MS-1 from Du-24 *Shenting* for 1 *cun* downwards, along the median line: for neuropsychiatric disorders such as insomnia, memory disorders, depression, psychosis, epilepsy, convulsions, and diseases of the head.
- MS-5, from Du-20 *Baihui* to Du-21 *Qianding*: for the same neuropsychiatric disorders, with accompanying lesions of the lower part of the body at the central nervous system level (paralysis of the lower extremities, urinary incontinence, etc.).

Joined by:

- MS-2, from BL-3 *Meichong* for 1 *cun* downward, parallel to the median line: for cases with chest symptoms and breathing disorders.

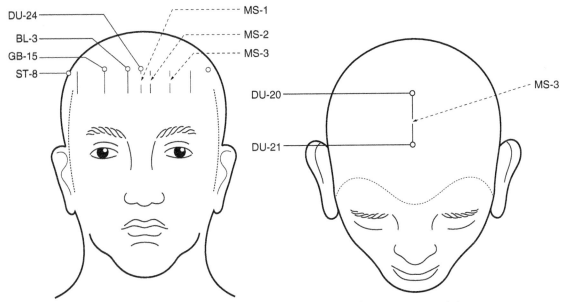

Figure 12.5 Principle points which relate to psychic disorders using the scalp acupuncture technique

- MS-3, 1 *cun* from GB-15 *Toulinqi*, for 1 *cun* downward, parallel to the median line: for cases with abdominal symptoms and digestive disorders.

Electrostimulation-*Dianzhen* (电 针)

Electrostimulation of somatic points is not commonly used in the treatment of emotional disorders. Its use is mentioned in more serious psychiatric cases with the presence of delirium and hallucinations.[12]

Used with scalp acupuncture, it has been presented as a valid alternative to the electroconvulsive treatment used for schizophrenia.

If electrostimulation is used with scalp acupuncture, the intensity tends to be greater than with somatic acupuncture; the type of wave is generally continuous, with medium frequency (normally, it is low for somatic acupuncture and high for analgesia).

Dense-disperse waves are used in treatments that are repeated at short intervals, since this avoids the development of tolerance (this method alternates

---

[12] On this issue see the text on schizophrenia edited by T. Dey, 2000, where one can find discussions borrowed from 14 articles published in the 80s (p.105–109) and where it is said: 'In case of hallucinations one can use, as an addition to common psychotherapy, the following points: *Fengchi* GB-20, *Tinghui* GB-2 and *Taichong* LIV-3, all bilateral, to drain the minister fire of liver and spleen bladder, to purify the heart and *shen* and to calm the orifices of the eyes and ears.' (p. 72).

periods of high frequency, 50–100 hertz, with periods of low frequency, 2–5 hertz, 16 or 24 times per minute).

Electrostimulation is contraindicated in cases of:

- poorly controlled hypertension
- uncooperative patients or those unable to communicate
- spastic pathologies or those with rigidity
- use of a pacemaker.

Case Study 12.1

Drinks and Depression

This woman came to me for the first time at the suggestion of her baker; 10 years have passed since then, and approximately once a year she comes in for a treatment course consisting of 8–10 appointments.

She was 54 years old then and entering menopause. Well groomed, with lively eyes, she was however, both overweight in her body and heavy in her thoughts.

She complained of joint pain in her hands, neck, and knees and had been prescribed a tranquilliser and an antidepressant, which, however, she did not take.

Diagnosis and Therapeutic Principles

Over time, her main symptoms had been: tiredness, interrupted sleep, constipation, palpitations, headache, heaviness in the hypochondria, nausea, and bad moods. Various therapeutic principles were followed, such as nourish the *yin* and drain empty fire, extinguish wind and resolve dampness in the channels, and pacify liver *yang*, but the main task always consisted of freeing the liver *qi* stagnation.

Treatment

It became progressively clearer even to her that the periods of physical malaise corresponded to those moments in which she felt more unhappy and irritable. She spoke of not having major reasons for being unsatisfied, but in those periods she angered easily and suffered above all from the lack of appreciation by one or another person that was close to her, who disappointed her by not recognising how much she was doing for them or offended her by not listening to her advice.

The periods of therapy generally help her get past these impediments: 'Acupuncture removes the black cloud, I have less rancour, am less anxious, more optimistic; otherwise I become fixated on things, and I also become forgetful'. Her relatives tell her that she becomes less impossible, and the amount of Lexotan that she takes goes down from 50 to 20 drops or is completely suspended.

At times she seems to be looking for advice, but it is only a sham: she asks for detailed instructions for the bus but always comes by taxi, she does not follow any suggestions regarding diet or physical activity, she has never used moxa at home as I had suggested, and she is a long way from accepting any hint that she needs to work on herself.

Three years ago I see she is particularly gloomy, and with great embarrassment she tells me that she may have a 'drinking problem'. In the morning she drinks one or two martinis at the bar 'to calm her anxiety'. I answer that in order to understand if and how big a problem this is she should try to abstain from any alcohol for 7 days. Since she tells me at the next appointment that it had been impossible for her, I propose a treatment using points from the Acudetox protocol, even if there is time for only four appointments before I leave for a holiday. A cycle of treatments similar to those she already knows can be given upon my return if needed.

I use the five auricular points, leaving the needles in for 20 minutes, with treatments on alternate days.

I do not ask about the progress of the treatment; during the third treatment she says that she is dizzy and very nervous, but I do not comment. During the fourth treatment she says that she feels like a new woman, she no longer drinks, has lost 4 kilos in weight and is truly satisfied.

Follow-up

A year later she returns, worried because she has started drinking one or two beers in the morning. Three treatments using the Acudetox protocol points are sufficient to stop the habit. She feels well also because 'I think of the glass of beer and the thought dissolves'.

She calls me again after 8 months because she has again started to drink a beer in the morning and we once again have four appointments with the auricular points, in this case, however, followed by a more complex treatment.

Comments

This is not the place to comment on the effectiveness of the Acudetox protocol, which, among other things, has been modified in this case given the different setting, but the experience does provide a number of points for further thought.

In this case, the outcome was positive, the results with regard to the alcohol dependency were probably facilitated by the fact that the woman was very motivated, frightened by the idea of becoming an alcoholic, and furthermore she had a prior trust in my therapeutic proposals.

The cyclic recurrence of the same situation brings us back to a well-known point, which we risk overlooking at times: the disappearance of the symptoms does not coincide with the resolution of the causes the pathogenic conditions that originally produced them.

Points with Diverse Applications

13

The *Ren Mai* and *Du Mai* points that recur most frequently in pathologies with prevalent psychic components are revisited here independently from the specific clinical patterns in order to clarify their diverse therapeutic effects and differentiate their usage.

Heart and pericardium points are then discussed together in order to establish their specific actions and compare them, so as to avoid excessive repetition in the text.[1]

PRINCIPAL POINTS OF THE *REN MAI* AND *DU MAI* IN RELATION TO *SHEN* DISORDERS

The *qijing*, the extraordinary or curious channels, function as a reservoir of energy that can supply *qi* and blood to the main and secondary channel system in cases of deficit or accept them in cases of abundance.

The *Ren* and *Du Mai* are the deep paths along which *qi* moves in its *yin* and *yang* aspects. They also form a circuit called the 'small circulation', along which are found the primary sites where *qi* is stored, accumulated and transformed: including the *dantian*, or 'cinnabar fields', in front and the *mingmen*, or 'gate of life', behind.[2]

---

[1] The most important texts for reference on points are: the detailed and complete *A Manual of Acupuncture* by Deadman and Al-Khafaji, 1998; the text from the excellent publishing house Huaxia, *Acupoints and Meridians*, 1996, which also showing classical prescriptions; the two atlases of the Shandong and Beijing academies, *Anatomical Atlas of Chinese Acupuncture Points*, 1982, and *The Location of Acupoints*, 1990.

[2] *Dan* 丹 'cinnabar', is mercury sulphide, one of the most important substances in alchemy practices. *Ming* 命 means 'destiny, fate; life; decree, ordinance'; the life which comes to us from the pre-heaven, from that which comes before our birth.

Being energetic fields on which the internal practices work, their location does not coincide precisely with specific anatomical locations: 'Dantian is an area in which true qi accumulates and is stored. Over time the masters of qigong placed it in various locations. In summary, it can be clarified into the upper, middle and lower dantians. The majority of qigong masters call the upper dantian niwan (mud pill) and they place it at the Du-20 Baihui point on top of the head; the Huangting Neijing ('Classic of the Yellow Court') calls it zuqiao (portal of the ancestors) and places it at 3 cun inside the EX-HN-3 Yintang point between the eyebrows. The middle dantian is located in the Ren-17 Shanzhong point between the two nipples and is called jianggong (scarlet palace), but a few locate it in the umbilicus. The lower dantian is located in the lower abdomen below the umbilicus, usually in the upper two-thirds of the line that joins the umbilicus with the pubic symphysis. An area is referred to rather than a specific point, and a few believe it is located at Ren-1 Huiyin or KI-1 Yongquan'.[3]

Ren Mai

The Ren Mai is the sea of yin, and has a nourishing function.[4]

Its action on alterations of the psyche is linked to the function of its points in nourishing yin and blood, the residence of shen, and their ability to regulate the movements of qi in cases of constraint, knotting and converse rising.[5]

We note that the points of the Ren Mai, kidney, and stomach that are at the same level often have similar actions, so that they can be used in association to reinforce the therapeutic effect.

Ren-4 Guanyuan

Meeting point of the spleen, liver, and kidney, mu point of the small intestine.

Principal Actions

— Nourishes yin and blood.
— Reinforces yuanqi, tonifies the kidney and benefits jing.
— Regulates uterus and small intestine.

---

[3] Chinese Qigong, 1988, p. 31. On practices for the nourishment of like and a hint on the 'three gates' see also Chapter 1. The lower dantian 丹田 may correspond to Qihai Ren-6 or to Guanyuan Ren-4. Sometimes Shenting Du-24 is considered to be the access to the 'dung ball' niwan 泥丸. (The term niwan may also be a transliteration of 'nirvana' and it recalls the egg laid by the female dung-beetle at the end of a gallery dug in cow and hearse droppings. The female covers the egg in excrements that will serve as food for the maggots, her offspring.)

[4] The character ren 任 means 'to occupy oneself with, to take care of'. See also in Chapter 3 the note relative to yi and zhi and to the heart, which 'takes care' of things according to Chapter 8 of the Lingshu. The same character ren 任 preceded by the radical 'woman' means 'to give birth, pregnant'.

[5] On this issue see: the protocol for anxiety used in a public structure (Chapter 23); the comments by Jin Shubai in Chapter 20 and case studies 5.1, 7.4, 9.1, 9.2, 9.4, 10.3, 10.5 and 11.3.

Notes

By nourishing *yin* and blood it calms the *shen* when this is agitated due to lack of an abode.

Ren-6 *Qihai*

Principal Actions

— Tonifies *qi* and reinforces *yang*.
— Regulates *qi* and guides it downward.

Notes

It acts on confusion of the *shen* because it regulates disorderly movement of *qi* and moves it down.

Ren-12 *Zhongwan*

Mu point of the stomach and the middle *jiao*, *hui*-meeting point of the *fu*, meeting point of the stomach, small intestine and lung channels.

Principal Actions

— Tonifies stomach and spleen.
— Regulates stomach *qi*.

Notes

It is important in *shen* disorders both because it tonifies the middle *jiao* and therefore deficiencies of *qi* and blood, and also because it invigorates and regulates *qi*, whose functions of transforming and transporting are often compromised by the emotions.

Ren-14 *Juque*

Mu point of the heart.

Principal Actions

— Regulates heart *qi* and calms the *shen*.
— Moves down conversely rising *qi* and opens the chest.
— Clears heat and resolves phlegm.

Notes

Because it regulates *qi* of the heart, of which it is the *mu* point, and moves down knotted or conversely rising *qi*, it acts on alterations of the *shen* especially in cases of lateral costal symptoms of emotional origin; these include irritation, pain, heaviness or burning sensations referred to the stomach, the heart or the 'opening of the stomach'; in the classics they are often called *xinfan*, or 'restlessness in the heart'.

Ren-15 *Jiuwei*

Luo point of the *Ren Mai*.

Principal Actions

— Invigorates heart blood and *qi*.
— Calms the *shen* and resolves phlegm.
— Regulates and moves down lung *qi* and opens the chest.

Notes

Being a *luo* point, it is useful in moving *qi* when there is constraint and knotting of *qi* with sensations of oppression and heaviness, or in cases of phlegm that obstructs the heart with dimming of the *shen*.[6]

Ren-17 *Shanzhong* (or *Tanzhong*)

Mu point of the pericardium, *mu* point of the upper *jiao*, *hui*-meeting point of *qi*, point of the sea of *qi*, meeting point of the *Ren Mai* with the spleen, kidney, small intestine and *San Jiao* (Triple Burner) channels.

Principal Actions

— Regulates and tonifies *qi* of the upper *jiao*.
— Moves down *qi* and resolves phlegm.

Notes

It is used in cases of conversely rising *qi*, constraint and phlegm, which can manifest as a weight on the chest, a knot in the throat, breathlessness, or obstructed flow of breast milk.

Stimulation often produces an initial sensation of strong irritation or oppression, followed by a feeling of relief and opening.

Needling is directed downward or at times, in a 'chicken feet' manner – in other words, directing the needles also to the left and right respectively at a 45° angle to the midline.

---

[6] In the *Jiayijing* ('The systematic classic of acupuncture and moxibustion') and in the *Zhenjiu dacheng* ('Great compendium of acupuncture and moxibustion') the point *luo* of the *Ren Mai* is instead *Changqiang* Ren-1. We also recall that *Jiuwei* Ren-15 is the *yuan* point of the *gao* 膏 area, under the heart.

Ren-22 *Tiantu*

Meeting point of the *Ren Mai* with the *Yin Wei Mai*, point of the window of heaven.

Principal Actions

— Clears heat and resolves phlegm.
— Regulates *qi* and frees constraint.

Notes

This is an important point for resolving plum-stone *qi*, *meiheqi*.

Du Mai

The action of *Dumai* on *shen* is related to the kidney function of nourishing marrow and brain.[7] The internal path of the *Dumai* passes through the brain, whose role in relation to the mental faculties is clearly recognised in Chinese medical tradition.

Being the sea of *yang*, its points act both on emptiness of *yang* and on its excess above. Its important functions in alterations of the *shen* are those of tonifying *qi* and *yang*, clearing heat, extinguishing wind, and opening the portals of the heart that have been dimmed by phlegm.

The points of the *Dumai* on the head are often repeated in classic and modern prescriptions for cognitive or psychiatric disorders. Of the 13 *gui* points of Sun Simiao, three are on the *Dumai*: Du-26 *Renzhong*, Du-16 *Fengfu*, and Du-23 *Shanxing*, later substituted for Du-24 Shenting by Gao Wu.[8]

Du-4 *Mingmen*

Principal Actions

— Tonifies kidney *yang* and warms the fire of *mingmen*.
— Nourishes *yuanqi* and benefits *jing*.

Notes

Located at the same level as the *shu* point of the kidney, BL-23 *Shenshu*, and BL-52 *Zhishi* (also called the palace of essence, *jinggong*), these three points can be tonified together to support the kidney in its role as the origin of *yang* and

---

[7] The character *du* 督 contains the radical 'eye' and means 'to supervise, direct, govern'.
[8] With regard to the role of the brain see also Deadman and Al-Khafaji, 2000; for a discussion on the 13 *gui* points see Chapter 8 on *diankuang*-madness; on the use of certain points in severe mental disorders see the contributions by Zhang Mingjiu (Chapter 19) and by Jin Shubai (Chapter 20).

residence of *yuanqi* and *jing*. In this sense, direct moxa with small cones of the size of rice grains is very useful.

Du-8 *Jinsuo*

Principal Actions

–Calms the liver and extinguishes internal wind.

Notes

Located at the same level as the *shu* point of the liver BL-18 *Ganshu* and that of BL-47 *Hunmen*, it shares many qualities with them and these three points can be used at the same time in cases of agitation of liver *yang*.

Du-11 *Shendao*

Principal Actions

–Tonifies heart and lung.
–Clears heat and extinguishes internal wind.

Notes

Located at the same level as the *shu* point of the heart BL-15 *Xinshu* and that of BL-44 *Shentang*, it shares their action of nourishing the heart, clearing heat and calming *shen*. These three points are often used at the same time.

Du-14 *Dazhui*

Meeting point of the three *yang* channels of the hand and foot, point of the sea of *qi*.

Principal Actions

–Disperses external wind and extinguishes internal wind.
–Clears heat and circulates *qi* in the *yang* channels.
–Regulates and tonifies *qi* and *yang*.

Notes

This is a very useful point in many cases, such as *shen* disorders associated with stagnation of *qi* in the occipital, neck or upper back areas (for example, in neck pain linked to stress), or when one chooses to act on the *Du Mai* treating a high point together with a low point (for example, with Du-26 *Renzhong*, Du-24 *Shenting*, or Du-20 *Baihui* and with Du-4 *Mingmen* or Du-1 *Changqiang*), or for tonifying *qi* and *yang* – for example in retarded development in children or to support defensive *qi*.

Du-16 *Fengfu*

Meeting point with *yinweimai,* point sea of marrow.

Principal Actions

— Extinguishes wind and calms the *shen.*
— Benefits the marrow and the head.

Notes

The *Dumai* enters the brain at this point and from here also the descending branch of the *Dumai* emerges.

Du-20 *Baihui*

Meeting point of the three *yang* channels of the hand and foot and the liver channel.

Principal Actions

— Resolves phlegm that has dimmed the portals of the heart and calms *shen* agitation.
— Extinguishes internal wind and guides *qi* upward.

Notes

It should be dispersed or bled when there is fullness above and emptiness below. It should be tonified or stimulated with moxa to raise the *qi.*

    Its action on confusion or agitation of the *shen* can be reinforced by the four extra points that surround it, EX-HN-1 *Sishencong.*

Du-24 *Shenting*

Meeting point of the *Dumai* with the bladder and stomach channels.

Principal Actions

— Resolves phlegm, opens the portals and calms the *shen.*
— Extinguishes wind and benefits the brain, nose and eyes.

Notes

Its action is similar to that of EX-HN-3 *Yintang* and these two points may be used in association to reinforce their action. This point may be reached with the needle starting from Du-23 *Shangxing* or from Du-20 *Baihui*, or one can start from Du-24 *Shenting* to reach the top of the head; the first stimulation is generally considered to be more intense and energetic whereas the second acts by eliminating the excess above in a milder fashion; however, this also of course depends on the way of stimulating of the needle.

Du-26 *Renzhong*

Meeting point of the *Dumai* with the *Yang ming* channel of hand and foot.

Principal Actions

— Opens the orifices and calms the *shen*.
— Frees the channel and benefits the brain, face and spinal column.

Notes

Its name, 'the centre of man', refers to its position between heaven and earth: it is, in fact, located between the nose/breathing and the mouth/food.

This point brings *yin* and *yang* back together when they are about to separate, manifesting as sudden loss of consciousness, or its serious weakening or alteration (such as convulsions or coma, dimming of cognitive function or demented, delirious or manic states).

EX-HN-3 *Yintang*

Extra point.

Principal Actions

— Opens the orifices that have been dimmed by phlegm and regulates the channel.
— Extinguishes wind and calms the *shen*.

Notes

Even though it has never been included in the *Dumai* points, this point was already discussed in the first classics.

It is a fundamental area in the contemplative traditions of many cultures and one of the most used for regulating the *shen*.

It is also a point that tends to be perceived in various ways; in fact, in comparison with other points, patients speak of it more often or ask us to have it repeated.

BACK *SHU* POINTS AND CORRESPONDING POINTS OF THE LATERAL BRANCH OF THE BLADDER CHANNEL

The *shu* points of the back have a direct relationship with the energy of their related organs and viscera.[9]

Located on the back, they guide *yang* energy inwardly – in other words to the *yin*.

They are used in this sense mostly in chronic pathologies of the five *zang* and their various related aspects (sense organs, tissues, emotions, etc.).

They also, however, have the ability to clear heat from the organs.

The selection of back *shu* points is closely related to the patient's reactions on palpation (painfulness, contraction) and may change during the course of a treatment after stimulation of the distal points.

On the external branch of the bladder channel, at the level of the five *shu* points of the organs, we find the points that contain the names of the 'psychic souls' within their names: BL-42 *Pohu*, BL-44 *Shentang*, BL-47 *Hunmen*, BL-49 *Yishe* and BL-52 *Zhishi*. However, these points, despite the suggestiveness of their names, do not actually seem to be used for disorders related to the particular psychic aspects, either in the classics or in the modern clinic.[10]

In treatment they are often associated with the related *shu* point and possibly with the *Dumai* point that is found at the same level. The EX-B-2 *huatuojiaji* points may also be taken into consideration.

HEART AND PERICARDIUM POINTS

Discussions on the heart and pericardium are found throughout the history of Chinese medicine, starting from the first discrepancy: the absence of a pericardium channel in the most ancient texts, found at Mawangdui.[11]

The structure of the 12 channels, including their names and directions, was already defined by the time of the *Neijing*, but the heart channel is not needled in order to avoid the dispersion of *shen*. Rather, it is said that the heart, being the residence of the *shen*, is defended against attack from external pathogens

---

[9] The character *shu* 輸 means 'transport' and is formed by the radical 'vehicle' and by the phonetic part 'boat'.

[10] In *Suwen*, Chapter 61, there is precise reference to their action of eliminating the heat.

[11] The texts found in the Mawangdui tomb, dated 168BC, were composed between the 3rd and 2nd century BC, but their content is more ancient. For a discussion on the evolution of the theory of meridians see also Giulia Boschi, 1997, Chapter 10.

by the pericardium, *xinbao* (heart wrapping), which envelops the heart and has no independent structure.[12]

All the points on the heart and pericardium channel calm the *shen* and have a greater or lesser ability to clear heat. In the clinic, the use of points on these two channels overlaps in many ways, but both channels and individual points also have well-defined characteristics.

The pericardium-*xinbao* is the ministerial fire, *xianghuo*, and envelops the heart protecting it from pathogens.

The pericardium channel descends through the middle and lower *jiao*, is paired with the *sanjiao* and is *jueyin* together with the liver.

Its points have a more specific effect than those of the heart in regulating and moving *qi* at the level of the chest and abdomen (they also regulate the *qi* of lung, stomach and liver). They are better indications in cases of febrile diseases, when external heat has penetrated into the *Yang Ming* and the more internal levels (with damp-heat in the stomach-intestines and heat that agitates the nutritive level and the blood).

The heart, rather, is the sovereign fire, *junhuo*, the ruler of the *zangfu*. The heart is the residence of the *shen*, whose clarity and brightness come from the heart; all emotions go to the heart. The points of the heart are therefore fundamental in treating disorders of the emotions and of the *shen*.

Furthermore, the heart has a specific relationship with the uterus through the *baomai* (uterus channel) and acts on heat in the skin.[13]

All the points have indications in emotional disorders, with symptoms such as restlessness, palpitations, and insomnia, but the choice of points will depend on the identification of the specific pattern: concomitant wind or phlegm, blood stasis, emptiness of *yin* and liquids, penetration of heat into the blood, involvement of stomach *qi*, etc.

---

[12] As a reference to *xinbao* we quote some of the arguments under debate: the *Lingshu*, Chapter 71, says: 'The heart governs the five *zang* and the six *fu*, it is the place where the *shen* is held, as an organ it is solid and cannot host the pathogenic *qi*. If pathogenic *qi* settles in it, the heart is damaged; if the heart is damaged the *shen* moves away, if the *shen* moves away one dies. This is why, when pathogenic *qi* settles in the heart, it is actually in the pericardium. The pericardium is the channel governed by the heart.'; in the *Nanjing*, Chapter 35, it is specified that: '*Xinbao* has an internal–external relationship with *sanjiao*, both have a name but no shape'. Later texts adopt different interpretations: 'In the *Nanjing* it is said of the pericardium that it has no shape, but in the *Neijing*, where it speaks of the 12 officers [*Suwen*, Chapter 8, where *tanzhong* is called officer, carrying out the ordinances of the prince and minister] the name pericardium is absent, it is called instead *tanzhong*. *Tanzhong* is the 'nest' of the heart; the heart is preserved in a nest, as wrapped in a casing. This is why *tanzhong* corresponds to the pericardium and one cannot maintain that it has no shape.' in: He Mengyao, *Yibian* ('Elements of medicine').

[13] ' If menstruation do not come, the *baomai* is closed. *Baomai* belongs to the heart and is connected to the centre of the womb. If the *qi* rises and constricts the lung then the heart *qi* can not pass underneath, so the menstruation does not come.' *Suwen*, Chapter 33. E: 'Pain, itching and ulcers are caused by the heart', *Suwen*, Chapter 74.

Jing Point and Wood Point – P-9 *Zhongchong* and HE-9 *Shaochong*

The action of the *jing*-well points of the heart and pericardium is very similar: both of them clear heat and extinguish internal wind, open the orifices and restore consciousness.

The *jing*-well points are very powerful: they are the place where *qi* changes from *yin* to *yang* or vice versa and the *qi* that runs through the channels spouts from them. Here *qi* is close to the surface and is influenced quickly and powerfully.

They strongly disperse pathogenic factors and are used in acute conditions, and especially mainly if due to fullness or heat above (often with bleeding); they act on the *shen* in cases of serious comprising of consciousness, in cases of fainting and of coma, and also in cases where the *shen* is altered or dimmed and in *diankuang* patterns.

In the classics, many *jing* points are also used for *shen* disorders due to emptiness such as fear, timidity, sighing, insomnia and sleepiness.[14]

Ying Point, Fire Point – P-8 *Laogong* and HE-8 *Shaofu*

Being *ying*-spring points, both these points eliminate pathogenic factors and heat in particular.

HE-8 clears heat from the heart, from its paired *yang*, the small intestine, and from the bladder, as the paired channel at *taiyang* level.

P-8 *Laogong* has a more specific action on febrile diseases with heat at the level of nutritive *qi* and blood, and it drains fire of the pericardium and stomach.

Shu and *Yuan* Point, Earth Point – P-7 *Daling* and HE-7 *Shenmen*

P-7 *Daling* and HE-7 *Shenmen* are both earth points, the child element of fire in the generating-*sheng* cycle, and they therefore perform a draining and dispersing action on heat. They are, however, also *yuan*-source points, the place where *yuanqi* surfaces in the channels. These two aspects reflect their functions.

---

[14] See also the chapter on the categories of points in Deadman and Al-Khafaji, 1998. Remember that the *jing* points also treat the inside: 'When the illness is in the organ puncture the *jing* points. [...] The five organs correspond to the winter, in winter puncture the *jing* points.' *Lingshu*, Chapter 44.

P-7 *Daling* has greater properties as a dispersion point and is very effective for clearing heat at the level of the blood; furthermore it regulates *jueyin* and stomach.

As a *yuan* point, HE-7 *Shenmen*, which regulates the heart, is more effective in opening the heart's portals and tonifying both its *qi* and blood.

Jing Point, Metal Point – P-5 *Jianshi* and HE-4 *Lingdao*

P-5 *Jianshi* regulates *qi* and moves its stagnation at any level: it is one of the primary points for transforming phlegm, in particular when it dims and obstructs the portals of the heart.

HE-4 *Lindao* calms both the *shen* and muscles and tendons (it is often cited in the classics for sudden loss of voice).

He Point, Water Point – P-3 *Quze* and HE-3 *Shaohai*

These are points in which the flow of *qi* deepens and are water points. Both cool *qi* and regulate it: they are, in fact, water points and *he*-sea points, in which *qi* enters more internally and 'joins with the sea'.

P-3 *Quze* is more indicated when heat has penetrated to the nutritive *qi* level and into the blood, or in cases of damp-heat (also of stomach and intestines): it is used for disturbed *shen* due to heat that has penetrated deeply or, for example, in skin disorders with psychological components.

HE-3 *Shaohai* has a superior action on heat with phlegm, such as in patterns of madness-*diankuang*, in epilepsy, or in weakening of consciousness due to dimming of the *shen*.

Xi Point – P-4 *Ximen* and HE-6 *Yinxi*

Being *xi*-cleft points, both these points resolve acute symptoms and – being *yin* channels – they have specific indications in blood disorders.

P-4 *Ximen's* ability to invigorate and cool blood makes it a primary choice in cases of *shen* agitation due to febrile diseases.

The *xi* point of the heart HE-6 *Yinxi* rather has the specific function of nourishing *yin* and fluids, thanks to which it is mostly used for empty heat – for which it is a main point.

Luo Point – P-6 *Neiguan* and HE-5 *Tongli*

Being *luo*-connecting points, they invigorate and regulate *qi*, with a specific action in emotional disorders.

P-6 *Neiguan* has a greater action in moving all types of stagnation, opening the chest, regulating the stomach, and in moving down *qi* that rises conversely.

HE-5 *Tongli* has the specific property of regulating heart *qi* and heart rhythm. Furthermore it clears heat, in particular when it transmits to the small intestine and – through the *Tai yang* – to the bladder, or when it agitates the blood of the uterus.

Luo Points on the Paired Yang – SI-7 *Zhizheng*, TB-5 *Waiguan*

SI-7 *Zhizheng* clears heat from the heart and calms the *shen* (it is suggested in the classics for madness-*diankuang*, fear and dread, sadness and anxiety, and *zangzao* syndromes).

TB-5 *Waiguan* rather has a greater action on the exterior, on the *Shao Yang* and on stagnations of *qi*: it disperses wind-heat, transforms damp-heat, regulates the *Shao yang* and moves and regulates *qi*, especially in the sides of the body.

Treatment with Emotions in Classical Texts

14

Throughout the history of Chinese medical thought there has been a full awareness that there are cases in which it is preferable or necessary to use other methods than medicines or needles. During the Ming Dynasty, for example, we find the statement: 'Excess of emotions cannot be cured with medicines; it must be cured with emotions, which are a medicine without form (*wuxing* 无形]).'[1]

A modern text specifies that this type of therapy is suitable both in psychological and in somatic pathologies when emotional factors are of primary importance: 'From the viewpoint of its tangential meaning, any technique that acts by influencing the psychic activities of the patient in order to achieve a therapeutic result can be called 'psychic therapeutic method' (*jingshen liaofa*). When the treatment regards a person in a conscious state, situations where psychic factors do not influence the results of the therapy are rare'.[2]

Terms such as *jingshen liaofa* (精 神 疗 法)'psychic therapeutic method' or the more classic *yiliao* (意疗) 'mind-therapy' mostly refer to the use of words as an instrument of analysis and 'rectification' of ideas in order to free up the flow of *qi*, to avoid destabilising explosive emotional outbursts and to maintain a tranquil heart.

Another Ming Dynasty quotation develops this thought in a very articulated manner:

> Euphoria, anger, anguish, thought, sadness, fear, fright: all seven originate from emotions-*qing*. The emotions are the conscience-*shi* (识) of the *shen*, we perceive them but cannot define them, they leave no trace that we can follow,

---

[1] Wu Kun, *Yifangkao* ('Studies of medical prescriptions'). The same concept can be found in the Qing period: 'The influence of emotions and desires can not be cured with medicines, the illnesses of the seven emotions must be treated with emotions.' In: Wu Shiji, *Liyue pingwen* ('Rimed discourse on new therapies').
[2] Wang Miqu, *Zhongguo gudai yixue xinlixue* ('Ancient Chinese medical psychology'), 1988.

they are activated by contact with the environment and when they get stuck it is difficult to free them and medicines have no effect. Then how can we eliminate their powerful grasp? Even if we managed to make already stagnant *qi* flow freely and already injured blood move, considering that there are a hundred pressing and continuous thoughts that have not been transformed how can we guarantee that in the future they will not knot again causing new suffering? The only proper way is that of removing [incorrect] conscience-*shi* using the correct conscience, expelling the emotions with principles-*li* (理). This is what is meant when it is said that one must treat disorders 'of the heart' with medicines 'of the heart'. If one manages to free the stagnations, melt the knots, create a certain distance between the emotions and the environment in order to avoid their combining so that one is able to maintain a state of stillness, then the heart-sovereign resides tranquilly and stably and the seven emotions have no consequences.[3]

This approach shares with a number of current therapies the use of analytical methods or those based on cognitive restructuring.

THE PHYSICIAN AS A GUIDE

The physician's role included that of counsellor, teacher and guide: 'Zhu Danxi, with regard to all the patients who came to be treated, worked to protect their spirit, guide their minds, open their hearts, was tireless in imparting lessons regarding all human endeavours, in reproaching, in exhorting and in encouraging'.[4]

These qualities are attributed to Zhu Danxi as a great physician, but they were also returned to during successive eras, in which the debate about the function of medicine was even wider.

If one desires to treat disease, he must first treat the heart; only by correcting the heart can one help to re-establish the normal state. If one manages to make the patient avoid thoughts that are full of doubts and preoccupations, if one eliminates absurd ideas, resentments, remorse regarding oneself and others, there is a sudden liberation, following which the heart is spontaneously cleared and the illness cures itself. If one manages to do this, the illness ends before medicines are taken.[5]

In modern texts, just as in the modern clinic, the importance of analysing the situation together with the patient, whose cooperation should be requested, is generally underlined:

---

[3] Miu Xiyong, *Bencao jinshu* ('Explanation of the Bencao').
[4] Chen Menglei and others, *Gujin tushu jicheng, yibu quanlu* ('Collection of images and ancient and modern books, complete register of works on medicine').
[5] Xu Xun, *Dongyi baojian* ('The precious mirror of medicine'), chapter 'Neijingpian'.

> In certain circumstances the stimulus of the type of language used can produce a great influence with regard to psychological and physiological activities. It is important to use the tool of words, adopting a heuristic method of guiding and inspiring the patient, making him aware of his illness by analysing its origins and mechanisms and liberating him from oppressive thoughts regarding it, increasing his trust in the battle against the disease in such a way as to make him actively cooperate in the therapy.[6]

Nevertheless, the same text immediately goes on to remind us of the pathological relevance of hidden mechanisms: 'The doctor must attempt to penetrate as deeply as possible into the interior world of the patient, because it is often in the depths of his heart that the secrets that are the crux of the disorder are hidden'.[7]

These last passages would be expressed in a modern context as consolidating the functions of the Self, processes therapeutic alliance, repression and the recognition of contradictory impulses.

'ALTER THE EMOTIONS AND CHANGE THE NATURE'

Specific attention is also dedicated to emotional aspects and to attempts at modifying character and behaviour. Often defined as 'shift the emotions and change the nature', these methods consist in distracting the thought towards different goals, people and objects, and in transforming habits, conceptions and ways of thinking.[8]

'People who are consumed by an excess of thought, if only they manage to shift their attention they can recover their lives even when they are in the most serious of conditions.'[9]

'Constraint-*yu* of emotions is due to sentiments and hidden thoughts, tangled and unexpressed [. . .] its cure completely depends on the patient's ability to shift the emotions and change his nature.'[10]

The therapeutic indications at times consist of 'psychophysical hygiene' instructions that pertain to internal practices, but can also translate into simple suggestions such as taking a trip, or remembering the importance of tranquillity, the liberating pleasure of music and reading, or the relief that comes from an enjoyable, carefree evening.

---

[6] Zhu Wenfeng, *Zhongyi xinlixue yuanzhi* ('Principles of psychology in Chinese medicine'), 1987, p. 148.
[7] Zhu Wenfeng, 1987, p. 155.
[8] 'Transforming emotions and changing nature', *yiqing bianxing*, recalls the title of Chapter 13 of the *Suwen*, 易 精 变 气 *Yijing bianqi* 'Transforming the *jing* and changing the *qi*'.
[9] Kou Zongshi, *Bencao yanyi* ('Development of the meaning of the Bencao').
[10] Ye Tianshi, *Lingzhen zhinan yian* ('Guide cases in clinic'), and similarly: 'The illnesses caused by a lack of satisfaction can only be cured by distracting the soul. Thus one must find something that is loved by the patient in order to shift his attention. The illness will be spontaneously solved.' In: Wei Zhixiu, *Xu mingyi leian*, ('Continuation of the Clinical cases of famous doctors').

'If there is tiredness *yang qi* is weakened, then it is worthwhile to distract oneself with a trip in a carriage or on horseback.'[11]

'Recent illnesses that are still light and superficial often heal with tranquillity, peace and serenity without the need for medicines.'[12]

'In emotional disorders, reading and listening to music in order to free oneself from oppression and eliminate worries, is often more useful than medicine.'[13]

'Bad moods are resolved by liberating the chest with a chat or with laughter.'[14]

The pathogenic role of the gap between desire, aspirations, internal movements and external constraints is also clearly delineated, amongst other things.

'Not even a good medicine can heal if there is no harmony with the surrounding environment, if aspirations are not satisfied and if anguishing thoughts linger in the depths.'[15]

Zhang Zhongjing, a great scholar of the *Neijing*, but also an attentive observer of individuals and their suffering, had earlier noted: 'Emotional disorders are only resolved by emotions; in women it is necessary that desires receive satisfaction and only in this way are they resolved'.[16]

In a number of cases, the necessity of accommodating the desires of the patient in the initial stage of treatment is underlined. 'What does using the *yi* (意) of the patient mean? If the patient loves eating cold things, you must give him cold things, if he loves hot, you must give him hot. In accordance with the nature of the patient, you must use a method of accommodation, in this way you will not annoy him and will achieve good results; otherwise he will lose faith in the doctor, no longer listen to his words or agree to take his medicines.'[17]

GOING AROUND THE OBSTACLE

When speaking of *dian* (癲) and *kuang* (狂) disorders, we note that in more serious cases it may be necessary to entice the patient:

> To treat wind in the heart it is first necessary to attract the patient through emotions and then use medicines, only in this way will there be easy results. Of what does attracting through emotions consist? If for example, the disorder is due to an excessive yearning for profits, you attract him with the prospect of becom-

[11] Li Dongyuan, *Piwei lun* ('Treatise on spleen and stomach').
[12] Qi Shi, *Lixu yuanjian* ('Mirror of the treatment of emptiness of the origin').
[13] Wu Shangxian, *Liyue pingwen* ('Rimed prose on principles and methods).
[14] Ye Tianshi, *Lingzhen zhinan yian* ('Guide cases in clinic').
[15] Li Zhongzi, *Yizong bidu* ('Essential readings of the medical tradition'), chapter 'Bushi renqinglun'.
[16] Zhang Jiebin, *Jingyue quanshu* ('The complete works of Jingyue'), chapter 'Furenguan'.
[17] Chen Shiduo, *Shishi milu* ('Secret notes on the stone chamber'), chapter 'Yiliaofa'.

ing rich; you deceive him with the prospects of benefits and favours. Therefore, one first acts to stabilise the emotions and only later treats with medicines; this is essential for success in the therapy.[18]

The following is a clinical example where this method of coaxing is applied:

Wang Shishan treated the following case: A criminal committed suicide by jumping into a river while he was being transported shackled in chains. The policeman that transported him was falsely accused by the family of having threatened him in order to extort money from him and in this way, to have induced him to depart this life. Forced to make a large financial compensation, he became ill from worry and resentment, started acting like an idiot or drunk, rambled on and made senseless speeches – in other words, he lost his mind. Shi Shan examined him and said: 'This man's disorder is caused by worries following the financial damages; to cure him he must feel joy. Is it possible that medicines are not able to treat him?' He told the relatives to have false coins made of tin and to place them next to him. The patient, seeing them, was happy; he picked them up and did not want to put them down. From that moment, the illness improved progressively and the patient in the end was cured.[19]

There are examples that exist where a form of behavioural conditioning is used, including methods that accustom the patient to the objects of their phobias, through procedures of exposure and desensitisation.

A typical example comes from the works of Zhang Zihe, in which 23 cases of emotional aetiology are described, 10 of which are treated through the emotions. The case regards a woman who, ever since a thief had entered her home a year earlier, has become frightened and almost faints as soon as she hears any noise, so much so that everyone has to walk silently and not make any noise. Since therapy with heart medicine had not been effective, a different treatment is now used instead.

He asks two women to hold her still on a high chair and he tells her to look at a low table in front of her. He then strikes it with a piece of wood, the woman becomes frightened, and he says: 'I hit a table with a piece of wood, why do you become frightened?' After the fright has attenuated a little he strikes the table again another three to five times, then he hits the door and the window behind her. He then says: 'Little by little the fright has calmed down'. The woman starts laughing and says: 'What kind of therapy is this?' He responds: 'In the *Neijing* it is said fright-*jing* then peace-*ping*. When there is fright [one must] calm and pacify, *ping* also means "often, normal", if one sees something often he no

---

[18] Xu Chunpu, *Gujin yitong daquan* ('Great compendium of ancient and modern medicine'), Book 49, chapter 'Xinfengmen'.
[19] Zhixiu, *Xu mingyi leian*, ('Continuation of the Clinical cases of famous doctors'), chapter 'Diankuang'.

longer becomes frightened. Tonight I will have someone bang on your door until dawn. Fright is *shen* that overflows above'.[20]

Techniques of suggestion, with regards both the doctor and the symptoms, are also used.

> Yang Bengheng treated a noble who suffered from cataracts and had become very irascible due to this and who looked at himself in the mirror continuously. No doctor was able to cure him, therefore Yang was called, who examined him and said: 'Your illness in the eyes will heal spontaneously, but since you have taken many medicines the poisons have already been transferred to your left thigh and in the space of a day and a night they will emerge; you should worry about this instead'. The man passed all his time observing and massaging his left thigh, out of fear of the illness. Over time the eyes healed, but the poison never manifested in the leg. He then called the doctor to request a bill. The doctor said: 'Doctor (*yi* 医) signifies thought (*yi* 意). In your impatience and hurry to heal, you continued to look at yourself in the mirror. The heart manifests in every moment in the eyes. In this way you caused fire to flare upward, how could your eyes heal? Therefore I deceived you, causing you to concentrate on your thigh so that fire would descend downward, and in this way the eyes healed.'[21]

CONTROL OF EMOTIONS THROUGH EMOTIONS

The necessity of taking into account the social, relational and emotional aspects of the patient in the diagnosis and structuring of treatment is already well represented in the *Neijing*, but it is well known that the possibility of treating an emotion through the emotion that dominates it in the controlling-*ke* (克) cycle is also discussed in this work.

One of Zhang Zihe's cases in which laughter (heart) resolves anger (liver) is famous:

> The wife of Commander Xiang became ill: even though she was hungry she did not desire to eat, she was often subject to outbursts of anger during which she yelled, insulted, and cursed everyone around her. Treated for 6 months by many physicians without results, her husband had her examined by Zhang Zihe. The doctor said: 'This illness is difficult to treat with medicines'. He then arranged for three courtesans to make themselves up and assume poses like actresses. The woman broke out in great laughter upon seeing them. The next

---

[20] Zhang Zihe, *Rumen shiqin* ('Confucian responsibilities towards family and parents'), Chapter 26. The sentence refers to Chapter 74 of the *Suwen*, '*Jing zhe ping zhi*' 惊 者 平 之.
[21] Wei Zhixiu, *Xu mingyi leian*, ('Continuation of the Clinical cases of famous doctors').

day he ordered them to stage a fighting match and again the woman laughed. Besides this, he also arranged that two women with very hearty appetites stay with her, who would comment on how delicious the food was as they ate. In this way, the woman not only started to desire food again, but wanted to taste everything. After a few days, her anger started diminishing, her appetite increased and the woman was cured without having used any medicines. Later she had a child.[22]

In other cases fear is used to control euphoria, like water dominates fire:

A certain Yin Zhuan, after having passed the exams to become a government official, having obtained the most prestigious title, requested permission to return home. During the trip, having arrived at the Huai River, he became ill and consulted a famous doctor. The doctor told him: 'Your illness is incurable and you will die within a week. If you hurry, you will make it in time to reach your home.' Yin Zhuan, hearing this, became desperate and hurried home with all means available. Having arrived home, after seven days nothing had yet happened to him. His servant said to him: 'There is a letter that a doctor told me to give you after your arrival home'. Yin Zhuan opened the letter, which read: 'You, sir, won the competition to become a government official and following the excess of joy your heart was injured. In this case, medicine would have had no effect, so I therefore frightened you with the prospect of death. At this point, the illness is over by now.' Yin Zhuan felt great admiration for the doctor.[23]

Reciprocal control of emotions can also be achieved through other channels; for instance, examination of the clinical cases found in the classics provides evidence of a recurrent use of *yang* emotions to move *yin* emotional states or, vice versa, the use of *yin* emotions to calm *yang* conditions. In many instances we see that the goal of the physician consists of provoking feelings of anger or joy specifically because they are emotions that move *qi* the most: the disorder derives, in fact, from a constraint of *qi*, or from sadness, thoughts and feelings of oppression, which can therefore be freed up by a *yang* movement.

In such cases there is a sort of psychodrama being played out, but using all the methods of everyday life. 'According to the principle of reciprocal control of the five emotions, all methods may be used as therapy, from music to farce, up to and including threats, deceptions and insults.'[24]

There are also cases in which the doctor risks his life and sometimes loses it, as is detailed in the 'Annals', a work that predates the *Neijing*:

[22] Zhang Zihe, *Rumen shiqin* ('Confucian responsibilities towards family and parents'), chapter 'Neishangxing'. See how at the end there is a reference to a son, from the start it is thus implicit that it is a case of sterility.
[23] Yishi teji ('Selection from the history of medicine').
[24] Xu Yongcheng, *Yuji weiyi* ('Subtle principle of the jade mechanism').

The king of Qi became ill with masses in his chest and sent for Doctor Wen Zhi from Song. Wen Zhi arrived and, having examined the king, said to the prince: 'The king will recover from his illness, but even if he recovers he will put me to death.' The prince asked why and Wen Zhi responded: 'The king can only be cured with anger, and I, having provoked the king's anger, will have to die.' The prince begged him: 'If you cure the king's illness, my mother and I will beseech the king to save you even at the cost of our own lives and the king will be forced to listen to us, therefore I beg you to have no fear and not to hesitate!' Wen Zhi said: 'Alright, in order to cure the king I am willing to give my life.' Through the prince he made appointments with the king three times and all three times he did not show up at the appointments, already provoking the king's anger. When he finally arrived, he went up onto the platform of the king's bed without even removing his shoes and asked the king about his illness while he tramped on the king's clothes. The king became so angry he could not speak, at which point Wen Zhi spoke to him using premeditatedly insolent phrases in order to increase his anger. The king broke out in a series of curses and his illness was immediately cured. Being angry with Wen Zhi, he ordered him put to death. The protests and prayers of the prince and the queen were in vain, and as he had foreseen, Wen Zhi died in a boiling vat.[25]

OBSESSIVE THOUGHTS AND ANGER

The majority of clinical stories with results that are outside of normally systematised treatments seem to relate to situations in which feelings of pain, anguish, obsessive thoughts and fixed ideas have become pervasive and crippling.

Liu Zhen's sister was the wife of King Bo Yang of Qi and the couple had a very close emotional bond. After the king was killed on orders of his brother, the wife became ill from her pain and no doctor was able to cure her. Yin Chun was very good at drawing very realistic portraits of people. Liu Zhen asked him to paint a picture in which the defunct king was depicted together with his favourite courtesan in the act of looking at themselves in the mirror while removing their clothes as though preparing to go to bed. Liu Zhen then secretly sent a servant to show the painting to his sister. She, seeing the painting, spat on it and cursed: 'He deserved to die earlier.' Together with the end of her feelings of marital bliss, her illness also was slowly cured.[26]

Han Shiliang treated a woman. She and her mother were very united by a deep affection, so much so that following the daughter's marriage the mother died, and the woman became ill at the thought of her mother. All treatments

---

[25] *Lushi chunqiu* ('Annals on spring and autumn'), chapter 'Zhizhong'.
[26] *Nanshi* ('History of Southern dynasties'), chapter 'Liezhuan'.

were ineffective. Han said: 'This illness is due to excess thought, therefore medicines cannot cure it, it must be treated with magic.' He bribed a sorceress, telling her what to say to the woman. One day the husband said to his wife: 'You think of your mother with so much nostalgia, but you do not know if she still thinks of you in her grave. I have to make a trip; in the meantime, go to the sorceress and ask her about your mother.' The wife agreed and called the sorceress. Among incense and prayers, her mother's spirit descended. The sorceress assumed the mannerisms and voice of the mother, and for the woman it was like having her in front of her and she broke out in tears. The mother reprimanded her saying: 'Do not weep. I died prematurely because your life limited mine and my death is entirely your fault. Now that I am in my grave I wish to revenge myself and your illness is in reality all my doing. During my life I was a mother to you; now I am your enemy.' After her words, the woman's expression altered and she burst out in anger: 'I have become ill due to my mother and she, in turn, wants to damage me. Why should I continue to think about her?' After this she was cured. This is called eliminating the object of adoration.[27]

A young man named Wang was sick; he loved to be alone, shut in a dark room, he would not even go near the light of a lamp, and if from time to time he went out the illness worsened. Since the best doctors were not able to cure him, Jian Hang was called. After terminating the examination, the doctor, instead of writing a prescription, asked the young man to give him one of his works in verse and he started to recite it in a coarse voice and making errors in all the punctuation. Wang burst out, asking what he was reading and the doctor, without paying any attention to him, increased the volume of his voice still more. Enraged, Wang ripped the paper from his hands, saying: 'You are not a professional and do not understand; reading without pauses between the phrases makes it nonsensical!' He then sat down near the lamp to read, completely forgetting his aversion to light. The doctor explained the case saying: 'This patient was ill from constraint-*yu*; with anger the constraint was resolved.'[28]

A woman from a wealthy family suffered from excessive thoughts, for two years had not been able to sleep and no doctor could cure her. Her husband called Zhang Zihe to examine her. He said: 'Her pulse on both sides is moderate, therefore the disorder is in the spleen and the reason is that the spleen governs thought.' He therefore arranged with the husband to act in a way so as to provoke anger in the woman. For a number of days he asked to be paid with high fees and abundant libations, always leaving without having treated her. The woman became very angry and sweated, and that night she managed to sleep. The treatment went on like this and for seven days she did not wake up, until she was cured, her appetite improved, and her pulses returned to normal.[29]

---

[27] Zhang Jiebin, *Leijing* ('The classic of categories'), chapter 'Lunzhilei'.
[28] *Nanbu xianzhi* ('Chronicles of the Southern counties'), chapter 'Lijian hangyishi'.
[29] Zhang Zihe, *Rumen shiqin*, ('Confucian responsibilities towards family and parents'), chapter 'Neishangxing'.

The Space Shared by the Patient and the Acupuncturist

15

A profession in which one is occupied with illness and suffering is a delicate vocation. It is particularly so for us Western acupuncturists, who work on an energetic level attempting to find our way between a conventional medical system, therapeutic traditions that are not in fact ours, and often complex requests by patients.

Although the decision to practise a type of medicine like that of Chinese tradition may derive from an evaluation of its clinical effectiveness, it also consists of other important factors, even if these are apparently marginal in comparison: the use of theoretical models and thought processes different to those currently dominant in the biomedical worldview, the particular attention to the relationship between the practitioner and patient, the peculiarity of a therapeutic treatment that is given through the medium of a needle.

Those who have practised acupuncture for a while will already be aware that experience settles many doubts while it creates others, and those who also teach become aware that for the younger students and colleagues difficulties often crop up that are not closely linked to diagnosis, the choice of points or the use of a technique.

Being doctors, we are paid to make a therapeutic change in the situation, and we feel gratified when this happens. However, patients are patients precisely because they suffer, and their state of being unwell can be invasive for us as practitioners; being submerged by this leaves us no room to breathe, whereas recognition of the ways in which it is transferred to us helps both us and those across the table from us.

A sure starting point – but also a point of arrival – is therefore not to take anything for granted, but to stop, listen to the patient, and to yourself, and consult with colleagues.

The text that follows is based on a study of the classics, which are extremely observant and suggestive in this sense, and from which selections of the more incisive passages are quoted. However, in addition it makes specific reference to psychoanalytical thought, the discipline that in today's Western culture – in which we live and participate – has most thoroughly investigated the risks and the richness of the dynamics of the therapeutic relationship. This basic explanation makes no reference to specific theories, but rather recognises a broad psychodynamic outlook in which, for example, the existence of the unconscious is a presupposition.

This a concept that, among other things, seems not far from Zhan Jiebin's reflections on what we would define as 'projection':

> The seven emotions of man originate from attraction and aversion; if there is excessive inclination towards one of them then there is imbalance, the prevailing of one and the defeat of the other, shen (神) and zhi (志) easily end up in disorder. If shen and zhi are unbalanced the pathogens establish themselves in turn, then ghosts-gui (鬼) are generated in the heart. Therefore he who has aversion inside sees aversion, he who has envy sees envy, he who has suspicion will see suspicion, he who has trepidation will see trepidation, and this not only in illnesses, but also in dreams when asleep. This means that if zhi has aversion for something it comes to think of it as on the outside, qi and blood are disordered internally and it is as though there were spirits and ghosts.[1]

Examples of the attention to the internal world and the role of relationships are found in passages that underline the elements of empathy and harmony between doctor and patient. 'Medicine-yi (医) is intention-yi(意); when one has a patient in front of him he must use intention for evaluating. I do not have great ability in this sense, but always, from my youth to old age, when I see sick people I calm the qi, contain the heart, share the breath and start to transform my body into that of the patient. [...] The negative arises; lamentations and the poisons of worry and confusion come.'[2]

---

[1] Zhang Jiebin, *Leijing*, chapter 'Zhuyou' ('Charms'). In the comment to Chapter 13 of the *Suwen* on transforming the *jing* and changing the *qi* ('Yijing bianqilun') Zhang Jiebin speaks also of those who cast charms and spells, who do not prescribe medicines, who force people to remain seated or recommend magic water. He maintains that illnesses are not caused by spirits, but that spirits come from emotions.

[2] Yu Chang, *Yimen falu* ('Principles and prohibitions of the medical practice'). *Yi zhe, yi ye* is a word riddle between 'medicine' and 'intention, thought, idea, attention' (on the meaning of *yi* see also Chapter 3 on the different *shen*). Zhang Jiebin criticises the relying on intuition and maintains, more strictly, that: 'In the past they used to say *yi zhe yi ye* 医者意也 medicine is intention-*yi*, if the intention is clear there will be success, instead I say *yi zhe li ye* 医 者理 也, medicine is a principle, if the principle is transparent the heart is luminous-*ming*. It was said that the eyes of Bian Que could see through and catch a glimpse of the principle-*li*, so those who want to learn the *shen* of Bian Que must be clear about the principle, and those who want to clarify the principle must search for it in the classics, and only after one must draw from the ideas of famous doctors.' In: Zhang Jiebin, *Leijing tuyi* ('Illustrated supplement to the classic of categories').

REGULATE THE SHEN

From this viewpoint it makes little sense to sanction what is 'proper' or to propose definitive solutions; it is, however, possible to look at some areas we need to pay attention to regarding the dynamics of relationships and the physical and mental space in which we operate, and furthermore to pinpoint a few 'good manners' that should be observed in order to minimise patient anxiety and the difficulties inherent in certain situations, with their not very helpful effects.

A number of specific aspects will therefore be examined, remembering however, that these are only details and that the true heart of the job consists in mentally keeping a small amount of space in relation to what happens in the consulting room, inside of us, inside of the person in front of us, and between the other person and ourselves.

Specifically because of the role of emotions in affecting the movements of *qi*, the importance that they assume as causes of illness and the recognition that soma and psyche are interdependent, the classics pay particular attention to the procedures of acupuncture. The *Neijing* discusses many times the *shen* of the doctor, that of the patient, and that of the acupuncturist, together with those factors that are today termed the 'doctor–patient relationship', the 'therapeutic alliance', and empathy.

We therefore firstly recall that passage in which it is quite clear that the doctor must: know the 'internal practices' and the properties of medicines, possess technical ability, be able to make a diagnosis, but as a first prerequisite must have the ability to regulate *shen*: 'There are five requisites for a good acupuncturist; many ignore them: the first is to regulate *shen*, the second is to know how to 'nourish life' (*yangsheng*), the third is to know the properties of the substances, the fourth is to know how to prepare stone points of various sizes, the fifth is to understand diagnosis of organs, *qi* and blood'.[3] 'Regulate *shen*' can refer to all the *shen* that is in play: the *shen* of the therapist, of the patient, and of the situation that is generated.

In our daily work everyone has his own personal style that is built in the course of contact with teachers and through direct experience, but all of us, in fact, follow a number of rules. Even if these regulations are generally implicit, in reality every act contains choices and consequences and it is therefore useful to bring into focus that space in which the acupuncture treatment takes place. In the first place, we are speaking of our own mental space, of the relationship between two people, in which there is a specific dimension of the body in a certain time and place.

Acquiring an awareness of a number of dynamics can be of assistance both to the health of the doctor and to the effectiveness of the treatment.

---

[3] *Suwen*, Chapter 25.

People turn to Chinese medicine for various reasons: to find a way to confront a disease which presents less risks of side effects, to reach a better integration of body, psyche and energy, or to find a different relationship with the healer.

The doctor, on the other hand, often finds himself faced with a patient in whom the somatic and psychic aspects are tightly interwoven, with thoughts that turn inwards upon themselves, a suffering that is not expressed, and a body that suffers in consequence.

We find traces of this in the classics when they remind us that in order to have a cure the abilities of the doctor are not sufficient; it is necessary to have the intense cooperation of the patient: 'It is useless to talk of the power of medicine to those who believe in ghosts and demons. It is useless to speak of needles with words of praise to those who detest them. It is useless to impose a treatment on one who does not wish to be cured, he will not heal despite all the efforts of the doctor.'[4]

Even taking into account that this passage essentially describes the cultural–historical movement away from shamanic medicine, nevertheless 'demons and ghosts' may be taken to be a form of thought that sees the illness as a pure external accident. The element of relationship, with its possibilities of therapeutic effect but also its risks, assumes particular importance in such cases, in which the patient cannot conceive of the illness as the expression of imbalance – the result of energetic chaos deriving from the interaction between internal and external forces.

STUMBLING BLOCKS, TRAPS AND SPIDER WEBS

We may not notice, but during treatment there are moments that leave us somewhat at a loss: an unexpected question from the patient, a gesture on our part that differs from the normal treatment procedure, or the intrusion of an extraneous thought or feeling.

Cases are not so rare in which we feel that, despite the accuracy of the diagnosis and of the choice of the points, something has not worked, or that something does not make sense from the first encounter, or we suddenly swerve in the therapeutic procedure and everything goes wrong. Here are a few example situations, very different from each other:

---

[4] *Suwen*, Chapter 11. 'Ghosts and demons' is the translation of *gui mo* 鬼魔 The *Neijing* presents an idea of man and illness that deeply differs from the shamanic tradition: we notice that *shen* in its meaning of 'spirit, ghost' (*guishen* 鬼神) is quoted only to stress the idea that it has no role in acupuncture (*Suwen*, Chapter 25), or to deny the fact that it could be one of the mysterious causes of illness (*Lingshu*, Chapter 9). Instead we find the term *shenming* 神明, clarity of the *shen*, luminous *shen*). About demonological medicine see also the second chapter by P. Unschuld, 'Medicine in China', 1985.

- A patient who loved and admired us before, becomes extremely critical about us or the therapy (in other words, very angry).
- We become deeply infected by the patient's feelings (we end up suffering from his same symptoms).
- We feel absolutely indispensable, totally inept, extremely irritated, or mortally bored (feelings that although different from each other share a more than 'reasonable' pervasiveness).
- We have the overall impression that the patient is actually asking for something different from his explicit requests, or in any event we do not understand what he is really talking about.
- The patient attaches himself to us without remedy, or recuperates from one symptom and develops another (in other words, does not heal), or asks for advice and then invariably does not follow it.
- Despite our intentions and without being aware of it, other figures are suddenly present (relatives who interfere and impose themselves by telephoning or appearing at the office).

First of all, though, we perhaps need to stop for a moment and think of our own part in these situations, and also consider a little bit why we chose this profession.

Being a therapist often implies fantasies of omnipotence, being a doctor has the taste of power, and taking care of others holds our own need to be taken care of.

In this sense, everyone goes forward with their own search for the truth about themselves in various ways, but it can be useful to list here a number of dynamics that should ring alarm bells when they appear. For example:

- I always feel required; patients fill my time ever more, 'because they really need me'.
- The patients do not understand what I am doing for them (maybe not even my colleagues), they underestimate my abilities and efforts – in short, I am a 'misunderstood victim'.
- Overwhelmed by the bad health of the patient, I gasp and grope.
- Treatments work well or even excellently up to a certain point and then wane, in such a way that there is never a complete resolution.
- There is a certain type of patient or situation that I really cannot tolerate (he/it bores me to death, or is exhausting, or immediately irritates me).

These dynamics may indicate important 'holes' or 'knots' if they are regularly repeated – in other words, if different patients and situations tend to produce the same dynamics then it is definitely worthwhile to take a closer look at our inner selves.

Just keeping in mind that we are humans and therefore imperfect, already spares much confusion and suffering, but a further effort to identify one's own deficiencies and fears can become a precious tool for developing more sensitivity in identifying the disturbances and deficiencies of patients.

The injunction to 'know thyself' that runs through different cultures in time and space is expressed in the *Neijing* as: 'He who uses needles understands the other through himself'.[5]

Chinese tradition advises that one should maintain 'an empty heart', since that which is full does not permit movement or the free flow of *qi*. However, suffering invades and fills, and someone who puts himself in the position of attempting to cure another is easily exposed to the risk of 'contamination' – so much so that in traditional cultures the healer is protected by rites, which act as containment against the dark forces and as a structure to use these forces to produce a new balance in the individual and the community.

In our society, disease and pain tend to be expelled both from the mind and from the social fibre, and the doctor too easily finds himself stuck, or overwhelmed by 'strange' mechanisms to which he can respond only by creating barriers of indifference, distance and coldness.

THE NEEDLE, THIS STRANGE OBJECT

Treatment with acupuncture takes place at an energetic level, the body is a 'powerful' presence in it, and a fundamental part of our clinical work consists of touching the patient, both in a diagnostic sense and through the insertion of the needle; this situation is decidedly delicate.

In the *Neijing*, the discussion on the method of needling is taken up a number of times, from different perspectives, but always extremely intensely and suggestively.

The act of needling must be preceded by the preparation of the doctor; this means both being clear about the clinical situation – in other words, knowing 'the state of the organs and the balance of the nine pulses' – and being able to 'govern the *shen*'. Since the arrival of *qi* cannot be controlled but only accepted, as the archer acts only when the flock of birds rises in flight, so too it is necessary for the acupuncturist to have the mind in a state of stillness, to needle in a fluid way, to observe that which 'is called hidden' in the patient, 'of which the form is not known', and then at the opportune moment to act rapidly.

> In order to practise good acupuncture, in the first place one has to govern *shen*, and not needle before having determined the state of the organs and the balance of the nine pulses. When the moment comes one has to act rapidly and manoeuvre with extreme attention, the needling must be smooth and regular; in a calm state of mind we observe the reactions of the patients – in other words, that which is said to be hidden, that of which we do not know the form:

---

[5] *Suwen*, Chapter 5.

> *qi* arrives like a flock of birds, it spreads as if in a millet field, its movements
> are like a flight of birds whose origin you do not know, in the same way the
> physician must be ready to shoot his arrow like an archer in ambush when the
> moment comes.[6]

We also find this uniqueness of the moment – described in terms that are certainly closer to the recent chaos theories in physics than to the consequentiality and the predictability of classical physics – in the chapter 'Explanations of the Needles', dedicated to the method of needling:

> As though on the edge of a cliff, careful not to fall, the hands as though holding
> a tiger, grasp it firmly, the *shen* does not allow itself to be distracted by things,
> observe the patient with a calm mind without looking left or right, to do it well
> one must needle straight, without deviations, one must rectify his own *shen* in
> order to rectify the *shen* of the patient, the doctor must look him in the eyes, if
> the *shen* is fixed *qi* flows with greater ease.[7]

The obtaining of *qi* constitutes a fundamental moment in the therapy: the illness may be the same, and the same point stimulated, but the results differ according to the level of experience, awareness, and practice. 'If *qi* arrives there is a therapeutic result, the certainty of the result is as clear as seeing a blue sky after the wind has swept away the clouds.'[8]

The needle sensation – even if it is hard to describe by both the patient and the practitioner – is, however, in itself very precise, and both recognise that changes take place during the treatment. The needle acts without introducing external substances, it touches something deep, called *qi*, and produces changes through a minimal stimulation. This process, which is so hard to describe in words, is full of unusual connection.

We cannot forget that this presupposes a major renunciation on the part of the patient: they quite properly defend themselves, in a situation which is at the least unusual, through comments that express anxiety and unease and at the same time try to take some of the tension out of the situation (comparisons to pincushions, hedgehogs, or Saint Sebastian are frequent). However, remarks about the meanness and sadistic tendencies inherent in the practice of acupuncture can be more undermining for us, and, in fact, the handling of such comments is not simple. The use of an instrument that penetrates the body and produces strange physical sensations adds to the already numerous and complicated internal experiences that can characterise the doctor–patient relationship.

---

[6] *Suwen*, Chapter 25. See also Chapter 12 on stimulation methods and Chapter 16 on the psychic action of acupuncture.

[7] *Suwen*, Chapter 54.

[8] *Lingshu*, Chapter 1. In this passage there is a reference to *qizhi*, the 'arrival of qi', *qizhi* 气 至, which corresponds to 'obtaining the qi', *deqi* 得 气. For its description refer to Chapter 12 on stimulation methods and to Chapter 16 on the psychic action of acupuncture.

Acupuncture is defined as an act that interrupts the continuity of the body, but is this really true? The point-hole can also be the space through which the needle reaches the *qi*. In effect, the Chinese term for the acupuncture points is *xue* (穴), meaning 'hole, lair'. This term is often used in connection to the question of locating the points and is translated as 'dimple, depression'. However, it also means a passage, a privileged path – so perhaps it is not by chance that in the classics it is written: 'When you get the point, the needle rushes into a hole'.[9]

In this sense also, acupuncture must be a gentle act.

SETTING AND TIME OF THERAPY

When everything goes well, the things that happen during an acupuncture treatment have a different quality and intensity to those of normal life. This 'happening' is facilitated by the fact that it is situated in a different time frame to that of daily life, and in a separate territory, which includes certain things and excludes others.

All psychotherapeutic treatments – from the healing rituals of various traditions to Freudian analysis or group psychodrama – fix rules to regulate the time, place and method of performance. This establishment of the workspace, or *setting*, has the function of regulating and containing, with regard to both the patient and the therapist.

In the doctor–patient relationship in modern China the rules may appear obscure, but even we foreigners can easily perceive their existence and consistency. We have seen how the classics affirm that in order to 'govern' the *shen*, to 'rectify' it and to 'fix' it, calmness, attention and concentration are necessary, but in other passages we also find more specific indications about the quality of the treatment: 'When he needles, the doctor has to be in a state of deep calm, has to come and go only together with *shen*, act as though he had doors and windows shut, *hun* and *po* are not dispersed, *yi* and *shen* are concentrated, *jing* and *qi* are not divided, the voices of the people around him are not heard, so that *jing* is collected, *shen* is united, and *zhi* is concentrated on the needle.'[10]

This space – both mental and physical – must be protected, 'like with doors and windows shut', so that 'one does not hear the voices of people around him'. These concise phrases, as always in classic Chinese texts, work by analogy – that is, they stand for a situation in which one protects himself from everything that is distracting, whether these are real stimuli or mental

---

[9] *Lingshu*, Chapter 4. For this change of perspective, which now appears obvious to me, I owe my thanks to Salvo Inglese, a colleague with no specific knowledge of acupuncture but with a curious and alert spirit.
[10] *Lingshu*, Chapter 9.

recollections. The delimitation of a space in which to pause facilitates the calm state of the therapist, avoids dispersion of *hun* and *po*, *jing* and *qi*, *shen* and *yi*, and allows concentration of intention on the needle.

The therapeutic act is performed inside a space–time framework, the *setting*; frames are boundaries, they delimit and limit, but – as artists well know – they are also that which gives relief to the painting. As often happens when something that grows is in play – whether a child or a project – the placing of boundaries allows the creation of a stable base so that a greater level of freedom may be reached later. It is mainly a question of keeping in mind that the therapeutic process is also influenced by factors such as place, time, manner of speech, external elements and so forth.

It would, however, make little sense to define absolute rules, even if only for contingent reasons: we perform acupuncture in very different environments (a doctor's office, a hospital, and the study of an independent professional generally have different characteristics), the structure of the office/study varies (one or more rooms, the presence or absence of a nurse), other therapeutic methods may be used in a complementary manner, and in any case, our training is different from that of others.

Remembering, therefore, that our main resource is always our attention, we can focus on a number of specific features that help us identify potential traps more easily. This process is similar to that of tongue diagnosis; first of all, we need to know that looking at the tongue can tell us something, then we learn to recognise and differentiate between the signs, and lastly, we use their meaning to draw inferences for treatment.

The *setting* consists of a mental attitude and relatively tangible influences on it regarding both space and time. Without entering here into the marvellous geomantic art called *fengshui*, we can nevertheless recognise that *qi* is also in the light, colours, the emptiness and fullness of a physical place in which the doctor and patient encounter each other, the sounds and smells of the place, and the movement and gaze of the acupuncturist.

The greater the easiness the better for the movements of *qi*; all of us know, for example, that being disturbed has a negative influence, although we have not always clearly stated to ourselves what level of disturbance we feel is allowable. It is important to decide how much disturbance to allow – in other words, how much we will allow what is outside to get inside. Whereas in psychotherapeutic sessions any external or telephone interruptions are excluded, this rule is not so rigid in the acupuncturist's study, but it is nevertheless fundamental to define precisely which annoyances to allow and then to maintain that limit firmly.

Depending on the structure of the clinic, the acupuncturist may or may not remain in the same room as the patient; however, the essential thing is to be aware of how much, and most of all 'how', to remain there.

If we think of the four methods of investigation (*sizhen*) and the eight rules of diagnosis (*bazheng*), that is, the methods through which we observe and evaluate *qi*, it is evident that this work is also done on a level of non-verbal communication where the code of indirect signals is in effect. Within the limits of our ability, we note the classic signs of the pulse, tongue, colour, odour, etc. but also what happens upon the insertion of the needles, that which the patient repeats a number of times and that which he does not say: the hesitations and blocks, the tone of voice, the facial expression, the body posture and gestures.

An accurate history, which also takes into consideration the social and emotional events in the life of the patient, is obviously fundamental: 'The one who diagnoses must be informed about the material and social conditions of the patient. Those who fall from a good social position may become ill even if they have not been invaded by external pathogens. In order to make a diagnosis it is necessary to inquire about eating habits and living environment, about emotions, and whether there have been intense joys or traumas and the time of their occurrence. In fact, all of these things injure *jing* and *qi*. When *jing* and *qi* become exhausted the body disaggregates. Anger injures *yin*, euphoria hurts *yang*, *qi* rises upwards, fills the vessels and [the *shen*] departs the body. He who diagnoses illness must understand its beginning and the point of arrival, understand its roots and branches. When he takes the pulse and asks about the symptoms, he must also take into account the differences between men and women. Regret due to the distance and separation of a loved one causes accumulations and constraint of the emotions; worries, fear, euphoria, and anger empty the five *zang* organs; *qi* and blood are no longer contained. The unrefined doctor cannot understand these processes, in this case how can we speak of true medical art?'[11]

Therefore, one cannot be in a hurry, there must be sufficient space for listening, both to the words and to whatever else may emerge: 'During the treatment one should withdraw to a quiet and secluded place, and ask the patient in an ample and complete manner about all aspects of the illness in order to understand its meaning. He who manages to grasp the *shen*, is successful; he who lets it go, is lost'.[12]

However, even words need to have a limit: if the patient relaxes into conversation he is easily distracted and the space for more intense events diminishes; the mind remains in the sphere of words and concepts and the work of the needles on *qi* is impeded; worries and sorrow cannot leave and remain as they were.

Our words and gestures have the same importance, since they can give meaning or increase confusion, especially since what we say and our way of acting are expressions of internal attitudes and movements, which at times are decidedly complex.

Because acupuncture is a treatment on an energetic level, it generally makes sense to concentrate on non-verbal avenues of perception and altered states

---

[11] *Suwen*, Chapter 77.
[12] *Suwen*, Chapter 13.

of consciousness, but it is also true that some people need to 'systemise' things through words, and in such cases it can be useful to suggest an energetic evaluation or to provide some explanations about the treatment.

In any case, while safeguarding that space in which the patient becomes aware of changes in a less 'rational' and more directly somatic way, a number of areas in which verbal communications are valid must nevertheless be maintained. For example, speaking of the problems that must be confronted, estimating the time necessary, specifying that the needles are sterile and asking explicitly whether there are doubts or questions are signs of respect towards the patient and a first step towards building the therapeutic alliance, showing that we understand both his natural diffidence and his just as natural curiosity.[13]

On the matter of words, it is also necessary to remember that overextended conversations – those in which the patient lets himself go and tells another all his miseries – run the risk of a rebound effect. The patient's narrative draws the doctor into the most painful parts of his intimate life; the expression of his deepest and at the same time most wretched fears may, however, be followed by closing up, and upset by feelings of anger linked to feelings of embarrassment and impotence. Also, without proper training, it is difficult to respond effectively to this overflowing river of words, but the simple tactic of spreading out the same narrative over a number of appointments can avoid patients feeling defrauded or deceived rather than understood and relieved.

The conclusion of treatment deserves particular attention, since the end of the relationship is a separation, with the more or less difficult procedures that this entails. The possibility of further contacts, for example, should be specified, but – especially in cases of serious somatising or chronic illnesses – the possibility of living with a number of disorders should be raised. At times, the patient may even adapt the prayer (attributed to various sources) 'Lord, give me the patience to tolerate the things which I cannot change, the strength to change the things which I can change, and the wisdom to see the difference.'

The time of the treatment therefore has qualitative variables: it may be an intense time, an empty time, or indeed empty in other ways. There is also, however, a simple quantitative variable, which is related to the theme of limits: we recall that the more the length of the treatment is precise and defined, the more it will fulfil a function of containment.

In psychotherapy, the therapist and patient both know the exact amount of time reserved for their encounter, implicitly recognising in this that there is time, but also that the time is not unlimited.[14] As acupuncturists we can expect

---

[13] It is worth remembering that the patient, however in need, is always an adult with whom we also have a relationship as equals. If we are too focused on reassuring the patient we might end up reinforcing any tendency to being passive and discouraged, whereas if we also mention difficulties we appeal to his health resources while still reassuring him.

[14] We recall that the agreements regulating the setting are stricter and more defined when the therapy is of an analytical–expressive type – that is, when we work at the level of unconscious phantoms.

and demand that the patient respect the time of the appointment more or less strictly, respect this time ourselves (or not respect it, even though we expect the patient to do so), we can decide to make a more or less constant amount of time available, and we can have the thoughtfulness to let the patient know.

The clarity of the limits, with its function of containment, in any case touches on all the various behaviours that are part of the therapeutic relationship, about which explicit and well-defined agreements may be made. Among these, we cite the rules of payment, punctuality at appointments, telephone calls outside office hours, the degree of involvement of third parties, the question of relatives in therapy, the initiatives regarding other doctors and treatments, and so on.

The essential thing is that these limits be very clear to us, although generally it is not necessary to be explicit about these rules with the majority of patients. Unfortunately, however, with a number of patients we discover too late that something has gone off beam, we find ourselves suddenly so entangled that we do not know where to turn, and at that point it becomes evident to us that we should have paid more attention at the start.

The problem is that when the psychic pathology is serious the manipulative dynamics act on the relationship at unconscious levels, and are therefore not manifest or readily recognisable; for this reason a preliminary definition of the rules of the relationship is fundamental.

DYNAMICS OF THE THERAPEUTIC RELATIONSHIP

We can compare the definition of the place, time and behaviours to the more external manifestations, *biao*, while the root, *ben*, relates to the fact that in the encounter between patient and acupuncturist the emotional components of each of them come into play, with all the complexity of their inner worlds.

It is at this level that the real 'therapeutic alliance' is constructed: since none of us is omnipotent, the people involved in the therapy must work together, on a basis of trust, in order to change the state of things that causes the suffering.

In the classics, the situation in which the patient does not heal and the clinical pattern is very severe is taken into consideration and an explanation is found in 'unlimited desires and endless worries':

> 'What happens when the form-*xing* is faulty, the blood is consumed and we don't achieve any results?' Qi Bo responded: 'It is due to *shen* not carrying out its action.' Huang Di said 'What does this mean?' 'Acupuncture is *dao*. *Jing* and *shen* do not proceed further, *zhi* and *yi* are not in order, and the illness is incurable. If *jing* is exhausted, *shen* is escaping, nutritive and defensive *qi* do not gather, it is because there are unlimited desires and endless worries, then *jing*

and *qi* loosen up and are ruined, defensive *qi* departs, nutritive *qi* flows out, *shen* leaves and illness does not heal.'[15]

A modern translation of this description consists of saying that a sick psyche can destroy any resource in the depths and be stronger than any therapeutic treatment.

Those dynamics that can lead to situations, emotions, and ways of acting in which we get stuck and confused originate from this deep level.

There are certain relationships (for example, the working relationships of teachers, preachers, magistrates and doctors) that possess a number of specific intrinsic characteristics: they are asymmetrical, delimited, relationships, aimed at an objective. So that considerations concerning the dynamics of the relationship are also specific.[16]

Psychoanalysis works with the dynamics of transference and countertransference, but in fact these processes are active in all human relations, and in particular in those situations in which one of the two protagonists is suffering and therefore is often more fragile and confused.

Transference, also called 'transfer', is that process in which a person transfers on to present relationships (in particular those with the therapist) aspects which belong to other people or to other moments and situations.[17] Traces of what was lived in the past appear in every relationship, but this mechanism becomes 'pathological' – in other words a cause of non-health – when it impinges upon and substitute in a repetitive and forceful way for the diversity of reality, when the rigidity of the responses does not allow any movement. We no longer have fun (and 'having fun' is also 'to diverge', 'to go off in another direction').

If psychotherapy, as a form of listening which transforms the patient's suffering, fully uses these mechanisms of transferance, for us acupuncturists it is important to recognise their presence and have some idea of what to do. Being by definition an unconscious movement, this process camouflages itself adeptly: the first thing to do is to remember that it exists.

We might suspect a transferance dynamic every time we perceive some disconnection between the real situation and the words or the behaviour of the patient, which turns out to have little to do with the 'actual' situation. It is as though there were a duplicate scenario so that we do not understand why the patient is saying certain things, or why certain things 'that don't make sense' are done. Or it may be the case that we do something and at the same time we

---

[15] *Suwen*, Chapter 14.
[16] With regard to certain relational dynamics see also the number of 'The European Journal of Oriental Medicine' dedicated to the therapeutic relationship (vol. 2, 1996) and my articles *Il corpo, la mente e noi* ('The body, the mind and us'), 1994 and *The Space Shared between Patient and Acupuncturist*, 2000, Chapter 16 on the psychic action of acupuncture and the comments to various clinical case studies such as 5.1, 8.1, 10.3, 10.4, 11.2, 15.1, 15.2 and 16.2.
[17] The transference 'in psychoanalysis is defined as that process with which unconscious desires emerge around certain objects in the space of a definite relation with them and mostly in the field of the analytic relationship. It is a repetition of childish prototypes, which is experienced with a strong sense of actuality.' In: Laplanche and Pontalis, 1967, p. 609.

have the feeling that we have not chosen to do it completely 'freely', as though the patient had somehow pulled us there.

Obviously, the therapist may also perform the same process of bringing into the present relationship things that do not belong to it. Without being aware of it, there can be something in the patient, or in the relationship, that takes us to another person or situation in the past, that touched us deeply, so that our emotional and behavioural response relates – at least partially – to these.

The problem is that transference is unconscious also for the therapist, and we therefore attribute our feelings of, for example, impatience, anger, sadness or disappointment to contingent reasons. We can, however, verify if there is a transference dynamic when emotions are too strong or in some way strange with respect to what we would expect in that situation, or if there is an alarming repetitiousness in our responses.[18]

ABSTENTION, EMPATHY AND NEUTRALITY

Faced with so much potential confusion, the acupuncturist has no choice but to refine his *shen*, maintain awareness of the existence of these dynamics and develop the sensitivity that can trace them in their various disguises. The response consists of avoiding them.

If a comparison can help us to understand without being presumptuous, we can lead this 'avoidance' back to the concept of abstention in *wuwei* behaviour: the 'non-action' of Chinese thought. One of the major Daoist texts states:

> When water is calm, it can reflect the beard and eyebrows, and its surface is so still that it can serve as a level for a carpenter. If the stillness of the water allows it to reflect things, then what can the spirit not do? How calm is the spirit of the saint! It is the mirror of the universe and all living things. Emptiness, stillness, detachment, carelessness, silence, non-acting are levels of the universe's equilibrium, the perfection of the way and of virtue.[19]

In the unconscious dynamics of relationships the patient 'provokes' the doctor to make responses that do not belong to the present condition but rather to a transferred situation; by abstaining the doctor avoids this operation, which tends to identify the present reality with an old story.[20]

---

[18] While the transference is this primary emotional experience linked to the patient, the countertransference is instead the emotional response we oppose to the patient's transference. The latter is one of the main tools used by the therapist to orient his actions within the therapy.

[19] *Zhuangzi*, Chapter 13, trad. it. Adelphi, 1982, p.114. For a discussion on *wu wei* 无 为 'non-acting', *dao* 道 'path', *de* 德 'power, virtue', see also Chapter 1 on classical thought.

[20] In this sense psychoanalysis speaks of 'abstinence': the patient must find the smallest possible quantity of substitute satisfactions to his symptoms. The analyst abstains from satisfying the patient's requests and from actually acting the roles that the patient tends to impose on him.

While maintaining an understanding sympathy, we cannot function like a friend or relative – relationships that belong to another sphere, that of reciprocity; we do not allow ourselves to become entangled in the patient's emotional games, we refrain from responding in the way he expects, and we abstain from returning the sentiments that the patient projects on us.

The wheel turns because it has an empty centre, *qi* circulates because the space is not completely filled; so we too must keep an emptiness that is not filled with what the patient expects us to do, or even with what we feel.

> The *shen* of man is revealed in its most true form in an intermediate space between intention-*yi* and non-intention. The doctor purifies his heart and concentrates his *shen* in the moment of the encounter, he perceives it, but it is not good for him to concentrate too much on defining it, in this case his personal intention is reawakened, the patient's *shen* and that of the doctor become confused, then he is prey to doubt and it is difficult to form a hypothesis.[21]

Upon contact with the destructive power of suffering, this attitude of non-adhesion allows us to truly 'be there' – mentally, affectively, and emotionally – and 'being there' means not being overrun: the emperor stands still as a mountain when the battle rages, an adult who is taking care of a child gathers and recomposes its frustrations and bad anger, the analyst acts as a 'container' for that which is too ugly for the patient to stand, and the doctor offers the support of empathy.[22]

Without specific psychodynamic training we cannot and must not interpret; attacking the defences of a patient is merely dangerous, and permitting deep processes of identification and regression is senseless. 'Being there' means, rather, using in a positive sense that non-specific transference which acts in the doctor–patient relationship, and which turns the doctor into 'the most used remedy in general medicine'.

---

[21] Shi Dinan, *Yiyuan* ('The origin of medicine'), chapter 'Wangse xucha shenqilun' ('Examining the *shen* in the inspection of the colour'). See also the discussion on memory and desire in Chapter 1 on classical thought.

[22] The concept of 'therapist as container' is developed by Winnicott, 1960: the analyst must let the patient develop his 'real', avoiding any invasiveness in certain phases of the therapeutic regression. The optimal function of the therapist in these conditions is that of an object 'sustaining' a role basically close to that of the mother, for those patients who did not receive maternal care. His intuition and his empathic comprehension are much more useful than verbal interpretation, with its disturbing effects experienced as intrusive. Bion highlights the 'intuitive daydreaming of the mother', whose *reverie* allows her to draw on herself the primitive, fragmented and dispersed experiences of distressing moments projected by the child, and thus recompose them. The intuition of the mother acts as a 'container' organising the projected content. On the consequences at the level of thought organisation see also Chapter 12 of *Apprendere dall'Esperienza* ('Learning from experience'), 1972. The analyst is used as a 'container' of those aspects that the patient can no longer bear to experiment on himself.

This 'being there' has two elements at the same time: empathy and neutrality.

A therapeutic relationship is obviously founded upon a feeling of trust and an alliance in the job, but it develops through empathy – in other words the 'ability to understand, listen to and share the thoughts and emotions of another person in a specific situation'.[23] Empathy includes a number of elements, all of which are fundamental: availability, attention, seriousness, warmth, acceptance, kindness, sympathy and support.

In a more specific way, empathy is defined as:

> Identification. Placing oneself in the psychological structures of another in such a way that thoughts, feelings and actions of the other person are understood and, in some way, foreseeable. Carl Rogers defines empathy as the ability to accompany another person wherever their feelings lead them, no matter how strong, deep, destructive or abnormal these may appear. Fenichel defines empathy as a process of temporary identification.[24]

Neutrality, which certainly does not mean indifference and coldness, is one of the aspects of an 'empty heart'. Jung, when commenting on the position of Switzerland regarding war, 'invites us to consider his nation (intended as a function) in the same way as the line which, in the symbol of the *dao*, runs between *yin* and *yang*' – in other words, not staying outside of the conflict, but in the middle.[25]

The suspension of moral judgement facilitates the abilities of listening and accepting, and permits the transformation of what would normally be a difficulty caused by being unknown to each other into an advantage, that of opening a new space.[26]

The concept of neutrality is also closely linked to the normal inclination to believe that the doctor, through his own experience, has managed to acquire a psychology of 'good sense' such that makes him able to face the psychological or relational problems of his patients. Even if at times it so happens that advice and encouragement do help, unfortunately the use of empirical methods acquired through daily experience is too fragile a guide to rely on. Since we do not know the underlying dynamics,

---

[23] Translation from N. Zingarelli, *Vocabolario della Lingua Italiana*, 1994

[24] L. E., Hinsie, R. J., Campbell, *Dizionario di Psichiatria* ('Dictionary of Psychiatry'), 1979, p. 244.

[25] P. F., Pieri, *Dizionario Junghiano* ('Jungian Dictionary'), 1998, p. 468. And he continues: 'In this sense neutrality expresses the condition assumed by the Ego during the psychic tension between opposites, so as to allow the transformation of the whole psychic apparatus.'

[26] In a more specifically psychoanalytic sense we read in Kernberg, 1984, p. 122: 'Neutrality is not a lack of warmth or empathy, it means keeping an equal distance between the forces which determine the intrapsychic conflicts of the patient. [...] Every psychotherapy asks the therapist at least the capacity to express authentic warmth and empathy, but empathy is not only an emotional, intuitive consciousness of the central experience of the patient in a definite moment; there must also be the ability to feel an empathy with that which the patient can not tolerate in himself.'

the possible advice (which in any case was probably already offered by other people with good sense) comprises, in fact, shots fired blindly.[27]

For example, even without going into the merits of complicated questions like emotional relationships or paths of self-realisation, it is quite difficult to find a patient who does not know it is unhealthy to eat in a hurry, or would not consider the practice of *qigong* useful, but notwithstanding the fact that he feels unwell he does not change his lifestyle. In reality, habits do not generally depend on simplistic factors like 'willpower', but rather are the result of very complex processes, the balance of which moves along lines and levels that are quite a bit deeper than cognitive–rational thinking.

Since, however, our role is supposed to be that of healing, we still have the problem as to how we should act when we observe behaviours that are more or less pathogenic.

First of all, the clearer is our vision and the more we have adapted certain internal practices the greater is the chance for the patient to open up. Our perception of this and its resonance happen at a different level to that of speech and verbal advice, and can have greater incisiveness.

On a cognitive level we can try to consider together with the patient what other solutions can be set into action, to determine what different behaviours can be thought of and put into practice more profitably. We can also prescribe an exercise, or a diet; any modification of a specific behaviour can be prescribed just as with medicines – but what, when and how to prescribe them must be defined extremely precisely. Life cannot be prescribed.

Those cases in which the person in front of us explicitly asks for indications on diet, exercises, lifestyle habits, etc., are obviously of a different order; these are cases in which, among other things, the knowledge offered by Chinese medicine is very rich and valuable.

THE PATIENT INSIDE OF ME

Every treatment has aspects of caring and taking charge, but also has elements of limits and separation.

The tendency of the patient to let himself go and that of the therapist to take care of him can slide into an excess of closeness, with unconscious processes of identification that lead to a sort of fusion with no way out. In other words, my participation is definitely a great help for the cure, but what good is it for

---

[27] On this issue see Balint, 1957, who speaks of the uselessness of the 'apostolic mission or function', referring to the vague idea that each doctor has of how his patients should act to face their illnesses, from which stems a sort of need to convert to his faith incredulous patients. As reassuring, it is not negative in itself, but it is dangerous when applied grossly and unconsciously.

the patient to have a person near him who feels his emotions and experiences his unwellness?

Excessive distance has no space for therapeutic change, as it is constructed by maintaining a rigid detachment or by distancing the complications of the emotions through indifference and coldness.

There are always blind spots in the mind of the therapist, and we must take them into account and do what can be done so that they do the least damage possible. We can look into ourselves for the motivations, or better yet the needs, that we try to address by practising this profession.

It may be, for example, that:

- old wounds still hurt too much, and I try to heal them by continuously taking care of others suffering;
- I can be aware of my existence only through the requests to which I respond with availability and sacrifice;
- the state of aid or victim is an instrument which allows me to exercise control over the situation;
- I cannot allow myself to see the other, his difference, so I assume the role of the omniscient doctor, invading ever bigger spheres in other's lives;
- any lack or any imperfection is intolerable for me, and immediately evokes judgements and punishments.

He who cures is not a teacher–guru–priest, nor a mother, nor a judge, but can possess fragments of all of these, and of much, much more.

And when we do not refuse these motivations, they have the richness of manure, which stinks a little, but also fertilises.

Case Study 15.1

Like a Buoy in the Sea

A 70-year-old woman came to me for the first time 6 years ago complaining of lumbar–sacral pain and a pain with functional impediment in the first finger of her right hand. Examination revealed a herniated disk at L3–L4 with degenerative disk pathology at L5–S1 and arthritis with a bone nub in the finger of her right hand; she has taken anti-inflammatory drugs daily for years.

These initial symptoms cleared up fairly quickly, but she returns periodically ever since then for a course of therapy that lasts a few months, with treatments every 1 or 2 weeks.

Over time she had vision disorders, heartburn, chest constraint, knee pain, numbness in the arm and trouble in falling asleep, have followed one after the other, with diffuse anxiety as a steady element.

Treatment had followed the underlying diagnosis, which was stagnation of *qi*, plus painful obstruction in the channels due to cold and dampness, internal heat, *yin* deficiency, restlessness of the *shen*, etc.

A childless widow, she works full time, and on weekends sets off by herself to her house in the mountains. She has short hair, is well dressed, and wears coloured earrings. Notwithstanding her age, you would not call her old, perhaps also because she still has the typical features of theatricality of a girl–woman.

She speaks willingly, even if often too fast to be understood. She tells of her nephews, of events that have touched her in recent days, of what her late husband (who had died many years earlier), or father, or the friend that had died more recently, meant to her.

Although she constantly took aspirin in the past, which – as she herself recognises – acted as a sort of lifejacket, this aspect has now been under control for some time, but cannot be defined as 'resolved' since apprehensions and agitation, and pain in the arm or in the lumbar region, appear at times, especially when she 'has less desire to go out and do things'.

Her involvement in a number of *qigong* practices was superficial and of limited duration and my exploration of the possibility of working at a deeper level was unsuccessful. Clearly others might have succeeded where I had failed, but I believe that this case may offer a number of points to reflect upon beyond the immediate results. In those cases in which the resolution of symptoms is only temporary, various issues present themselves, which while pertaining to diverse levels can be the cause of difficulties in different ways.

Beyond the interference caused by transference, it is never simple to understand our behaviour in these complex circumstances characterised by the cyclical reappearance of symptoms and coming for treatment: we suspect that our actions collude with the difficulty in changing and therefore validate a process that is, in point of fact, pathological.

In everyday practice we may have doubts, for example, about our attitudes and conduct with regard to patients who do not pursue a path that we have judged will be beneficial for them, such as the practice of *qigong*.

We then ask ourselves how intransigent we should be and whether it makes sense to be so.

A non-judgemental position can be maintained if we as doctors adopt a vision of the world and the person in which our acts of assistance are kept free of prejudgements about the receiver, or can simply derive from adhering to the Hippocratic principle that the work of a doctor must respect the choice of his patients.

Another aspect present in these treatments that are characterised by the lack of resolution is the frustration of the doctor, who, over time, sees his attempts at a cure fail. It is obviously unacceptable to express this sentiment through direct anger or aggressiveness; however, when one is tired the internal constraint of *qi* this situation can produce runs the risk of resolution in a sadistic manner, in which the practitioner shifts his impotence onto the patient ('it is your fault; it's all in your head').

The intense countertransference dynamic that often acts in these cases produces a condition in which the physician finds himself experiencing the same deep feelings of the patient; the non-healing of a person with *qi* stagnation who is continuously frustrated in realising his desires can in effect be a form of passive resistance, which invalidates the doctor's efforts and makes him feel as the patient does.

This type of communication is decidedly indirect and involuntary, and being aware of it does not completely clear away the fog in which we move; however, it allows us to maintain a calmer heart while working and permits us to evaluate the results of the therapy with greater objectivity.

At times the results seem be limited to a containment of biomedical intrusions, with a reduction in drug usage or recourse to investigations, but if this is accompanied by a gradual reduction in treatment frequency this can itself be a sign of a greater possibility of living with the fear which undermines life at the root.

In the case which I have just presented I confronted all these doubts and uncertainties, the sense of uselessness and futility, and, naturally, the feelings of impatience and anger. All this related to me personally and showed the need for further reflection.

I had the sensation that I acted as a sort of buoy for the patient, anchored to the bottom of the sea, to grab hold of when you are too tired in the water, or when the waves crash too strongly and you wish to recover your strength. However, the continued use of aspirin, which had started to cause her to bleed, would probably have been more damaging, and possibly this latest mourning for her friend might have had more serious consequences.

Even the role of 'being there' can often be more complicated than it seems, however. For example: it is the first treatment after a number of months, I have returned to Milan after a rather long absence and when she describes the way in which she perceives the actual presence of her departed loved ones I make a remark which is equivalent to a direct reassurance.

She immediately takes advantage of the situation: she tells me a long story about a friend who had asked her to do her a big favour and to whom she did not respond, and she asks me to justify her in a not so implicit manner. As usual, I remain silent about this. She tries again and I again maintain my silence. At the end of the appointment she says: 'I thought you would tell me that I had behaved properly'. I respond: 'I am sorry, but I can say nothing'. In effect, absolution and condemnation have nothing to do with the therapeutic support. However, she insists: 'I thought you would tell me I was right'. And I: 'But how can I do that? It is not my position to judge whether you have behaved well or badly'.

This sentence made explicit the difference between my role and a relationship of reciprocity, in which the other person can become an ally, accomplice or judge.

In effect, however, it was (I hope) a remedy to my previous error of 'reassuring' her, when I had carelessly deviated from the usual sequence: initial greetings, 5 minutes of various narratives on her part (with minimal intervention by me if the conversation about her nephews or other people became too long), five more to update the somatic picture, measuring of her blood pressure (a ceremony which counterbalances her hypochondriac fears), 20 minutes of needles (during which she remains alone, or in any case silent even if I am next to her, for example, in those cases where moxa cones are necessary), confirmation of the next appointment, and goodbyes.

I have mentioned these details to give an idea of actual proceedings in applying the concept of support, which does not include my telling the patient that she is right, or agreeing with her, or justifying her, and certainly not telling her what to do. She well knows my sympathy and affection for her; the help that I can give her is not to sink, break or disappear, and possibly not to swing back and forth too much.

Case Study 15.2

The Little Girl Who Would Not Eat or Sit Still

This case is incomplete, but is presented here because it contains a number of relevant features.

The young girl is 7 years old and has an acute intelligence, great sensitivity, and numerous natural talents, which are held in high consideration by her family.

She is thin, has lively eyes, a thin face and a slightly dull complexion.

For years she has eaten almost nothing and still accepts only a limited number of tastes and textures of food.

Furthermore, her incessant activity and absence of rest periods in her untiring movements have been notable since she was very little. Those who are close to her find themselves in a perpetual state of pre-alarm because her manner of moving around and touching things places the things around her, and probably her own safety, at risk.

Diagnosis
Emptiness of spleen *qi* with hyperactivity.

Therapeutic Principles
Tonify the *qi* of the middle *jiao*.

Treatment Rationale
Points may be chosen such as:
• ST-36 *Zusanli*, SP-6 *Sanyinjiao*, BL-20 *Pishu*, Ren-12 *Zhongwan*.

Comments
From the point of view of diagnosis it is fundamental not to confuse hyperactivity with signs of fullness, but rather to recognise the deficiency of spleen *qi*, which manifests in significantly altered appetite and eating habits, in the various signs

and symptoms and – as Julian Scott says – in the practice of appropriating and utilising other people's energy.

With these children, who are skilled manipulators, it is imperative to know what one is doing: to recognise exactly what is happening when the needle is inserted, whether it is causing pain or not, and to know clearly when *qi* arrives, how it arrives and where it goes (see Chapter 12 on methods of stimulation in this respect).

It is important to let them know that we know; that at least in this case their deceptions did not work. This experience of being contained is in reality a huge relief for the child, because someone else is taking charge of placing limits.

In this case, all this happened between the two of us entirely through facial expressions made 'back and forth', and I believe that in some way it worked, because the child returned for her second appointment without complaining. This young girl made an interesting comment after her first treatment, which was related to me by her mother: she said was tired and that she 'felt old'. This phrase could be describing a sensation that in some way is similar to a state of peace – a 'truce' in the condition of hyperactive *qi*.

The mother later preferred not to continue the therapy because she felt that, on the one hand, the request for a bland diet at school might help make up for the eating problems and, on the other, that the child's brilliant scholastic results would be sufficient to overcome the difficulties with the teachers.

Events Related to Acupuncture

Chinese medicine works on *qi*; the action on its imbalance – be it constraint, disruption, stasis or deficiency – produces changes at all levels.

Change can consist of a healthy recovery with the disappearance of symptoms, but as the needles affect the state of the energy the changes in the system can manifest themselves in many ways.

First of all there is the perception of the action on *qi*, which can range from an experience of peacefulness during the session to more complex internal sensations.

If everything works out well the feeling of well-being will concern not only the regression of the symptoms related by the patient, but also other aspects that have not been reported, producing 'unexpected effects' that will confirm the diagnosis and the therapeutic choices.

The following notes are simply some work jottings through which attention will be drawn to certain aspects. They are by no means complete or conclusively elaborated.

Although, on the one hand, acupuncture is often presented as non-symptomatic medicine, it is fundamental to keep in mind both what the expectations of the patient are and what our role is in relation to the illness and the patient's requests.

The same attention must be paid to the therapeutic relationship in cases of chronic illness with a fatal progression, but this too is an aspect on which the community of acupuncturists has only just begun to reflect. The following notes are presented as a starting point for further thought.

IMMEDIATE EFFECTS

The most evident immediate effects of acupuncture usually have two aspects: pain and agitation. The intensity of acute pain is generally more or less reduced and the acupuncture session calms the patient both physically and mentally (often falling asleep).

A slight modification of perception is frequently experienced during the session, which has a strong impression on those who have never experienced different states of conscience. This sensation is often accompanied by disorientation, but it also feels somewhat pleasant, which is an important opening to the work that will be conducted.

A similar quality characterises that specific sensation of physical and mental lightness that often follows a session.

There is a frequent manifestation of intense emotional and physical responses, such as sighing, tears, sobbing, shivers and a variety of different sensations of shifting, filling and emptying involving different parts of the body. Sometimes there is a possibility of perceptual distortion, the most common being alteration of the sense of smell, colour, or of body position, but a more complex hallucination might also occur. (For example a patient with *qi* and phlegm constriction who is treated with a stimulation of *Yintang*. Afterwards, she sees her head as though from the outside. It opens and a figure emerges from it. It appears small against a sea background. It then comes closer, turns and reveals itself as being the patient herself but in her old age and almost bald.)

The acupuncturist and the needle are the vehicles for the connection between the *qi* of the patient and that of the universe. The doctor works by means of the *qi* and therefore has to make sure that the needle works (i.e. that the *qi* moves). These movements of the *qi* and emotions must be controlled, or at least one must avoid being overwhelmed by them.

Let us briefly reiterate some of the basic qualities needed by the acupuncturist: when treating the patient the heart must be open, truthful, unwavering, calm and empty.[1]

To have an 'empty heart' means also to undergo that laborious process whereby one casts off habits of prejudice that bias and stiffen us; this is the prerequisite for developing *shen* (or *ling*) comprehension – that is to say the clear, deep, immediate comprehension that replaces the 'thousand thoughts' and hypothesis.

UNEXPECTED EFFECTS

In clinical work there are a number of non-specific and uninvestigated therapeutic effects.[2]

---

[1] See Chapter 12 for notes on stimulation and use of needles to influence *qi*. See Chapter 15 for clinical references and considerations on the therapy space shared by patient and acupuncturist.
[2] See also the comments concerning the child treated for headache whose behaviour at school changed (case study 15.2).

For instance, it is quite common for patients to report improvements in a specific symptom that they had never spoken of and that therefore had not been specifically treated.

A typical case, already presented, is that of the man who thought he was going to die (see case study 12.1) and who also had a pain in the elbow that I came to know about only after he got better. At that time the tennis elbow was obviously not a major concern and so he had not mentioned it, but the general treatment of the *qi* had clearly regulated the *qi* of that channel also, with a consequent resolution of the symptom.

Similar characteristics can be observed in the case of a 43-year-old patient who comes to me after the umpteenth episode of violent and abrupt colicky pain for which she had previously visited the emergency ward. The pain is piercing, radiates from the right scapula, and is accompanied by nausea, vertigo and sweating. From a rather hasty interview, for I had included this as an urgent visit, I find only a tendency to bitter mouth and constipation, while she considered her menstrual cycle to be regular. However, she reported that her menses after the first session were very different from previous ones, that is, 'without the usual delay, immediately flowing, with no nocturnal flooding, not painful'.[3]

There are also frequent effects in the sexual area that have not been targeted directly. Both men and women often report that they had been suffering diminished or absent desire or various difficulties in accomplishing the sexual act satisfactorily only after the situation has improved. In most texts such cases concern an emptiness of *yang*, but actually they can often be attributed to a simple *qi* deficiency caused by constraint or stagnation.

The case of the woman who felt her throat closing (see case study 10.4) and who rediscovered sexual pleasure after treatment is typical of an absence of libido associated with constraint of the *qi* and emptiness of *yin*.

Stagnation of *qi* was the primary cause for the impotence of a man of 35 who had turned to acupuncture for cervical pain. He spoke about a 'body the does not follow the mind' only in response to direct questions during the first interview and at the end of the therapy, when the cervical pain had disappeared. It seems that his sexual activity has become much more satisfactory even though it was not one of the central points in therapeutic strategy.

A deficiency of the *qi* was the principal cause of weakness in a 45-year-old singer who was worried that her vocal cords and strength would become insufficient to sustain public performances. In this case too the improvement

---

[3] *Diagnosis*: Stagnation of liver and gall bladder *qi*. Treatment: 1st session: *Neiguan* P-6, *Zhongwan* Ren-12, *Tianshu* ST-25, *Riyue* GB-24, *Yanglingquan* GB-34, *Taichong* LIV-3. Three other sessions follow in a short period and one session per month for 10 months, with slight changes in the points. During this year there have been four episodes of dull yet slight pain. Follow-up, after 1 year: there are no more biliary symptoms and the menstrual cycle is regular.

of her general conditions and the disappearance of her propensity to fatigue/tiredness coincided with renewed desire and pleasure.[4]

Unexpected 'psychological effects' are extremely frequent. It is quite common for patients to report a general improvement because they feel in a better mood, because they have slept better than they had done for a long time, because new energy has 'magically' appeared, or because they feel strangely peaceful or have made a decision – and all of this without the problems of mood, sleep, fatigue or agitation being the stated reason for the visit. In some cases the patients were not even aware of these problems.

A typical example is that of the 34-year-old woman who comes to me for treatment because of recurrent lumbar and sacral pain, which for the last 6 months has turned out to be rather disabling in her everyday life. During the eighth session, when the symptoms have almost disappeared and the therapy is halted for the summer holidays, I ask her if she has noticed any other more general effects. The answer is that she feels calmer and that her mood has become more calmer, for example she is not agitated when giving an important dinner and does not worry, as usual, about the fact that she and her husband have not yet decided where to go on holiday.

Of course they are not revolutionary, but nevertheless these changes in everyday behaviour and thought are not at all simple and obvious; in this case the action of inducing qi and blood to circulate in the jingluo included moving the liver qi and had effects on qi and emotions in general.[5]

Bearing in mind these cases, it can be noted that the shift in the energetic state occurs most often in syndromes involving stagnation of liver qi (see case studies 2.2, 4.1, 10.5, 15.2). In fact, when pathological changes are consolidated (i.e. when there is a fullness of fire or of phlegm, blood stasis, or emptiness of qi or yin) the condition is such that the psychological symptoms actually disturb the patient and are therefore recognised and treated more directly. Unhappiness, frustration or discontent lead to suffering/resentment – in the double sense of the body suffering from something and of acrimony towards the world. In terms of conventional psychiatry, stagnation of the qi corresponds mainly to somatic disorders. To use different terminology, for example Jungian, the unfulfilled

---

[4] *Other symptoms*: insomnia, fatigability, easy crying, feeling the cold, semifluid faeces or constipation, skinniness, frequent throat pain with a growth of the laterocervical lymph gland, recurrent bronchitis in remote case history.

Diagnosis: Deficit of lung, spleen and heart qi.

Treatment: Points are chosen among: *Lieque* LU-7, *Taibai* SP-3, *Zusanli* ST-36, *Feishu* BL-13, *Pishu* BL-20, *Renying* ST-9, *Yintang* EX-HN-3, *Tiantu* Ren-22, *Tanzhong* Ren-17, *Qsihai* Ren-6, etc.

[5] *Diagnosis*: Obstruction of qi and blood in the *Shao Yang* channel (the pain spreads to the inferior limb, laterally).

Treatment: Points of gall bladder on the inferior limb, local points chosen among the *Baliao* BL-31-34 and the *huatuo jiaji* EX-B-2, *Taichong* LIV-3.

Follow-up. After 5 months: she was well both physically and emotionally, but in the last days, perhaps due to the increase of work at the end of the year, she felt the usual pain, yet more moderate.

expression of one's self and the constraint in the development of one's potential bring with them signs of somatic and psychological distress.

REQUESTS IN PSYCHOLOGICAL CONDITIONS AND CHRONIC ILLNESS

Working on rebalancing the *qi* can be the starting point for effecting a change in both internal attitudes and external behaviours.

There are cases in which the person turns to acupuncture in situations of anxiety or depression: Chinese medicine is quite effective but it is always good to remember that it is proper medicine, and resorting to it may lead to a medicalisation of the problem, of the disorder, of the difficulty of life. It can be an expression of a tendency to 'psychologise' the pains of the body: suffering does not automatically call for therapy.

Those who resort to non-conventional medicine are often conscious of their emotional and psychological movements or somehow feel a need for a change at this level even though their view of the situation is not completely clear. The patient finds in the treatment with Chinese medicine a space for these emotional and psychological aspects.

It is worth remembering that symptom presentation is often influenced by the context of the clinical interaction: a type of medicine such as acupuncture seems to be located somewhere between the context of general medicine, where the patient might, for example, worry about palpitations and interpret them as a dysfunction of the heart, and a psychiatric or psychoanalytic context, where the patient can give greater expression to feelings of anguish.

Moreover treatment with acupuncture has a diachronic structure, so that in different sessions it can facilitate the emergence of the physical or the emotional aspects of the problem. Even the time when the patient has the needles in place is space for a sort of decantation, as if solid and liquid were separating, enabling the perception of emotions to occur precisely.

The energetic perspective of acupuncture allows an integration of the different physical and mental manifestations, and this may be the reason why the patient initially chose this approach, or it may emerge and take form during the therapy. For instance, an appeal that suggests some psychological elements may be just mentioned in passing, or it can be tacit, as often happens with youngsters and teenagers.

In clinical practice it is particularly important to be conscious of the nature of the patient's request. This may range from a very specific one to an expectation that is almost unlimited both in time and in symptoms (see case study 16.1 as an example). At one extreme is the case of someone who comes to us for an acute backache or a frequent headache and, once the pain is treated successfully (or unsuccessfully), stops seeing the doctor. The trust we build up during the treatment course might mean that the patient returns in similar circumstances when medical help is being sought, but it again involves a limited intervention.

In other circumstances the patient's request might grow into a wider demand in which the acupuncturist, or Chinese medicine itself, become a point of reference by which the person orientates his life. This latter role is a risky one. Chapter 15 discussed in detail the various aspects of the dynamics of relationships, and the importance of abstinence and neutrality; here I will relate only a short episode that has greatly impressed me. A patient who was sent to me by a colleague for a potential psychotherapy treatment, in the midst of a dream association, connects the stomach with a fracture, a trauma that my colleague would have mentioned while observing his tongue. The most likely reconstruction is that the colleague had spoken about a 'split' in the stomach area of the tongue (the central crack) and that this had set off a multitude of interpretations that led to a connection with a trauma caused by lack of affection. The episode in itself is neither positive nor negative, but rather an example of how an initial input can create unexpected images or ideas.

The brevity of a therapy is not in itself a parameter by which to determine the 'boundaries' of the request and consequently of the relationship: chronic pathologies that need continuous treatment can be similar in nature. Here also it is often useful to maintain a certain distance and neutrality. In the case of patients with degenerative diseases, cancer or HIV, it is essential that the illness does not pervade all of their life, for we cannot take the chance of their equating their pathology with their living.

The relevance of psychological strain is also quite evident to the patient, even when it is not continuously expressed. Anxiousness and insomnia, despondency and fear are well known companions. The acupuncturist takes care of them daily, making sure that there are no stagnations and knots in the *qi*, while tonifying it and nourishing the *yin*.

It is very difficult for the therapist to know the real causes of the illness or to know their possible developments, but he/she can become an instrument for the patient to draw upon when and how he wants. The instrument consists both of the specific knowledge acquired by the doctor (acupuncture, *qigong*, prescriptions, dietetic guidelines, etc.) and of his/her 'being there'.

The empathic component, although essential, must be accompanied at all times by a basic feature of civilisation – that of respect: in fact, in these situations of fragility, any interference can easily turn into abuse.

Case Study 16.1

Being Able to Say No

A 21-year-old woman is directed to me for a headache that she speaks of as being continuously present in her life, but which has become more frequent at the age of

16 when she began using oral contraceptives. She has a nice face with a sweet smile and a peaceful expression, although she sometimes looks frightened. Her father had died the previous year after a long illness and she worries about her mother, who is quite depressed and lives alone in another city.

She works in the social sector, usually with great pleasure and satisfaction, but this activity is now becoming extremely tiring because she is dealing with a difficult case in a very manipulative family.

The headache appears during the day, it is bilateral, located in the eyes, forehead and temples, and is continuous with stronger stabs of pain accompanied by nausea; the fits take place once or twice every week and they tend to be more frequent just before her menstrual period and during the first days of it.

Cold, humidity, chocolate, fried food, long waits and weekends are all factors that worsen the situation.

The interview reveals other relevant information: her abdomen is often swollen while her bowels, which were constipated, have been regular since she adopted a vegetarian diet in the last year; she often feels cold, especially in the hands and feet, but she is very thirsty and is often subject to mouth ulcers; her sleep is good.

The tongue is slightly pale, with curled up edges, but not red, the coating is thin and yellow. The pulse is thin and wiry.

Diagnosis

Stagnation of liver *qi*, heat in the *yangming*, and fullness of the gall bladder.

Therapeutic Principles

Facilitate the circulation of the *qi*, eliminate the heat and regulate the *qi* in *yangming*, liver and gall bladder.

Treatment

Nine sessions: the first four every 5 days, the fifth and the sixth after 7 and 10 days, and the last three once per month.

- GB-20 *Fengchi*, ST-8 *Touwei*, ST-36 *Zusanli*, ST-44 *Neiting*, LI-4 *Hegu*, Ren-6 *Qihai*.

In the second session she says that she has noticed some signs of the headache, which then did not develop. This type of progress in which the painful symptoms become milder is quite common at the beginning of the treatments of severe headaches and it is usually a good prognostic sign.

She says she has resigned from her job and she is happy to have done so. In fact she had been thinking of it for a long time but could never get herself to do it.

After the second session she reports an episode of medium-strong headache with the simultaneous appearance of a cold and a slight temperature. Another crisis takes place after the third session, during the premenstrual time.

In the fifth session she declares that she has not had any headaches, even during her period, and she says she has returned to work because they had transferred the case of the family she could not handle to someone else.

She says that after the stimulation of GB-20 *Fengchi* she had for some hours a feeling, which then disappeared spontaneously, of 'having something in her throat'. In this session the insertion of the needle in GB-20 *Fengchi* causes a strong pain in the forehead, around GB-14 *Yangbai*, on the right. This disappears after the stimulation of GB-41 *Zulinqi* of the same side.

I therefore substitute the three stomach points with GB-41 *Zulinqi* and LIV-3 *Taichong* and I keep the same combination in the four following sessions:

- GB-20 *Fengchi*, GB-41 *Zulinqi*, LIV-3 *Taichong*, LI-4 *Hegu*, Ren-4 *Guanyuan*.

The knot in the throat no longer appears and the headache attacks are reduced to a few, occasional, mild episodes.

Comments

The stagnation of the liver *qi* was also evident in the curled up edges of the tongue and in the wiry pulse; when the *qi* cannot circulate freely a series of different 'contractions' arise: tension in various muscular areas, emotional constraint, curled-up edges of the tongue and 'contracted' vessels, so that the pulse is tense like a bowstring.

I chose to start working on *Yang Ming* because this was the level where I could see the most overt manifestations of fullness. I then orientated the treatment towards regulating the wood *qi*. Its stagnation was probably the source of the heat and of the uprising *yang*.

The best moment for changing the direction of the treatment was signalled by specific events: the stimulation of a point such as GB-20 *Fengchi*, so important in the regulation of the downward flow of *qi*, highlighted both an obstruction, which at first did not manifest (*meiheqi*, 'plum stone'), and a blockage in the channel (the pain in GB-14 *Yangbai*). This suggested the use of GB-41 *Zulinqi* for its capacity to move the *qi* and take it down, and of LIV-3 *Taichong* to regulate it.

I have reported this case because it is a good example of how constrictions can manifest themselves at different levels and of how the treatment acts on various expressions and alterations of the movements of the *qi*, be they a pain in the head or a difficulty in making decisions.

Obviously it could have been a pure coincidence, but the connection between the resolution of somatic symptoms and that of an equivalent 'freeing' action, like tendering a resignation, is quite a common experience.

Follow-up

After a few months the girl decides to go back to her hometown. When I hear from her again, 5 months later, she tells me that life is not easy and that she had some episodes of headache, but infrequent and bearable. In the last month the attacks have reappeared as a result of an accident with whiplash injury. They are as frequent and severe as they used to be, so she has decided to resort again to acupuncture.

Case Study 16.2

Chronic Diseases

There are many cancer or neurological patients who are now resorting to acupuncture and also a growing number of HIV+ persons who seek its help.

I do not have direct experience with treating cancer patients because I prefer to direct them to colleagues with specific expertise. However, I treat a number of patients with degenerative diseases and those who are HIV+, and I believe that in such situations the relationship aspects and the general care of the patient are fundamental but delicate matters.

In the case of HIV+ patients the situation varies depending on whether or not they are receiving drug treatment. In this respect much has changed over recent years with the introduction of protease inhibitors, but psychological factors are still relevant. Acupuncture has an important role here: it preserves an energetic balance that allows the body to react more effectively to the attacks of external pathogens; it reduces the consequences of the drugs, such as production of heat, accumulation of phlegm, stagnation of the *qi* or consumption of *yin*; it balances the effects of latent heat in the deepest layers; it soothes emotional disturbance caused by the diagnosis and by subsequent events.

In these situations it is also possible for feelings of guilt and punishment, which are inherent in the presentation of any disease, to become stronger and grow. As in all therapeutic relationships, it is important to maintain an attitude of empathy and neutrality, and to develop our earth nature – the element that dwells in the centre, and has the power of accepting all (the clean as well as the dirty things), of transforming, of nourishing and of helping to sprout.[6]

Here I will refer briefly to two cases that can illustrate certain psychological aspects of long-term therapy.

First, a 20-year-old student from Milan, suffering from a de-myelisation disease, has turned to a centre in Florence and a colleague directs him to me for the acupuncture treatment. He has now been coming to my clinic for more than a year, with weekly sessions (the initial request was twice a week) and some intervals, but it was agreed that the doctor in Florence would remain his main point of reference.

---

[6] With regard to this point the *qigong* and acupuncture master Liu Dong says that traditionally it was important for a student to have this earthly nature (*tuxing*), but that this could also be reached through transformation (MediCina seminar, December 2001). The role of the earth as a neutral element that makes any transformation and any definition possible is re-proposed by F. Jullien in *Elogio dell'insapore*, 1999. Here he traces its origin in the concept of *dan* 淡, 'tasteless', in Daoist and Confucian thought as well as in painting, literature, music, cuisine, gardens, etc.

The multiple sclerosis was diagnosed the previous year and the symptoms basically consisted in numbness of variable quality, gravity, duration and localisation, and as episodes described as 'muffled head, dulled perceptions, and sensations of losing my sense of balance'. The symptoms worsened with air humidity, the tongue had red dots with spots and a thick, white coating, and the pulse was deep and wiry.

The treatment focused on *Yang Ming* to tonify *qi* and blood (LI-4 *Hegu* and ST-36 *Zusanli*), alternating with that on *Yang Wei Mai,* the extraordinary channel greatly involved in locomotion (TB-5 *Waiguan* and GB-41 *Zulinqi*). It was also important to sustain the *yang* (Du-14 *Dazhui*, Ren-6 *Qihai*, KI-3 *Taixi*) and transform the phlegm (ST-40 *Fenglong* and P-5 *Jianshi*). At times the *shu* points on the back of the involved organs were chosen. On all occasions I used MS-7 (the sensitive area of scalp-acupuncture, with electrostimulation).

The young man was clearly thinking a lot and I decided not to dwell on his descriptions of his state of mind. Just before the summer break I asked him if he thought there were any 'general effects' of the treatment. He answered that he could perceive a change in his feelings: before he was more indifferent towards events. The people around him and his friends would say that he seemed to be far away and detached from matters pertaining to life.

This wider contact with the internal and external world could also derive from the work on the transformation of the phlegm, which is an important aspect of the pathology.

In autumn he asks me for some information and decides to start *taijiquan* and *qigong*, practices I had mentioned some months before.

In the other case, a patient suffering from the same disease, I made a similar decision and did not dwell on the psychological aspects, always remaining very neutral.

This patient, a 30-year-old insurance agent, had suffered from an obsessive–compulsive disorder since he was a teenager. He had resolved this problem two years previously thanks to three years of psychoanalysis, which he had started after being diagnosed with multiple sclerosis.

His pale complexion, feeble voice, quiet manner and limited thirst indicated coldness, but his disposition to constipation, red tongue with curled up edges and yellow coating, and rapid and flooding pulse signalled the presence of internal heat. The heat would manifest also as bad temper.[7] The diagnosis was one of hidden heat, false coldness and true heat, with consequent therapeutic indications.

The treatment is therefore based on therapeutic principles and points similar to those illustrated in the previous case. In addition it acts on the motor area MS-6 because there is impeded movement in the lower limbs, and focuses more on

---

[7] For example he answered the question I always pose before the beginning of the summer break: 'Would you say that acupuncture has had some generic effect?' in this way: 'Like benzodiazepine: I feel more pacified'. 'Would you say that it calms anxiety?' 'No, I am not anxious, I am short-tempered.'

nourishing the *yin* and eliminating internal fire using points such as BL-15 *Xinshu*, BL-18 *Ganshu*, BL-20 *Pishu*, SP-6 *Sanyinjiao*, LIV-3 *Taichong*, LIV-8 *Ququan*, etc.

In the seventh session, after one and a half months of therapy, the patient tells me he has decided to discontinue the treatment with antidepressants and he asks for my help. I mention to him the Acudetox method, pointing out how it can be repeated at short intervals. He halves the dosage of the serotonergic drug and the following week he suspends the treatment completely. I give just two detoxifying treatments using the five auricular points, without any need to change the weekly frequency of the sessions or introduce psychotherapeutic sessions.

SECTION IV

CONTEMPORARY CLINICAL CONTRIBUTIONS

This section on contemporary applications stems from the consideration that theoretical models are a result of experience and that, in order to maintain their validity, they must be regarded as areas of research.

Acupuncture is also a craft, a practical and direct knowledge that involves the things we observe while working with our patients, as well as those that we have studied and 'accepted'. However, there are also other elements playing a part, elements that come from more marginal perspectives and enable us to look at objects from various angles, to see them lit in different colours.

In different times and places various basic theories of the Chinese medical thought were put forward to meet a range of perspectives, which tended to highlight specific elements; the contributions presented here illustrate attempts to systematise the theories of reference and to verify them in the clinic so as to keep them alive.

Tongue and *Shen*
Barbara Kirschbaum

17

INTRODUCTION

This contribution by Barbara Kirschbaum refers specifically to diagnosis based on the tongue signs.

Here her profound knowledge background is combined with skills of acute observation and clear diagnosis.

In this short chapter she reminds us that the *shen*, being beyond *yin* and *yang*, cannot be considered in terms of strength and weakness; nor can it be judged directly from the tongue. However, from the tongue's appearance we can draw inferences about the abode of the *shen*, as it reveals the energetic conditions of the heart, home of the *shen*, the state of *yin* and blood, which nourish and root it, and the alterations of *qi*, liquids, essence and organs, which participate in the quality of the emotional and mental life.

The original contribution of Barbara Kirschbaum is followed by a brief recapitulation of the main signs referring to clinical patterns where the alteration of the *shen* is important.

The 'summary notes on the key signs regarding *shen*' are borrowed from her text and have been edited in collaboration with Margherita Majno.[1]

TONGUE DIAGNOSIS AND *SHEN*

The *shen* is beyond *yin* and *yang*; it cannot be measured and judged in terms of *yin* and *yang*. This means that the state of the *shen* cannot be seen directly on the tongue.

---

[1] For an overview of tongue diagnosis refer to her *Atlas of Tongue Diagnosis*, 2000 (German edition 1998), which illustrates the tongue signs through an excellent photographic documentation. The text *Applied Tongue Diagnosis*, is also being published. It combines tongue diagnosis, general differential diagnosis and clinical notes. The summary notes are also borrowed from her seminar 'Diagnosis of the tongue body', June 2001, MediCina. An excellent manual for diagnosis by examination of the tongue is also G. Maciocia, *Tongue Diagnosis in Chinese Medicine*, 1995.

Nevertheless the tongue body, the colour and the coating reflect the energetic conditions that ensure the stability and nourishment of the spirit.

The heart is the home of the *shen*. In order to fulfil this function the heart must be nourished by blood and *yin*. The mind can flourish only when blood and *yin* are in good shape.

When blood and *yin* are sufficient, sleep is good and the mental and emotional capacities are strong.

In the field of tongue diagnosis it is mostly the tip of the tongue that reveals the conditions of the heart. This is the topographic area that corresponds to the heart, thus reflecting its pathologies. Changes in the shape and colour of this region reveal disharmonies of the heart and alterations in the home of the *shen*.

There are signs that reveal clearly a lack of heart blood or heart *yin*.

The colour of the tongue body when the heart blood is insufficient will always be pale. If this deficiency lasts for long the tip will not only be pale but it will also have a deep indentation. This is due to the fact that the chronic lack of blood prevents the filling of the tip of the tongue, thus changing its normal shape. Those who have this type of tongue are often very anxious, have a tendency to be easily startled and have difficulties in falling asleep.

When the lack of heart blood evolves into empty heat, the tip of the tongue becomes red. Since heat troubles the spirit the person grows restless, suffers from palpitations and more severe sleep disorders. Thus the tongue reveals the alterations of the energetic state of the heart, which influence and disturb the *shen*.

When the communication between water and fire, between kidney and heart is disturbed, the clinical mental pattern can become very serious. If there is an underlying insufficiency of kidney *yin*, the heart *yin* will linger without nourishment. The kidney *yin* cannot rise to nourish heart *yang*. The resulting empty heart will produce night sweating, insomnia, anxiousness, deep mental restlessness, agitation and nervousness, and often an inability to concentrate. This process is reflected in a red tongue body, with a rootless coating and in an evident reddening of the tip.

The tongue signs are of great help when distinguishing empty fire from heart fire. If the heart fire is blazing, the tip of the tongue will be extremely red or curved upwards and the tongue body will be red and covered in a thick and greasy yellow coating. The mental agitation will be more evident and the patient will have a tendency to be more impulsive and agitated with thirst, insomnia and sometimes aphthae in the oral cavity.

The heart fire damages the fluids and this may lead to the formation of fire-phlegm that disturbs the heart. The consequence may be severe mental disorder, including psychotic forms. The patient may have hallucinations, incoherent speech, mental confusion and depression. This condition appears on the tongue through very specific signs; there is often a longitudinal crack in the centre of the tongue, with a yellow, dry and granulose coating. The red colour of the tongue and of the tip can be more or less evident.

Each human being has certain constitutional strengths and weaknesses. To understand this means finding a way to live suitably, using our energies according to their availability and accepting our 'vulnerable' areas.

It is worth highlighting the existence of signs which refer to constitutional disharmonies of the heart and which can, in time, affect the *shen*. An example is the long longitudinal cracks in the centre of the tongue body (they start on the last third and extend to the tip of the tongue or close to it). If this sign appears on a tongue body that is moderately or notably red it can indicate a constitutional tendency to develop heat in the heart. People with this sign might have a propensity towards hyperreactivity, worrying, self-doubt and mood fluctuations.

If this fact is taken into consideration it is possible to adopt precautionary measures such as meditation or relaxation techniques and to pay attention to avoiding overwork and excessive mental stimulation in order to prevent heart disharmonies and agitation of the *shen*.

These examples underline the importance of tongue diagnosis, especially when there is a necessity for the evaluation of energetic processes that deviate from the normal physiological functioning of the organs. This is particularly useful in relation to the heart since there are plenty of specific signs on the tongue reflecting its condition.

SUMMARY OF THE KEY SIGNS REGARDING *SHEN*

The examination of the tongue starts with the observation of its *shen*. The tongue has *shen* when it is lively, i.e. when it has a fresh and shiny look.

Next comes the evaluation of colour, shape, movement, coating and sublingual region.

In a normal tongue the colour is light red; dimensions and thickness are consistent with the constitution of the individual; the tongue body is soft, firm and mobile; the surface is smooth and moderately damp; there is a thin, white coating, equally spread and well rooted (at the last third it can be thicker); the sublingual vessels are not congested.

Colour

Paleness indicates emptiness (there is insufficient blood or the *qi* is too scarce to guarantee the flow).

A pale tongue is a sign of emptiness of the blood or of the *qi/yang*, with a specific relationship to the heart if the tip is pale (the heart manifests on the tip).

If the paleness concerns a thin, small or contracted tongue, this indicates emptiness of the blood (insufficient to colour and 'give a shape' to the tongue).

If it concerns a swollen tongue it reveals an emptiness of the *qi* or *yang* (their deficiency prevents an adequate transportation of the blood and transformation of liquids, which consequently accumulate).

If the tongue is pale and has a hollow last third it suggests a discontinuity of the *jing* (there is a lack of substance in the area of the kidney).

Edges with an orange tinge indicate emptiness of the liver blood.

Red indicates empty or full heat (there is an absolute or relative lack of movement of the *yang*, which carries the blood upwards).

The intensity of the colour is related to the strength of the heat (which also determines the dryness of the coating).

In physiological conditions the tip of the tongue is slightly red or has small spots (this reflects a good communication between *mingmen* and heart).

A red tip or a tip with very noticeable spots indicates heart heat.

If this happens all over the first third the heat is in the upper *jiao*.

The reddening of the edges or the presence of spots along the edges is an expression of liver fire (often the edges are also thickened), whereas the reddening in the centre is a sign of stomach heat or fire.

Intense red can also be caused by toxic heat that has penetrated the blood.

A red, short tongue with a thin or absent coating indicates emptiness of *yin*, chiefly of the kidney or liver.

A blue colour indicates blood stasis.

The colour can show itself in different ways: an inclination to purple in a dark red, a tinge of blue in a general paleness, congestion of the sublingual vessels, or red-bluish marks (which can pinpoint the locations of the stagnation).

If the tongue is pale-bluish, stasis can derive from an emptiness of blood, from emptiness of *qi*, which is insufficient to move the blood, or from cold that stops the blood moving.

If the tongue is red-purplish, the stasis is produced by heat that dries the blood.

Shape

Alterations in the shape of the tongue body and the presence of cracks result from chronic pathological conditions.

A tongue that is swollen and flabby and with marked edges is the result of emptiness of *qi* or of spleen or kidney *yang* (*yin* and liquids accumulate).

It the edges are raised 'like a step' or contracted, this indicates stagnation of liver *qi* (the tension deriving from the constraint of the *qi* also shows in the tongue muscles).

A long and/or pointed or curled tongue is usually a sign of heat in the heart (the force of the heat 'pushes' the tongue).

A short tongue reveals a severe emptiness of kidney and liver *yin* (fluids, blood and *yin* are not nourishing the tongue, which often loses its elasticity and mobility).

The case of a hollow at the last third is even more serious. This reflects emptiness of *jing* (the loss of substance is visible in the area of the kidney).

Indentation of the tip results from emptiness of blood or heart *yin* (there is a lack of substance to fill the area of the heart).

If the tip is swollen and red, it is a sign of phlegm-heat in the heart or in the upper *jiao*.

Cracks are a sign of emptiness of *yin* and their depth is related to the gravity of the emptiness (the liquids are consumed, there is a loss of substance and the tongue body collapses).

Transverse cracks on the edges indicate spleen emptiness whereas a central longitudinal crack denotes an emptiness of stomach and kidney *yin* (in this case the tongue is red and the coating is thin or absent).

A central crack that originates on the last third of the tongue and extends to the tip, or close to it, signifies a constitutional weakness of the heart (if the crack is light and the colour of the tongue is normal); that there is heart fire (if the crack is deep and the tongue is red), or that there is an emptiness of heart *yin* (if the coating is missing and the tongue or tip are red).

Coating

The coating originates from the stomach, like cloudy smoke rising to dampen the surface of the tongue; it is linked with body fluids.

A damp coating is a sign of emptiness of *qi* or *yang* (the *qi* is insufficient to move dampness).

The slippery quality of the coating indicates an accumulation of dampness (damp-cold if the coating is white, damp-heat if it is yellow, thick and sticky) and its thickening into a greasy coating denotes the accumulation of phlegm.

A dry coating suggests heat and dryness, exhaustion of the body fluids (if the coating becomes dark yellow, brown or black, the consumption of *yin* and fluids is serious).

If the coating is completely missing or there are only a few patches left it means there is an emptiness of *yin* (the fluids that should rise to generate the coating are lacking).

If the coating is absent from the centre of the tongue this indicates emptiness of stomach *yin*. If it is absent from the last third, the emptiness of the *yin* involves the kidney as well.

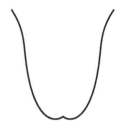

Figure 17.1 Tongue with indented tip: emptiness of heart blood.

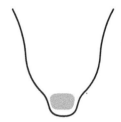

Figure 17.2 Tongue with pointed and red tip: heart heat-fire.

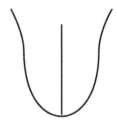

Figure 17.3 Tongue with longitudinal crack reaching the tip: constitutional imbalance of the heart.

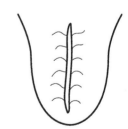

Figure 17.4 Wide longitudinal crack in the centre of the tongue, with thick yellow coating and red tip: phlegm that troubles the heart.

Stress Disorders: Considerations and Clinical Notes

Qiao Wenlei

18

INTRODUCTION

Qiao Wenlei was born in Nanjing in 1951. She joined the army when she was 16 and studied traditional medicine in a medical unit working as an acupuncturist. In 1973 she graduated in Western medicine in Shanghai. In 1977 she finished her TCM PhD in Nanjing, where she has been teaching at the International Acupuncture Training Center since 1987 (since 1996 as a professor).

She has worked for the Chinese government in hospitals and schools in Zambia, Malta, Germany, Italy, Scotland, Norway, Sweden and Finland.

Qiao Wenlei is an expert in scalp acupuncture and 'wrist–ankle' techniques and she has studied clinical areas such as stress disorders, dysthymic disorders, ictus sequelae and pain.

This contribution was written in Nanjing in September 2000 as a result of her experience with great masters and of her clinical work in China and Europe. It also stems from her attention to the manner with which we interact with the changing world and the ways in which pathologies develop.

Her theoretical interpretations are always consistent with the traditional system, but they also result from a careful consideration of today's clinical situations.

Whoever has worked with Qiao Wenlei knows her clear insight, her accurate interventions and her generous teaching, but even a written contribution such as the following is rich in theoretical observations and practical suggestions.

We remind the reader that the term 'stress' was introduced in biology by W. Cannon and received a univocal definition with H. Seyle who maintained that 'stress is the non-specific response of the organism to every demand'.[1]

According to Seyle stress is not a pathological condition but it may produce pathologies. It is a defensive and adaptive reaction – called emergency – characterised by an alarm phase with hormonal biochemical alterations, a resistance phase where the organism functionally organises itself in a defensive sense and a breakdown phase in which defences drop and one loses the capacity for further adaptation.

Later on, more flexible views were proposed which gave consideration to the relationship between the psychological system and the endocrine reactions, so that the response was also seen as dependent on cognitive evaluation of the significance of the stimulus.

When difficulties surpass the capacity for response the rope turns out to be too tense. The Chinese term for 'stress' is *jinzhang* in which *jin* is the same term as that used to define the tense pulse and *zhang* means 'stretched': the rope is so stretched and tense that it has lost its elasticity and there is no space for movement.[2]

STRESS SYNDROME

Since 1993 I have worked closely with European colleagues and I have regularly treated their patients. I have thus realised that there are a great number of cases in which pathologies and disorders are caused by stress.

The heavy pressures of contemporary society, the level of competitiveness, family tensions, but also physical events such as neck whiplash injury, cause emotional and body changes. Consequences can remain in the area of a physiological response but they may also become pathological, with clinical manifestations that can be mental or strictly physical (muscular tension before anything else).

In Western medicine Seyle was the first to describe the 'stress syndrome'. This text is expounded following his three-stage theory. There is no one-to-one correspondence with the 'classical' TCM syndromes but there is a strong relationship, which allows us to identify some of the main patterns.

In Chinese medical theory, the gall bladder has a fundamental role, which is even more important than that of the liver. Although the seven emotions are

---

[1] H. Seyle, *Stress without fear*, 1976, p. 12.
[2] The modern term is *jinzhang* 紧 张, translated as 'stress, tension, tense, nervous': the character *jin* 'tense, hard, narrow' consists of a phonetic part *jian* – which in ancient times meant 'hard' – and of the radical 'thread' (Wieger p. 82e, Karlgren p. 369); *zhang* means 'to stretch, to strain, string of a musical instrument' and it consists of a phonetic part *chang* and of the radical 'bow' (Karlgren p. 1173).

usually linked to the five *zang* organs, the gall bladder has peculiar characteristics that place it in the forefront of the exopathogenesis of illnesses.[3] If the gall bladder *qi* is strong enough it can withstand the stress deriving from external pressures and from the constant changes taking place around us, making it possible for us to face consequent emotional alterations.

The first manifestations are somatic, with weariness and muscular tensions principally located in the neck and shoulders, mainly along the *jinjing* (gall bladder sinew channel). Other psychological symptoms can be associated with an emptiness of the gall bladder and include diffused anxiety, a general state of alarm, restlessness.

When discussing the various stages and the connected syndromes, I will examine how the pathology can worsen with the production of fire and the involvement of the organs, manifesting also as respiratory and gastrointestinal disorders.

The primary elements suggesting the importance of the gall bladder are the following:

- The path of the gall bladder channel, *Shao Yang* of the foot, and particularly of its *jinjing*, the sinew channel which covers the lateral side of the foot and lower limb, the hip joint, the side of the chest, the armpit, breast, supraclavicular fossa. We remind the reader that its ramifications reach the anterior side of the thigh (*Yang Ming*), the sacral area (*Tai Yang*), the neck and the mastoid region, and that they extend to the top of the head, the temple, the nose and the outer corner of the eye.

These areas correspond to those where muscular tensions caused by stress appear and the *jinjing* pain is indeed characterised by the fact that it spreads along an area.[4]

- The association of the gall bladder with wood. Moreover it has an internal–external connection with the liver, with which it shares the task of keeping the *qi* circulation free and fluid.
- Its role in governing courage, judgement and the ability to decide, which also determines the correct development of the coordinating role of the liver 'general of the army who thinks about the strategy'.
- Its peculiarity as a curious or extraordinary *yang* organ, *qiheng zhifu*, which fills and empties itself as do all other *yang* organs, but also behaves like a *zang*, by storing *jingzhi*, liquid-essence.
- Its attribute of *xianghuo*, or 'ministerial fire', which has the role of supporting the spleen in its food processing, but can also damage the organ if it becomes too strong.

---

[3] See also Chapter 2 for a discussion on emotions and on the role of the gall bladder.
[4] The *jinjing* pathologies also have emotional causes. Pain, which is mediated by the CNS, is not only a response to external stimuli but also involves psychic factors (Huang Jinwei, *Muscle Region Therapy*, 1996).

- Its characteristic, linked to its being at a *Shao Yang* level, of acting as a pivot between the exterior and the interior.

CLINICAL MANIFESTATIONS

First Stage: Alarm Reaction

This stage corresponds to an intensification of epinephrine production by the adrenal glands in response to stimuli. It includes two syndromes that partly overlap, but in the second case the pattern is worsened by a stagnation of *qi*, with manifestations mainly at the level of digestion.

Emptiness of Gall Bladder and Heart

The insufficiency is mostly on the side of the gall bladder. The patient is constantly alert, with a vague anxiety ('as if he was always about to be arrested'), an extreme reaction to any external stimulus ('palpitations and jolts at each unexpected noise') and mental restlessness (*fanzao*). Sleep is uneasy and there can be signs of tachycardia and occasional increase in blood pressure.

Muscles are constantly contracted or there is a feeling of tension in the neck and shoulders, which is not necessarily distressing, but still produces a painful reaction to local pressure. The tongue is usually pale, and the pulse is thready and wiry.

There are not many patients in this stage because they usually start looking for treatment when they are in more advanced phases. But the disorder can be easily traced, for example in patients with a diagnosis of post-traumatic stress disorder.

Fullness with Stagnation of Gall Bladder and Accumulation of Phlegm

The gall bladder is a 'calm' organ, which contains liquid-essence, and its *qi* must flow fluently, as does the liver *qi*. Its stagnation produces phlegm-heat, which causes a stomach disharmony in which the *qi* counterflows and ascends.

The main symptoms are bitter mouth, nausea, changes in appetite and a feeling of oppression in the chest. The coating is sticky and yellow or white, and the pulse is wiry and slippery.

Second Stage: Resistance Phase

This is a protracted phase and the majority of our patients are seen in this stage.

Gall bladder and liver still maintain a primary role, with a pre-eminence of the gall bladder, but – as opposed to the first stage – the pathological mechanism involves a larger number of organs.

Gall Bladder and Heart

Symptoms are more severe compared with the previous stage. There is hypertension, rapid heartbeat, palpitations or more severe arrhythmias, changes in sleeping habits, anxiousness and restlessness, which indicate the suffering of the heart and the *zang* dominating the mind.

Lung

The breathing is superficial and fast. It differs both from the typical sighs of liver *qi* stagnation, which are deep and bring relief, and from the shortness of breath caused by kidney emptiness where the *qi* does not reach the organ. The shortness of breath is caused by the muscular tension of the gall bladder *jinjing* and by the obstruction of the great circulation between the gall bladder, liver and lung channels.

Spleen and Stomach

Here heat-phlegm attacks the earth, as in the first stage, but in a deeper way and with manifestations such as constipation or diarrhoea, sensations of swelling and abdominal distension.

There can also be an actual increase in the size of the abdomen because the stomach is always open, continuously working. Such patients always feel like eating, even though they have little energy and do not have any desires or interests.

The spleen *qi* is consumed because of overcontrol from the wood element, causing underfunctioning of the spleen and a tendency to overweight. The stomach overworks because of the fullness of fire transmitted by the gall bladder: the digestive process balances the excess of fire and when eating the patient experiences a temporary relief, feeling that the food has a soothing effect.

Third Stage: Exhaustion

Kidney

As in any long-lasting illness, whichever organ is involved the kidney also suffers because of the overwork and becomes deficient.

Moreover there is a specific relationship between kidney and liver, which share the same root, just as *jing* and blood have the same origin.

There are two main syndromes:

- Emptiness of *yin* with internal heat:
  Here there are signs of excitement, with manifestations of empty heat – particularly in the upper body – such as migraines, muscular pain and a hot face. At the same time there are signs of emptiness such as cold hands and weakness of the loins and knees. It is a frequent pattern during the menopause.

- Emptiness of *qi* and *yin*:
  This is a more serious syndrome because the *qi* is consumed; there are no signs of *yang* rising because there is relative excess and the patient appears very weak, with dyspnoea, severe asthenia and a disposition to fatigue.

OBJECTIVE EXAMINATION

Inspection and palpation also relate to a specific evaluation of the pain symptomatology. It is necessary to check for the presence of nodules, contractions and fibrosity in the painful areas, produced by a persistent stagnation, and to evaluate carefully the location and intensity of the muscular pain.

For each point we must define the response to pressure, for example:

+:   the patient verbally expresses the fact that the pressure produces pain;
++:   the facial grimaces and the eyes clearly reveal a more intense pain;
+++:   the whole body contracts because of the pain caused by the pressure;
++++:   the pain is so strong that the patient shouts and cannot stand the pressure.

TREATMENT

Main Points

Yanglingquan GB-34 and Upper-5 are used in all cases.

- *Yanglingquan* GB-34: *hui*-meeting point of tendons and muscles, *he*-sea point of gall bladder, point used to bring downwards that which stagnates in the upper part of the channel – it has an action on *Shao Yang*, on tendons, on *qi* stagnation, on damp-heat, on uprising *yang* and on wind, but also has a specific efficacy on the emptiness of the organ *qi*, with cowardice, fear and a state of alarm.
  The stimulation of this point immediately frees the breathing.[5]
- Upper-5[6]: the 'wrist–ankle' technique, *wanhuaizhen*, is particularly indicated for cases of muscular contraction and pain. The region related to Upper-5 broadly corresponds to that of the sinew channel of the hand *Shao Yang*.

---

[5] The results of a research conducted in China on patients with postural hypertension from various traumas indicate that *Yanglingquan* GB-34 increases the release of GABA in the cerebrospinal fluid, with a muscle-relaxing action on striated muscle. In: Zhao Yanling et al., *Needling Yanglingquan GB-34 for Relieving Spasm and its Influence on Gamma-Amino-Butyric Acid in Cerebrospinal Fluid*, 1998.
[6] For more detail on this methodology and on bleeding and cupping techniques see Chapter 12 on stimulation methods.

After introducing the needles in these two points we evaluated the patient again, checking the various painful areas and the intensity of the response to pressure. Usually there is less muscular tension and most of the painful areas have disappeared.

Secondary Points

Secondary points are those points that are still very sensitive after the insertion of the main needles. They usually correspond to important points such as:

- *Jianjing* GB-21: 1 or 1.5 *cun* needle, with slight inclination towards the head.[7] If there is a nodule the needle must be inserted in its centre and two others must be inserted slanting towards the first one. They are stimulated in order to 'open' holes and at the end they are made to bleed with the help of cupping.
- *Qubing* GB-7: 1 *cun* needle, perpendicular. Bleeding if there is heat in the upper body.
- *Fengchi* GB-20: 1.5 *cun* needle, directed towards the tip of the nose.
- *Wangu* GB-12: 1 *cun* needle, perpendicular.
- *Ganshu* BL-18: 1 *cun* needle, perpendicular. Bleeding if there is heat.
- *Danshu* BL-19: 1 *cun* needle, perpendicular. Bleeding if there is heat.

The two main points are supported by other points depending on the medical condition.

First Stage

Emptiness of gall bladder and heart:

- + *Qiuxu* GB-40 and *Shenmen* HE-7 (1 *cun* needle in the direction of *Neiguan* P-6).

Stagnation of gall bladder with phlegm:

- + *Fenglong* ST-40 and EX-HN-6 Ear apex (with bleeding).

Second Stage

With involvement of the heart:

- + *Jianshi* P-5.

With involvement of the lung:

- + *Shanzhong* Ren-17.

---

[7] The point unblocks the channels and harmonises the five *zang* organs: the *Zhenjiu dacheng*, ('The great compendium of acupuncture and moxibustion') by Yang Jizhou already mentions it as a crossing-point between four channels – foot and hand *Shao Yang*, foot *Yang Ming* and *Yang Wei*. It is said that it 'connects the five *zang*'.

With involvement of the spleen:

- + *Zusanli* ST-36.

If there is a swollen abdomen:

- + *Gongsun* SP-4.

If the patient gains weight and there is phlegm:

- + *Fenglong* ST-40 (or *Yinlingquan* SP-9 if there is pain under pressure, as is common in women).

If there is excessive appetite:

- + *Danshu* BL-19 and *Weishu* BL-21 with bleeding to eliminate the fire directly from the *zangfu*.

If there is nausea, with stomach *qi* rising:

- + *Neiguan* P-6.

If the liver *qi* is constricted:

- + *Taichong* LIV-3.

Third Stage

Emptiness of *yin*:

- + *Taixi* KI-3.

If there is constipation and dry mouth:

- + *Zhaohai* KI-6.

If there is ascending heat:

- + *Taiyang* EX-HN-5 (for example when there is migraine) or EX-HN-6 Ear apex (for example in case of hypertension): with bleeding.

Emptiness of *qi* and *yin*:

- + *Zusanli* ST-36;
- + *Sanyinjiao* SP-6, *Shenshu* BL-23, *Taixi* KI-3.

In addition:
If the patient feels pain all over the body:

- + *Hegu* LI-4 and *Taichong* LIV-3.

Regardless of the organs involved we use the 'four gates', to regulate the circulation of the *qi* and blood in the whole body and calm the mind by moving the *qi*.

If the patient feels the pain only on one side of the body:

- + *Hegu* LI-4, *Taichong* LIV-3, *Quchi* LI-11.

First we use the points on the healthy side, then those on the side with the pain: since in the latter side there already is stagnation (pain), it is necessary to conduct the *qi* first towards the healthy side and then towards the painful side, in order to encourage the circulation of the *qi*.

NB: Upper-5 can be used on both sides because it is not necessary to obtain the *qi* (*deqi*).

Bleeding

This is very important because the pain often depends upon blood stasis and there is blood stasis in every long-lasting symptom. It is also fundamental for the heat in the upper body, for example in cases of headache from ascending heat.

- *Qubing* GB-7 and *Taiyang* EX-HN-5: if the pain is lateral;
- *Baihui* DU-20: if the pain is located at the top of the head;
- *Shenting* DU-24: if the pain is located at the front;
- *Dazhui* Du-14: if there is itching or dermatological problems linked to stress, to eliminate the heat from the *yang* channels, calm the mind, and regulate the immune system;
- *Weizhong* BL-40: if the pain is dorsal, lumbar or located in the knees;
- *shu* points on the back: if there is heat in the organs, usually the liver, gall bladder, or stomach.

NB: If there is ascending heat and particularly when other treatments have had scarce results, it is essential to bleed Ear apex (at least eight to ten drops of blood), which calms the mind, resolves chronic migraine, relieves severe insomnia and reduces hypertension deriving from ascending *yang*.

Ear Therapy

- Liver, Gall bladder, Subcortex, Adrenal, Endocrine;
- + points according to the differential diagnosis (Heart, Spleen, Stomach, Large intestines, Kidney, etc.)
- + Subcortex if there is pain, or *Shenmen* if the pain is of a full type.

Scalp Acupuncture

This can be used but it is a second choice to body acupuncture.

- MS 1: if there are migraines, insomnia, mental disorders;
- MS 2: if there are thoracic symptoms, breathing problems;
- MS 3: if there are abdominal symptoms, digestion disorders.

'Wrist–Ankle' Technique

This method is principally used when – due to various reasons – we prefer to avoid *deqi*, that is, the obtaining of the *qi* through needle insertion.

- We can add Upper-1, which is useful for all emotional and mental disorders.

CLINICAL CASES

Case Study 18.1

37-Year-Old Nurse – Second Stage (Norway – May 2000)

The patient says that after separating from her husband 2 years ago, she has suffered from migraine on the left side, with a pain that reaches her eye, neck, shoulder and upper back. She always hunches her shoulders a little because this position relieves the pain.

After her divorce she had to change job because she could not stand the level of commitment, but her current part time job also seems to be too tiring. She also says that she has thought several times of committing suicide. One month ago a car accident worsened the situation although she has not suffered from a real whiplash injury.

Now she always feels tired, sometimes she has nausea or sour regurgitation while stools are normal. The pain, the mood and the difficulties in working worsen during the ovulation period.

The tongue is pale, with toothmarks, and with a white and thin coating. The pulse is fine and wiry.

The objective examination shows:
- *Qubing* GB-7: +++ on the left;
- *Jianjing* GB-21: ++ bilateral.

Diagnosis
Stagnation of liver *qi* and deficiency of spleen *qi*.

Treatment
(1 session/week)
   1st session:
- Upper-5 bilateral;
- *Yanglingquan* GB-34.
   When re-evaluating sensitive points:
- *Qubing* GB-7 ++ and *Jianjing* GB-21 + (*Qubing* GB-7 is less tense during the palpation, but the pain persists. The patient feels slight distress but no pain when we press the trapezius muscle).
   As a result we add to the two main points:

- *Qubing* GB-7 on the left, with bleeding;
- *Neiguan* P-6, *Taichong* LIV-3, *Sanyinjiao* SP-6;

that take into consideration the counterflowing *qi*, the constraint of the liver *qi* and the fact that the symptoms worsen during ovulation.

At the end of the session *Qubing* GB-7 is +, the patient says that she is feeling much better: she still feels heaviness in the shoulders and head, but no pain.

We explain to her she has to keep Upper-5 in place.

2nd session:

The pain is much relieved.

We repeat the treatment.

3rd session:

The patient says that she feels better, but that she is now in her ovulation period and has had a strong headache in the last hours.

We repeat the treatment using *Baihui* DU-20 instead of *Qubing* GB-7, with bleeding.

During the treatment, after the bleeding, the headache becomes less strong.

4th session:

The patient says that she feels well, that she has not had any more pain but only tiredness and a feeling of heaviness in the shoulders and head from time to time. She is thinking of returning to her normal job.

We repeat the treatment, eliminating *Qubing* GB-7 and adding *Zusanli* ST-36 to tonify the *qi*.

Case Study 18.2

37-Year-Old Teacher – Third Stage (Norway – May 2000)

The patient says that she is depressed, agitated, and has had a severe insomnia for the last 20 years (light, disturbed sleep, disturbed by many dreams). All symptoms have worsened in the last year, a period in which she changed many jobs because she did not like them. This has worsened the pressure and the stress. She increased her evening dose of tranquillisers because her sleep pattern was worsening, she was waking up early with obsessive thoughts about the harassment she would have to suffer from her boss.

She talks about a pain on the right side of the head, with temporal headache spreading towards the forehead.

She has a feeling of oppression in her throat and chest when she starts getting worried. She has palpitations and a short, superficial breath that gets better when breathing deeply. She eats too much when she feels agitated and anxious, she sweats during the night, has heat at the 'five hearts', lumbar pain, and a dry mouth when stressed. Her periods are every 25–28 days with a scanty, dark flow, which lasts 2 days.

The tongue is purplish with red sides, thin coating; the pulse is thready, wiry and weak in the rear position.

The objective examination shows:

- *Taiyang* EX-HN-9: ++ on the right;
- *Wangu* GB-12: +++ on the right;
- *Fengchi* GB-20: ++ on the right;
- *Jianjing* GB-21: +++ on the right;
- *Tianzhu* BL-10: ++ on the right;
- *Feishu* BL-13 and *Jueyinshu* BL-14: ++ bilateral.

Diagnosis

Emptiness of *yin* and internal heat.

Treatment

First session:

- Upper-5 on the right:
- *Yanglingquan* GB-34 bilateral;
- Upper-1 bilateral, to calm the mind;
- *Taichong* LIV-3 and *Taixi* KI-3 bilateral, to nourish *yin*;
- *Anmian* N-HN-54, to facilitate sleep;
- *Baihui* Du-20, *Shenting* Du-24 and *Taiyang* EX-HN-9 on the right, with bleeding, to eliminate heat.

At the end of the session the patient says that she feels much better and all the painful points show a two-point decrease in sensitivity.

We explain to her she has to keep Upper-5 and Upper-1 in place.

2nd session:

The patient says that her sleep is so much better that she has stopped the pills, that the pain is less and that she feels more relaxed. The sweating during the night and the other signs of internal heat are also improved.

We repeat the treatment without bleeding *Taiyang* EX-HN-9.

3rd session:

The patient says that she feels as if she has 'a new body'. The objective examination reveals only a +- response to the pressure of the painful points.

We repeat the treatment but we use only Ear apex, with bleeding, instead of the head points.

Notes

In order to retain the body fluids it is important to eliminate heat and not only to nourish *yin*.

After the stimulation of *Yanglingquan* GB-34, the breathing immediately becomes deeper and more free.

Patients say that the feeling of relaxation is not confined to the muscles but rather is a more general sense of well-being and peacefulness.

'WHIPLASH'

'Whiplash' injury is disturbance of the cervical vertebrae caused by trauma, usually following a car or sport accident. The tissues are stretched by a sudden and violent movement of the neck region and they produce acute pain and damage to the nerves roots.

The neck and shoulder muscles and the tendons are strained beyond their capability and the medulla oblongata and cerebellum can be damaged. This produces tension and pain. Sight and balance disorders can also arise.

If the condition lasts for long, mental and emotional stress can follow the physical one. Many patients say that a 'whiplash' injury has changed their lives.

Main Clinical Manifestations

- Stiffness and pain in the neck.
- Mental stress, anxiety and fear.
- Headache in the posterior, lateral or upper side of the head.
- Sight disorders such as double vision.
- Lumbar or dorsal pain, or pain all over the body.
- Tiredness and easy fatigue.
- Irritability.
- Coordination disorders of an ataxic type.
- Tensions, contractions, muscle nodules, increase in sensitivity in the areas of *Tianzhu* BL-10, *Jianjing* GB-21, *Fengchi* GB-20, *Baihui* Du-20, *Wangu* GB-12, etc.

Early Stage – Damage to The Sinew Channels, Jinjing

Traumas from car accidents or sports create contractions of tendons and vessels and they induce blood and *qi* stagnation in muscles, tendons, ligaments, fascias, etc. which belong to the *Jinjing,* sinew channels. This produces muscular tension and contraction in the occipital and cervical region. Pain can spread to the temples and to the top of the head, to the dorsal and sacral region and to the lower limbs along the pathways of the foot channels *Tai Yang* and *Shao Yang.*

Since the 'whiplash' involves not only the body but also the mind, it can increase mental stress and induce a state of constant fear. The mental state and the emotional changes usually worsen the muscular tension and vice versa.

Advanced Stage – Yin Deficiency and Disorders of the Shen

If the muscular tension and the emotional stress reach a chronic condition, they consume the body fluids and the *zangfu yin*, so that the patients who have experienced 'whiplash' often present with psychological disorders. The responses of the body to the stress include an increase in epinephrine secretion. This damage to the kidney and liver *yin* impairs their function of nourishing the tendons and bones.

Treatment

Main Points

- Upper-6 or Upper-5, depending on the region involved.

The 'wrist–ankle' technique is very well tolerated in the treatment of 'whiplash'. There are good results both in pain relief and in relaxing the muscular tension.

Points are located only in areas of the wrist and ankle and the insertion of the needle does not involve the traditional *deqi*, 'obtaining the *qi*'. Patients who have experienced 'whiplash' and its associated stress may tolerate this therapy more easily.

The needle can be left in place in the subcutaneous layers without causing any problems in limb movement. This helps if one cannot undertake daily treatment.

Secondary Points

If there is severe headache:

- occipital region: Upper-6;
- lateral region: Upper-5;
- top of the head: Upper-4 or bleeding of *Baihui* DU-20;
- temples and eyes: bleeding of *Tai Yang* EX-HN-5.

Bleeding is useful for eliminating heat, including empty heat and retaining body fluids. Moreover it moves the blood stasis, lowers the pressure and pain in the main and sinew channels, and reduces mental stress. It is used for both the first and second stages.

If there is muscular tension and contraction in the neck and shoulders:

- for symptoms in the area of *Tianzhu* BL-10 or *Dazhu* BL-11: Upper-6;
- for symptoms in the area of *Jianjing* GB-21: Upper-5.

If there is dorsal–lumbar–sacral pain:

- dorsal region or in the area of *Zhibian* BL-54 or *Huantiao* GB-30: Lower-5;
- sacral region: Lower-6.

If there is vision disorder or ataxic walking:

- scalp acupuncture MS-13 (region of the vision or MS-14 (region of the balance);

- scalp acupuncture is very effective in cases where the central nervous system is involved.

If there are emotional problems:

- Upper-1 and/or *hegu* LI-4 and *taichong* LIV-3 ('the four gates');
- *Hegu* LI-4: it relates to *yang*, it dominates the *qi* and raises it;
- *Taichong* LIV-3: it relates to *yin*, it dominates the blood, and lowers *qi*;
- *Hegu* LI-4 and *Taichong* LIV-3 are *yuan*-source points of all the *yin* and *yang* channels: their combination induces a movement of the *qi* towards the limbs, in order to dispel blood and *qi* stasis in the upper body and to calm the mind.

If there are symptoms from *yin* deficiency:

- *Sanyinjiao* SP-6 or *Taixi* KI-3.
- + the classical prescriptions *Liuwei dihuang wan* or *Qiju dihuang wan* to nourish the *yin* and improve the functions of the adrenal glands.

Case Study 18.3

42-Year-Old Woman (Malta, December 1994)

Main Problem
Headaches and stiff neck caused by a 'whiplash' injury from a car accident three months previously.

Clinical Manifestations
- Frequent headaches at the top of the head with a sense of distension.
- Stiff and aching neck, with limited movements of the neck and shoulders.
- Mental stress.
- High sensitivity in *Tianzhu* DU-10 (+++), *Baihui* DU-20 (+++), *Sishencong* EX-HN-1 (++) (all bilaterally), *Jianjing* GB-21 (+++ on the left, ++ on the right).
- Wiry pulse and dark red tongue with thin coating.

Diagnosis
Tension of the sinew channels and mental stress.

Therapeutic Principles
Release the muscular tension and calm the mind.

Treatment
First session:
- Upper-5 and Upper-6 bilaterally, then *Baihui* DU-20 with bleeding of about 10 drops, using cotton soaked in alcohol to facilitate the bleeding and prevent infections.

The patient immediately feels that the head was more relaxed and the neck movements are improved.

We leave Upper-6 in place.

Second session:

The patient is very optimistic: she says that this treatment is different from all the others she has tried. The muscular tension is now much reduced. She took the two needles out after 3 days.

- When pressing: *Tianzhu* Du-10 (+), *Baihui* Du-20 (+-), *Jianjing* GB-21 (++ on the right, +- on the left).

We repeat the treatment.

Two more sessions follow.

The general conditions are very much improved. When pressing: *Tianzhu* Du-10 (+-), *Baihui* Du-20 (-), *Jianjing* GB-21 (+-). The patient is clearly improved at both a physical and a mental level.

Case Study 18.4

47-Year-Old Woman (Norway, June 1999)

Main Problem
Headache and stiff neck for 3 years, following a car accident.

Clinical Manifestations
- Headache on both sides, frequent, with pain reaching the eyes, especially on the right.
- Swollen eyes following emotional changes.
- Pain and stiff neck and shoulders, with limited movements, especially on the right.
- Mental stress and irritability.
- Increased sensitivity in the areas of *Qubin* GB-7 (right++++, left++), *Taiyang* EX-HN-9 (right+++, left+), *Fengchi* GB-20 (right++, left++), *Jianjing* GB-21 (right+++, left++)
- Lumbar pain, week knees, easily tired.
- Double vision and sometimes ataxic movements.
- Night sweating, frequent flushes, sudden amenorrhoea after the trauma.
- Thready and wiry pulse, red tongue with thin coating.

Diagnosis
Yin deficiency caused by the long lasting muscular tension and stress.

Therapeutic Principles
Reduce the muscular tension and relax the mental stress, nourish the *yin* in order to balance *yin* and *yang*.

Treatment

First session:

- Upper-5 left permanently, bilateral;
- *Yanglinquan* GB-34, *Sanyinjiao* SP-6, *Hegu* LI-4 and *Taichong* LIV-3 ('the four gates').
- *Qubin* GB-7 with bleeding of ten drops.

At the end of the session the patient feels an internal relaxation of the body and the headache is much better.

We prescribe *Qiju dihuanwan* to nourish *yin*, eliminate heat and help the eyes.

Second session:

The patient has not suffered from headache, but her eyes are still swollen.

We repeat the points of the first session, adding:

- Upper-1 and the bleeding of *Taiyang* EX-HN-5 instead of *Qubin* GB-7.

There is an immediate reduction of the swelling of the eyes.

- We also stimulate manually MS-13 (visual area) for the double vision and MS-14 (balance area) for the ataxic movements (scalp acupuncture is used from the second session in order not to upset the patient in the first session).

Six more sessions follow:

- *Taiyang* EX-HN-5 with bleeding, *Shenshu* BL-23, *Ganshu* BL-18 with bleeding and cupping to eliminate heat and pacify liver and gall bladder.

The pain is definitely better, the patient's mind is calm and she has more energy.

Use of Points in Severe Psychiatric Pathology

Zhang Mingjiu

19

The following chapter is based on notes taken during a series of lectures by Prof. Zhang Mingjiu, acupuncturist doctor at the psychiatric hospital 'Nanjing Jingshenbing Yiyuan' (now 'Naoke Yiyuan'). The lectures were held in Nanjing in June–July 1988.

Zhang Mingjiu was born in 1927 and in 1987 he established the department of TCM at the Nanjing psychiatric hospital. There he treated patients with mental problems through traditional acupuncture and scalp acupuncture.[1]

Zhang Mingjiu has been a teacher and a friend for many of the doctors who now work at Nanjing University. On the 23rd of June 1992 he died at the hands of a patient who fell in love with his daughter. This episode made a deep impression on everyone.

I have decided to publish these notes even though they are incomplete and in need of expansion. I believe they contain elements that reveal a great technical knowledge and the precious clinical experience of a lifetime.

The shortcomings in the material are numerous and two factors called for further analysis. First of all, the terminology used in all the lectures was somewhat 'outside' that agreed with the TCM College, forcing us to come to terms with some imprecise translations. Secondly, the type of approach and

---

[1] The data of one of his studies on scalp acupuncture are published in: Zhang Mingjiu, *Toupizhen zhiliao huanjue 296 lide jingyan* ('Scalp-acupuncture in 296 cases of schizophrenia and hallucinations'), Zhongyi zazhi no. 6:52, 1987. An abstract and the final results can be found in the text edited by T. Dey, 2000, p. 110.

systematisation of the lectures is significantly different from the one most commonly used today.

Nevertheless I believe that the peculiarity of this methodology of interpretation and treatment is precisely what makes this chapter significant. As a result the text has undergone a very limited revision: the original structure, the clinical descriptions and the expressions used by the translator have been retained. No terminologies, hypothesis, connections and unconfirmed interpretations have been added.

SERIOUS *SHEN* DISORDERS AND THE CHOICE OF POINTS

During a brief introduction professor Zhang recalled how traditional Chinese medicine perceives the disorders of the spirit as closely related to the five organs and how disordered organs may produce changes in our spiritual areas.

He then referred to the *Jiayijing*, where it is said that in order to cure one must first look at the *shen*.[2]

He highlighted how the symptoms taken into consideration could be manifestations of physical or mental illnesses, for example septicaemia, intoxications, encephalitis, senile dementia, hysteria, schizophrenia, depression, etc.

Finally he specified that it is possible to use all the 46 points on the head and about 81 among the other traditional somatic points, all distal to the elbow and knee.

According to Zhang Mingjiu the criteria for choosing the points are the following: the experience of ancient masters, the location of the illness, the path of the meridians, the name of the points, one's personal experience, the relationship between the five *zang* organs, the connection between organ and *yang* organ and the belonging to a same channel (for example, *Shao Yin* of hand and foot).

Notes on Reading

- The following material is presented in accordance with the sequence and the terminology used in the lectures. Some comments can be found at the end of the chapter.
- The cited points refer to specific cases that are only roughly outlined.
- Traditional pharmacological prescriptions and differential diagnosis with reference to *zangfu* were added only because of our insistence and might therefore often appear extemporary.

---

[2] 'All acupuncture methods must have their root in the *shen*.' In: Huangfu Mi, *Zhenjiu Jiayijing* ('The systematic classic of acupuncture and moxibustion', AD259), Chapter 1.

- The depth of the discussion is not homogeneous owing to the lack of time towards the end of the lectures.
- Zhang Mingjiu's comments on individual points and the proposed translation of their names are placed in footnotes to facilitate their retrieval.
- When a point is followed by 'to...' and another point, it implies a reference to the technique of joining two points with one needle, also frequently used by Jin Shubai.
- When the point is referred to 'with moxa' it means the needle is heated with a piece of moxa.
- I have added the standard abbreviations to the Chinese name of points, whilst omitting the comments on prescriptions since they were inhomogeneous and generally limited to the prescription's category.

SHEN

This can be defined as an activity of the consciousness, the thought and the speech.

Consciousness

Consciousness means being able to recognise oneself and one's surroundings.

Disorders of consciousness generally result from an emptiness of heart *qi* or, sometimes, of *yin*.

Confusion of the Consciousness

Example. A patient who confuses dreams and reality, who thinks he knows something and at the same time feels like he doesn't know it, who believes he is living in a dream. He likes to drink and smoke. The treatment involves giving up or reducing smoking and drinking.

- *Meichong* BL-3, *Daling* P-7, *Yanglingquan* GB-34 (if the body is strong, revealed by looks, pulse and brevity of course).
- *Benshen* GB-13, *Shenmen* HE-7, *Sanyinjiao* SP-6 (if the body is weak).

Stuporous Condition, with Response only to Strong Stimuli

Example: a woman, following an argument with the husband, would always sleep when he was at home. She wouldn't even drink or go to the bathroom, whereas she would behave normally when he was not there.

- *Shangxing* Du-23 to *Shenting* Du-24, *Tongli* HE-5, *Yongquan* KI-1 (strong stimulation).

One session was enough to resolve the situation.

Lack of Response to Stimuli with Delirium or Confusion

The heart *qi* is dirty.

- *Baihui* Du-20, *Zhongchong* P-9, *Yongquan* KI-1 (in general).
- *Shenting* Du-24, *Suliao* Du-25, *Neiguan* P-6, *Zusanli* ST-36 with moxa (if the patient is weak).

Disorders of the Consciousness and of the Self

It can also refer to cases of double or multiple personality.
    Example: a man thinks he is a cat and imitates its behaviour.

- *Wuchu* BL-5 to *Quchai* BL-4, *Daling* P-7, *Zhiyin* BL-67.

Persecution Delirium

Example: a young man never went out of home and refused to see friends because he thought that everyone knew his thoughts and intentions. The reason for this was that he had stolen something and no one knew it.

- *Benshen* GB-13 to *Touwei* ST-8, *Shenmen* HE-7, *Dazhong* KI-4.

    Ten days with 2-hour sessions per day, without stimulation.

Possession Delirium

Emptiness of heart, gall bladder and spleen.
    This is more common among elderly people.
    Example: a woman shouted and insulted her husband. She was convinced that it was her own father who was doing this by using her body.

- *Baihui* Du-20, *Rangu* KI-2, *Daling* P-7, *Zhongchong* P-9 (with bleeding).

Thought

Disorders of the thought belong to the heart, sometimes involving large intestine, bladder and fire of the stomach.

Manic Thought

Ideas follow one another and continuously change. The speaking never stops, 'mouth and mind vie'.
    Example: a student, after having passed his exams successfully, goes around telling everyone about it and travels day and night until he is too tired to move.

- *Tianchong* GB-9 to *Shuaigu* GB-8, *Yintang* EX-HN-3 (with bleeding), *Hegu* LI- 4, *Taichong* LIV-3.

After four sessions the patient could sleep well and after eight the situation went back to normal.

Slow Spirit

Example: a woman was exhausted after having tended her dying husband and after his death she didn't want to talk or participate in any activity.

- *Xinhui* Du-22 to *Shangxing* Du-23, *Suliao* Du-25 (directed upwards), *Yongquan* KI-1, *Shixuan* Ex-UE-1 + *Jiawei xiaoyao wan*.

Poverty of Thought

The mind feels empty, there are few reactions to external stimuli, it can be a depressive psychosis.

Example: a 55-year-old professor who had always been curious and cultured found increasing difficulty in thinking, writing and teaching.

- *Sishencong* EX-HN-1 (towards *Baihui* Du-20, with moxa), *Shenmen* HE-7, *Hegu* LI-4, *Dazhong* KI-4 (30 sessions) + *Baizi yangxin wan* (also suggested for elderly people and children with mental retardation).

Incoherent Thought

Emptiness of heart *qi*.

Example: a university student keeps talking inconsistently, without any clear logic.

- *Baihui* Du-20 to *Chengling* GB-18, *Daling* P-7, *Dazhong* KI-4 + *Yangxintang* + *Tianwang buxin dan*.

Convoluted Thought

Example: a patient talks in a confused manner, interrupting and repeating himself. The reason for the visit is a cardiopathy, but he speaks about his parents, his work, and his everyday achievements.

- *Sishencong* EX-HN-1, *Fubai* GB-10 to *Touqiaoyin* GB-11, *Shenmen* HE-7, *Sanyinjiao* SP-6 (with moxa).

Obsessive Thought

This can also be an obsessive–compulsive disorder, with reiterated actions such as continuously washing the hands or repeatedly checking whether the door is closed.

Example: a woman was afraid every time she saw a sharp object because she thought she could kill her husband.

- *Qiangjian* Du-18 to *Naokong* GB-19, *Zhizheng* SI-7, *Ligou* LIV-5.

These are difficult cases; at times it might be better to leave the needles in place for 3–7 days; it is better to combine the treatment with 'mental therapies'.[3]

Emptiness of Heart qi and Gall Bladder

Incorrect Thought

Example: a 12-year-old girl, quite bright and good at school, was convinced that her mother wanted to kill her. Given the small results obtained with a 'mental therapy' it was decided to try with acupuncture.

- *Chengling* GB-18 to 17, *Houxi* SI-3, *Taixi* KI-3 + *Guipi tang*.

After five sessions the beginning of a transformation of the thought could be observed.

Delirious Thought

Ideas that do not correspond to reality; patients believe in things that do not exist.

- *Baihui* Du-20 to *Chengling* GB-18, *Shenmen* HE-7, *Dazhong* KI-4.

Other points are added depending on the type of delirium.

Delusion of Persecution

Example: a 25-year-old girl thought her mother wanted to kill her because she would tell her to dress more:
- + *Quchai* BL-4.

Delusion of Grandeur

Example: a man used to say that he was rich and graduated, but really he was quite poor and little educated:

- + *Tianchong* GB-9.

Delusion of Guilt

Example: a man thinks it is his fault if it rains or if a friend is ill, therefore he believes it would be better if he died:

- + *Toulinqi* GB-15.[4]

---

[3] When asked what he meant by 'mental therapy' or 'spiritual treatment' he answered: 'To talk'.
[4] *Toulinqi* GB-15 means 'falling tears'.

Delusion of Reference

Example: patients who think that everyone is talking about them, that the radio reveals their secrets or that fish swim away from them in disgust. These are difficult cases to treat:

• + *Luoque* BL-8.

Delusion of Jealousy

Example: a 60-year-old man is convinced that his wife has many lovers and follows her everywhere:

• + *Chengling* GB-18.[5]

Eroto-maniac Delusion

Example: a 24-year-old boy is very unattractive, has no education and does not have a job. Yet he is convinced that many women love him. One day he approaches a woman who had smiled to him, she hits him and he thinks it is a sign of her love:

• + *Sanyinjiao* SP-6.

Hypochondriac Delusion

Example: a 50-year-old peasant is convinced that he has a brain cancer and fatal lung and stomach diseases. He requests examinations in all the hospitals in Nanjing and spends all his money on medicines:

• + *Zhizheng* SI-7.[6]

Delusion of Denial

Example: a 36-year-old woman engineer had the feeling of becoming empty. She felt that her existence had no meaning, that her husband was not her husband any more and that her children were no longer her children; she had tried to commit suicide more than once:

• + *Zhengying* GB-17, with good results.

---

[5] G. Maciocia, 1989, refers to a personal conversation with Zhang Mingjiu to underline the importance of certain points in the treatment of various syndromes. The fact that there is no consistent correspondence (for example in a case of pathological jealousy, there is a reference to the combination *Benshen* GB-13, *Tongli* HE-5, *Yangfu* GB-38, p.446) proves that the points are chosen on the basis of individual conditions.

[6] *Zhizheng* SI-7, which means 'to sustain the right', is suggested by the classics for difficult cases when the doctor cannot find the cause and there is the possibility of leaving the needle in place.

Delusion of Interpretation

Example: a patient is convinced that men do not have two heads or two mouths because otherwise they would be constantly arguing:

- + *Xuanli* GB-6, with alternating results.[7]

Genealogical Delusion

Example: a student is convinced that his father is a stranger:

- + *Touqiaoyin* GB-11, with good results.

Speech

The heart governs the speech, the vibration of the sound belongs to the lung, the root is in the kidney.

Mutism

Stagnation of Heart and Liver qi

Example: a child had stopped talking because he was continuously ill treated by his quarrelsome and violent parents.

- *Tongtian* BL-7 to *Chengling* GB-18, *Tongli* HE-5, *Rangu* KI-2.

Echolalia, Echopraxia

Emptiness of heart and spleen.
Example: a 21-year-old boy would imitate the gestures of every stranger and follow him even to the bathroom. He often got beaten because people thought he was curious.

- *Qiangjian* Du-18 to *Naokong* GB-19, *Quchi* LI-11, *Zusanli* ST-36, with 10 daily sessions, 10 sessions in alternate days and 10 sessions every 2 weeks.

Speech Difficulties, Stuttering

Example: a patient who had undergone a great shock.

- *Baihui* Du-20, *Lianquan* Ren-23, *Tongli* HE-5, *Taixi* KI-3.

PO

This is the inferior spirit. it is stored, nourished and ruled by the lung.
It includes three aspects: appearance, movement and behaviour.
It relates to energy, strength and health conditions.

---

[7] *Xuanli* GB-6 means 'to correct'. In the text by G. Maciocia, 1989, the point is cited in relation to 'disorders of the will, lack of motivation, difficulties in speech' with a reference to Zhang Mingjiu (p. 445). The accepted meaning of 'delusion of interpretation' is to explain things through a private system of significance.

Appearance

This includes gesticulation, gestures, movements, grooming, styles and behaviours that should suit the customs of a particular society. If, after having treated the illness, there are still problems with appearances the patient can die.

Movement

Excited Locomotion

Heat in the liver, stomach, large intestine.

Hyperactivity in movement and speech, but the speech remains clear.

Example: a 50-year-old professor felt a deep emotional pain. He would sleep very little and talk continuously with everybody, yet he retained a clear logic; the gesticulation was too lively, the voice too high, the face was red and the pulse strong.

- *Sishencong* EX-HN-1, *Yintang* EX-HN-3 (with bleeding), *Hegu* LI-4, *Taichong* LIV-3 + *Danggui longhui wan*.

Stuporous Condition

Emptiness of the lung and spleen *qi* and cold.

Example: an 18-year-old boy had suddenly stopped talking and reacting; he would always be sitting without eating and going to the bathroom, and he would sleep with an 'air pillow' [catatonia].

- *Shangxing* Du-23 to *Shenting* Du-24, *Dazhui* Du-14, *Quchi* LI-11, *Zusanli* ST-36[8] + *Simo yin*.

Example: a girl was very weak and always drowsy.

- *Dazhui* Du-14, *Shenzhu* Du-12, *Shendao* Du-11, *Pishu* BL-20, using only moxa.

Negativism

Disharmony of heart and kidney.

This is frequent in young people who do the opposite of what they are asked to do. It stems from depression.

Example: a 16-year-old girl was being unsuccessful at school and she was consequently mocked and scolded. Her personality had gradually changed until she started doing the opposite of what she was asked to do, i.e. she would not study any more.

- *Wuchu* BL-5, *Shenzhu* Du-12, *Renzhong* Du-26, *Houxi* SI-3, *Neiting* ST-44.[9]

---

[8] *Shangxing* Du-23 means 'to clarify' and *Shenting* Du-24 'hall of the spirit'.
[9] *Wuchu* BL-5 means 'five places' and it connects with ever-present states of unhappiness; *Shenzhu* Du-12 is the 'pillar of the body'; *Renzhong* Du-26 is used for confusion, maniacal states; *Houxi* SI-3 for unhappiness, lack of peace; *Neiting* ST-44 to purify the heat, for example for toothache.

After three sessions the girl begins to describe her thoughts, she makes friends with the doctor [creation of a relationship] who can set up a 'spiritual therapy'. The situation is resolved in 10 sessions.

Stereotypy and Repetition

Example: a clever and well-behaved boy who starts getting bad results at school, especially in mathematics. He begins to repeat the sentence: 'mathematics is difficult', without stopping, even in his sleep.

- *Luoque* BL-8, *Naokong* GB-19, *Daling* P-7, *Yongquan* KI-1.[10]

Behaviour

Eccentricity

Loss of heart *qi*.

Example: a patient behaved in a strange way, he would take three steps forward and then two backwards, without considering obstacles.

- *Wuchu* BL-5 to *Quchai* BL-4, *Jianshi* P-5, *Yanglingquan* GB-34.[11]

Violent Behaviour Towards People and Objects

There could be delusions and hallucinations, with liver fire.

Example: a man was convinced that all yellow objects wanted to harm him, so he would destroy them all.

- *Baihui* Du-20, *Yintang* EX-HN-3 (with bleeding), *Hegu* LI-4, *Taichong* LIV-3 + modified *Sanhuang shigao tang*.

Self-Punishment

Disharmony of heart and kidney.

Example: a man thought that the only way to avoid suffering and death was to cut or burn the hand that had done something wrong.

- *Muchuang* GB-16 to *Toulinqi* GB-15, *Hegu* LI-4, *Taichong* LIV-3[12] + modified *Xiaoyao san, with dangshen, yujin, longgu*.

---

[10] *Luoque* BL-8 refers to 'connection–opposition', *Naokong* GB-19 means 'empty mind'. They are also useful for cases of mental retardation and senile dementia.

[11] *Wuchu* BL-5 means 'five places' and is connected to the feeling of being continually out of place; *Quchai* BL-4 means 'wrong, different, distorted': together they are useful in the treatment of cases where there are incorrect ideas or decisions; *Jianshi* P-5, 'intermediate messenger', calms the conscience and corrects it (when we speak of the heart the reference is actually to the sovereign, the pericardium, because the heart falls ill and dies). In relation to this case we asked: 'Does the symptom look similar to the obsessive–compulsive behaviour that we have looked at in the disorders of the *shen* and thoughts?' The answer was: 'the root is the heart, if the heart is hit the four soldiers cannot stand in good order'.

[12] *Muchuang* GB-16 means 'window of the eyes', because we must observe the eyes to understand; *Toulinqi* GB-15 means 'tears coming through'.

Wandering

Disharmony of kidney and liver.

Example: a man leaves home without realising why or knowing where to go (here we refer to cases with delirium and hallucination, not to be confused with cases of senile dementia):

- *Tongtian* BL-7 to *Chengling* GB-18, *Shenmen* HE-7, *Ligou* LIV-5[13] + *Chaihu shugan tang.*

HUN

This refers to sensation, as both perception and emotion.

Sense Perception

Illusions or Distorted Perceptions

These can also be experienced by normal people, especially if they are tired or frightened.

- *Touwei* ST-8 to *Benshen* GB-13, *Tongli* HE-5, *Guangming* GB-37.

Hallucinations

- *Baihui* Du-20 to *Chengling* GB-18, *Lingdao* HE-4, *Ququan* LIV-8, *Ligou* LIV-5.
- Auditory hallucinations: *Luxi* TB-19 or *Yifeng* TB-17.
- Visual hallucinations: *Yanglao* SI-6, *Guangming* GB-37.
- Olfactory hallucinations: *Yingxiang* LI-20, *Neiting* ST-44.
- Gustatory hallucinations: extra point under the tongue *Haiquan* EX-HN-37, *Yinjiao* Ren-7.
- Tactile hallucinations: *Neiguan* P-6, *Fenglong* ST-40.

Distorted Perceptions

- Distorted perception of space and dimensions: *Chengguang* BL-6, *Yanglao* SI-6, *Guangming* GB-37.
- Distorted perception of time: *Tongtian* BL-7, *Tongli* HE-5, *Xingjian* LIV-2.
- Distorted perception of body structure: *Xuanlu* GB-5, *Zhizheng* SI-7.
- Distorted perception of movement: *Xuanli* GB-6, *Hegu* LI-4, *Taichong* LIV-3.

---

[13] *Tongtian* BL-7 means 'communication of the heaven'; *Chengling* GB-18 means 'to sustain the spirit', it is useful for obsessive thoughts and dementia; *Shenmen* HE-7 is the 'door of the *shen*'.

Affectivity

Indifference

Emptiness of heart and spleen.
    Example: a patient without any type of reaction and emotion.

- *Wuchu* BL-5 to *Meichong* BL-3, *Lingdao* HE-4, *Ququan* LIV-8 + *Guipi tang*.

Pessimism

Emptiness of lung and spleen.
    Example: a patient who saw everything in a negative light.

- *Muchuang* GB-16, *Toulinqi* GB-15, *Suliao* Du-25, *Quchi* LI-11, *Zusanli* ST-36 + *Shenyang yiwei tang*.

Exaltation

Heat of heart and liver.
    Example: a patient who was extremely tense in his speech and behaviour.

- *Tianchong* GB-9 to *Shuaigu* GB-8, *Hegu* LI-4, *Taichong* LIV-3 + *Longdan xiegan tang* or *Banxia xiexin tang*.

Opposite Reactions

Example: a patient who would laugh at funerals.

- *Wuchu* BL-5 to *Quchai* BL-4, *Zhizheng* SI-7 or *Tongli* HT-5, *Ligou* LIV-5, *Sanyinjiao* SP-6 + *Qinggu san*.

Discrepancy Between Feelings and Their Expression

Example: a patient who would display enjoyment even when he was sad, like an actress.

- *Tongtian* BL-7 to *Chengling* GB-18, *Lingdao* HE-4, *Sanyinjiao* SP-6 + *Bazhen yimu wan*.

Emotional Instability

Disharmony of heart and liver.
    Example: a patient with strong mood fluctuations, from happy to depressed and vice versa.

- *Suliao* Du-25, *Zhengying* GB-17, *Hegu* LI-4, *Taichong* LIV-3, *Feiyang* BL-58[14] + *Fuling buxin tang*.

---

[14] *Zhengying* GB-17, 'correct action', it is a point for those who fail in their plans or make impossible plans, *ying* also means 'to nourish', and is useful for example in endocrine illnesses and tachycardia; *Feiyang* BL-58, 'flying *yang*', is useful because the patient feels unsettled.

Anxiousness

This can be caused by an emptiness of heart blood or by a disharmony of heart and kidney or by heart fire.

Example: a patient who could not stand still, sweated, had to move his feet continuously and was always doing something.

- To nourish the heart: *Yangxin tang*; to eliminate heart fire: *Qingxin liangge san*.

Aggression

Disharmony of heart and liver, with stomach and intestines heat.

Example: a patient spoke and acted with violence, without remembering it afterwards.

- *Tianchong* GB-9 to GB-8, *Ligou* LIV-5 (fire), *Renzhong* Du-26, *Taichong* LIV-3 + *Huanglian jiedu tang*.

Euphoria

Fullness of heart and emptiness of kidney.

Example: a patient appeared to be always happy, almost naive and stupid. He was also always frightened and with a lasting hunger that was not caused by stomach heat since he could not eat.

- *Baihui* Du-20, *Tongtian* BL-7, *Daling* P-7, *Yongquan* KI-1 + *Xiexin tang*.

Laughter or Weeping Without Reason

Emptiness of spleen *yang*, emptiness of kidney *yin*, heart heat.

- *Baihui* Du-20 to *Qianding* Du-21, *Daling* P-7, *Yinbai* SP-1 + *Ganmai dazao tang*.

Irritability

Emptiness of kidney *yin*, liver and heart heat.

Example: a patient would argue or cry in response to little stimulation.

- *Baihui* Du-20 to 21, *Renzhong* Du-26, *Houxi* SI-3, *Yongquan* KI-1 + *Shengtie yin*.

Paradoxical Emotions

Example: love and hate at the same time.

- *Chengling* GB-18 to *Zhengying* GB-17, *Wuchu* BL-5 to *Quchai* BL-4, *Lingdao* HE-4, *Ligou* LIV-5.

'This carries two meanings, linked to attention and will'. These were the words of a lecture given by Dr Zhang. There is also an extensive discussion on *yi* and *Zhi* in Chapter 3.

Attention

The heart is always involved, together with liver, kidney or spleen.

Disproportionate Attention

Example: a patient would notice and consider details such as the gestures or clothes of a stranger.

- *Shangxing* Du-23 to *Shenting* Du-24, *Tianchong* GB-9 to *Shuaigu* GB-8, *Hegu* LI-4, *Taichong* LIV-3 + *Qingshi anshen huatan yin*.

Divergent Attention

Example: a woman who could not follow a conversation; she would forget what had been said.

- *Chengling* GB-18 to *Zhengying* GB-17, *Lingdao* HE-4, *Taixi* KI-3 + *Yang xin tang*.

Floating Attention

- *Luoque* BL-8, *Naokong* GB-19, *Zhigou* TB-6, *Dazhong* KI-4 + *Wendan tang*.

Inadequate Attention

Example: having an exaggerated attention for small and useless things.

- *Wuchu* BL-5 to *Quchai* BL-4, *Sanyinjiao* SP-6, *Zhizheng* SI-7 + *Qingxin liangge yin*.

Will–Intention

This means deciding to do something and seeing it through.

Poor Will

Emptiness of spleen and kidney *yang*.

Example: a patient did not have any desires; he would not make decisions or plans.

- *Xinhui* Du-22 to *Shenting* Du-24, *Dazhui* Du-14 or *Mingmen* Du-4 (with moxa), *Tongli* HE-5, *Zusanli* ST-36.

Uncertain Will

Emptiness of heart and gall bladder *qi*.

Example: a patient who, before going out to buy something, would hesitate for hours because the street was too noisy.

- *Chengling* GB-18 to *Zhengying* GB-17, *Shenmen* HE-7, *Sanyinjiao* SP-6 + *Anshen dingzhi wan*.

Excessive Will

Fullness of heart, liver and gall bladder.

Example: a patient would do anything to fulfil impossible tasks. For example he had sold everything and risked his life to climb a mountain convinced that this would make him a king.

- *Baihui* Du-20 to *Tianchong* GB-9, *Wuchu* BL-5 to BL-4, *Hegu* LI-4, *Taichong* LIV-3 + *Yuejiu wan*.

ZHI

This has the meaning of intelligence and memory.

Intelligence

This consists of four aspects that are all necessary to solve a problem: attention, evaluation, comprehension and memory.

Congenital Dementia

- *Baihui* Du-20 to *Chengling* GB-18, *Lingdao* HE-4, *Dazhong* KI-4.

Secondary Dementia (Traumas, Fever, Intoxications)

- *Sishencong* EX-HN-1, *Dazhui* Du-14, *Quchi* LI-11, *Shenmen* HE-7, *Dazhong* KI-4, *Sanyinjiao* SP-6.

Pseudo-Organic Dementia

Often caused by organic factors, it usually has an abrupt beginning and a rapid course, like hysteria.

- *Shenting* Du-24 to *Shangxing* Du-23, *Houting* Du-19 to *Qianding* Du-21, *Lingdao* HE-4, *Zhongchong* P-9, *Dazhui* Du-14.

Memory

This implies recognising things and keeping them in mind.

Decreasing Memory

Emptiness of heart and spleen.

Amnesias

- *Baihui* Du-20 to *Houting* Du-19, *Naokong* GB-19 to *Tianzhu* BL-10, *Lingdao* HE-4, *Sanyinjiao* SP-6.

Paramnesias

- *Houting* Du-19 to *Luoque* BL-8, *Fubai* GB-10 to *Touqiaoyin* GB-11, *Lingdao* HE-4, *Xingjian* LIV-2.

Pseudoreminiscence, Confabulation

- *Baihui* Du-20 to *Zhengying* GB-17, *Wuchu* BL-5 to *Quchai* BL-4, *Daling* P-7.

COMMENTS

- Normally four points are used:
  - two points on the head, very often with the indication of a second point that the needle should reach, usually along a centripetal direction;
  - two points distal to the main joints, usually placed along one channel of the hand and one of the foot.
- The head points more frequently in use are:
  - *Baihui* Du-20 (at times reaching *Qianding* Du-21 or *Houting* Du-19 or *Chengling* GB-18), *Tianchong* GB-9 and *Chengling* GB-18 in case of a positive psychotic symptomatology;
  - otherwise *Shangxing* Du-23 to *Shenting* Du-24 if there are negative psychotic symptoms;
  - *Xinhui* Du-22 to *Shangxing* Du-23 for lighter negative symptoms;
  - *Zhengying* GB-17 to correct instability, lack of decision, wrong interpretation of reality;
  - *Wuchu* BL-5 is used for 'lasting discomfort and unhappiness', but also for inappropriate responses and multiple personality.
- The distal points that appear more often are:
  - *Lingdao* HE-4, *Tongli* HE-5, *Shenmen* HE-7; *Daling* P-7; *Zhizheng* SI-7;
  - *Taixi* KI-3, *Dazhong* KI-4, *Yongquan* KI-1; *Feiyang* BL-58;
  - *Taibai* SP-3, *Sanyinjiao* SP-6; *Zusanli* ST-36, *Fenglong* ST-40, *Neiting* ST-44;
  - *Xingjian* LIV-2, *Taichong* LIV-3, *Ligou* LIV-5, *Ququan* LIV-8; *Yanglingquan* GB-34.
- The points are often chosen in relation to the function expressed by their names.

- The courses of the channels or the specific actions of the points are also important: for example with auditory hallucinations the diagnosis is emptiness of kidney, but he also uses points on the triple burner and gall bladder. In olfactory hallucinations he uses *Yingxiang* LI-20 and *Neiting* ST-44. In visual hallucinations he uses points that are helpful to the eyes such as *Guangming* GB-37 and *Yanglao* SI-6.

SYNDROMES

This arrangement on the basis of syndromes was presented at the end of the course, possibly because we insisted that the subject be related to the common differential diagnosis patterns.

Looking at it today, I believe this summary to be a result of the attempt to integrate a point of view that privileges points and channels with the TCM syndrome-based systematisation. Moreover it aims at combining the former with a diagnostic organisation of conventional psychiatry that defines classes on the basis of the inclusion criteria (see DSM).

Zhang Mingjiu specified that in the clinical practice there are four types of patterns of emptiness and one of fullness that can usually be recognised. Each syndrome is characterised by four groups of signs, of which at least two must be recognised in order to develop a diagnosis.

He added that the syndromes are often mixed: if it is not possible to link the case to a well-defined category one should use the points in accordance to symptoms and signs.

Emptiness of Spleen and Lungs

This produces phlegm that disturbs the heart.

- Face with oedema and lack of spirit, little desire to eat and speak.
- Slow thought (spleen), olfactory hallucinations, frequent diarrhoea.
- Self-denigration, little self-esteem, pessimism (thought belongs to spleen, sadness belongs to lung).
- State of unconsciousness, with pale tongue and weak pulse.

Therapeutic Principles

- Warm and tonify the spleen and lung, calm the *po*, clarify the mind.

Treatment

- *Fubai* GB-10 to *Touqiaoyin* GB-11, *Tongtian* BL-7 to *Chengguang* BL-6, *Taiyuan* LU-9, *Taibai* SP-3, *Pianli* LI-6 (*luo*), *Fenglong* ST-40 + *Xiangsha liujunzi wan*.

Emptiness of Heart and Spleen Blood

This causes a loss of control of the *shen*.

- Pale face and lips, worrying, occasional incoherent speech.
- Hypersensibility, uncertainty, hesitation.
- Uncontrolled crying and laughing.
- Pale tongue, weak pulse.

Therapeutic Principles

- Nourish heart and spleen, calm the *shen*.

Treatment

- *Chengling* GB-18 to *Zhengying* GB-17, *Shangxing* Du-23 to *Shenting* Du-24, *Shenmen* HE-7, *Zhizheng* SI-7, *Taibai* SP-3, *Fenglong* ST-40 + *Yangxin tang*.

Emptiness of Liver and Kidney

This produces a full fire and agitation of the *shen*.

- Red face, dry lips, auditory or visual hallucinations.
- Absurd thought, naive behaviour.
- Uncertainty and hyper sensibility, night perspiration.
- Dark red tongue without coating, weak pulse.

Therapeutic Principles

- Nourish kidney, harmonise the liver, calm the spirit, promote the *zhi*.

Treatment

- *Tianchong* GB-9 to *S* GB-11 to *Yifeng* TB-17, *Erjian* LI-2, *Guangming* GB-37, *Taixi* KI-3, *Feiyang* BL-58 + *Yiguan jian*.

Emptiness of Kidney and Spleen *Yang*

This produces a weakness of the *shen*.

- Pale face and complexion, difficulty in speaking, slow thought.
- Fatigue, drowsiness, fear of the cold.
- Lack of appetite, facial oedema, auditory or gustative hallucinations.
- Swollen and pale tongue, weak pulse.

Therapeutic Principles

- Warm the spleen and kidney *yang*, calm the *shen* and *yi*.

Treatment

- *Baihui* Du-20 to *Shenting* Du-24, *Wuchu* BL-5 to *Meichong* BL-3, *Taibai* SP-3, *Taixi* KI-3, *Fenglong* ST-40, *Feiyang* BL-58 + *Zhenwu erxian tang*.

Full Heat of Liver and *Yang* Organ-*fu*

The heart is attacked by fire and poisons.

- Complexion is apparently strong, red face, halitosis.
- State of excitement, with hyperactivity of movement and speech.
- Constant hunger, constipation, dark urine.
- Dark red tongue, full and rapid pulse.

Therapeutic Principles

Pacify the liver, disperse the fire, calm the *hun* and *shen*.

Treatment

- *Qianding* Du-21 to *Muchuang* GB-16, *Tianchong* GB-9 to *Shuaigu* GB-8, *Dadun* LIV-1, *Fenglong* ST-40, *Ququan* LIV-8, *Chongyang* ST-42 + *Shigao tang*.

Stagnation of *qi* and Blood or Stagnation of Heart and Liver *qi*

Mixed syndrome of fullness and emptiness, with confusion of the *shen*.

- Dark face with a brown-red colour similar to coffee, blurred spirit like in a dream.
- Incoherent thought and speech, sometimes delirium and fever.
- Dry mouth and lips, loss of memory.
- Tongue with purple spots, thready, slow and choppy pulse.

Therapeutic Principles

- Harmonise liver and move blood, open the orifices, calm the heart.

Treatment

- *Qianding* Du-21 to *Zhengying* GB-17, *Touwei* ST-8 to *Benshen* GB-13, *Shenmen* HE-7, *Zhizheng* SI-7, *Ligou* LIV-5, *Taichong* LIV-3 + *Danzhi xiaoyao wan* (*Jiawei xiaoyao san*).

Clinic for Mental Disorders

Jin Shubai

20

INTRODUCTION

The following notes are drawn from the text *Acupuncture and Moxibustion in the Treatment of Mental Disorders* by Jin Shubai.[1]

Jin Shubai was born in the twenties in Shanghai and her work follows a family tradition. She first practised alongside her father, a pupil of Chen Zhilan, and then mostly in Long Hua hospital in Shanghai, accumulating an extraordinary wealth of experience in treating patients with mental disorders.

As is so often the case, the text that goes by her name is a collection of her teachings that were gathered, arranged and reviewed by her pupils.

The work comprises: an introduction on her thought and clinical experience in the treatment of mental disorders using acupuncture; four chapters on *dian*, *kuang*, *diankuang* and *yuzheng* (viewed as depression); and an appendix with the title 'Clinical observations on the treatment of hysteria with acupuncture' in which *meiheqi*, *zangzao*, *bentunqi*, epileptic-like symptoms, and *diankuang* are considered.[2]

I have decided to include certain parts of this book as comments and clinical examples of such syndromes. In fact the accounts are extremely clear and ably integrate classical knowledge with a wide experience of contemporary clinical work.

I consider the style in which Jin Shubai selects and uses points to be very useful for those alterations of the *qi* – particularly those revealed by psychic symptoms – that are almost cases of psychosis, but also for those seen in everyday medical practice.

---

[1] Jin Shubai, *'Zhenjiu zhiliao jingshenbing'* ('Acupuncture and moxibustion in the treatment of mental disorders'), Shanghai zhongyi xueyuan chubanshi, Shanghai, 1987.

[2] 'Hysteria' is a translation of *yibing*, a modern term in which *yi* refers to 'idea, thought' and *bing* is the radical 'illness'. Sometimes an English-sounding transliteration is used.

Jin Shubai identifies certain guidelines for diagnosis and treatment that stem from her clinical experience. She maintains that in order to make a diagnosis one has to first differentiate emptiness and fullness and diagnose *dian* and *kuang*.

Pathogenesis

In the pathogenesis of the *diankuang* disorders one can identify four main factors: *qi*, blood, phlegm and fire.

Qi

Emotions influence the movements of the *qi* directly.

Blood (Empty and Full)

Empty: this comes from delivery or from excessive menstruation, which causes insufficiency of the heart blood. If the heart is not nourished its *qi* becomes empty; this manifests as *yuzheng*-constipation or as a *kuang* or *dian* pattern with anxiousness, fear, sadness and crying.

Full: this is often caused by alterations in menstruation or retention of lochia that produce blood stasis; the stagnating and turbid *qi* rises, invades the pericardium and clouds it, causing mental disorders.

Phlegm

Jin Shubai recalls certain passages by Zhu Danxi and Zhang Zihe regarding *diankuang* (detailed in Chapter 8). She explains that there can be:

- emptiness, mainly connected with an insufficiency of the central *yang*: if the spleen does not transport and transform the liquids well they condense into phlegm, with a pattern of emptiness of the *qi* and knotting of the phlegm;
- constraint-*yu* of the liver and knotting-*jie* of the *qi*, with the invasion of the spleen and the production of internal phlegm, which disturb the orifices and cause *dian*;
- full heat produced by the consumption of rich food, tobacco, alcohol and hot flavours;
- the five emotions, which transform themselves into fire; the heat evaporates and the liquids condense into phlegm;
- gall bladder fire, which attacks the stomach and knots up as fire-phlegm: the persistent phlegm enters the heart following the fire, the heart *shen* is disturbed and *kuan* manifests.

Constraint of the Fire

'Excessive *qi* is fire': there is heart fire, stomach fire, liver and gall bladder fire and minister fire, but all disturb the heart *shen*.

If the heart fire is too strong there is euphoria, laughter and loquacity.

If there is stomach fire there is madness and foolish running about.

If there is liver and gall bladder fire the person insults everyone in the vicinity and swears constantly.

Excessively strong minister fire causes excessive sexual activity, dreams about copulating with spirits, etc.

Description

Dian Pattern

This is a *yin* pattern, mostly from emptiness.

The main symptoms are: depression, mutism, fear, insecurity, anxiousness, memory deficit, depressed mood, deep and thready pulse, pale tongue, face without light, dull expression, etc.

There may also be fullness within emptiness. If the origin is a *yin* liver and kidney emptiness down below, with the *yang* floating uncontrolled above, there can be perceptual distortions, visual, auditory and olfactory hallucinations, inconsistent thought patterns and mental confusion, emotional instability, a tongue with red edges and tip, and a thready, rapid and wiry pulse.

There can be thick accumulations of phlegm blocking the *Du Mai* and this manifests through dullness, mutism, stiffness of the limbs like wood, psychological retreat, a white and greasy tongue coating, and a tense and full pulse.

Kuang Pattern

This is a *yang* pattern, mostly from fullness.

Usually the symptoms are megalomania, enhanced memory, verbal aggressiveness, and insults aimed at relatives and strangers alike; in severe cases the patient undresses, climbs up somewhere high and sings. The face is red and the lips are dry, the eyes have a terrible light, the person is thirsty with a desire for cold drinks, and has constipation, a red tongue with yellow coating, and a slippery, large, deep, rapid pulse. This is full heat of *Yang Ming*.

There may also be emptiness within the fullness; the signs are a thin body, eyes lacking *shen*, a desire to cry but no tears, shrill voice, loquacity and anxiousness, uneasiness and agitation, insomnia, a red tongue with absent or white slippery coating, and a thready and rapid pulse, etc. – that is, fire signs.

Combination of Dian and Kuang Patterns

This is a combination of *yin* and *yang*. The symptoms vary. At the beginning there is usually a grey and greasy coating, rapid and wiry pulse, and signs of constraint and knotting of the liver and gall bladder. There are sudden crises with madness and verbal aggression, but usually it is controllable because the two pathogens *yin* and *yang* combine in the liver and gall bladder and it is not a typical *kuang* with strong pathogens in the *Ysang Ming*.

During the menstrual period it is possible for women to become extremely agitated, almost like *kuang*: the disorder is in the blood layer and the liver and gall bladder *qi* counterflows disturbing the heart *shen*.

There can also be obstruction of the *Du Mai*: the patient lies down rigidly, refuses to eat and does not speak until the pathogens *yin* and *yang* collide and there is a sudden suicidal or homicidal impulse.

If, during the menstrual period, the insufficiency of heart and spleen or the emptiness of the liver and kidney *yin* cause such agitation that the woman cannot stand nor sit, behaving as if she were being constantly chased, it is a *dian* pattern; if the *yin* emptiness with a fire excess is combined with the phlegm and there is verbal and physical aggressiveness together with relationship conflicts, this is the category of *diankuang*.

Therapeutic Principles

Regulate *yin* and *yang*, put the organs and channels back into communication.

Treatment

The treatment of mental illnesses by Jin Shubai is part of her family tradition, in which basically Gao Wu's principle was applied to regulate *yin* and *yang*: 'Those who are good at using needles conduct the *yin* from the *yang* and the *yang* from the *yin*.'[3]

This is why she says that in order to treat *dian* we should select the *Du Mai* – that is, we should take from the *yang* to the *yin*, and in order to treat *kuang* we should select the *Ren Mai*. In mixed patterns we select one or two important points of the *Ren Mai* and *Du Mai*.

Moreover, since the 'heart is the home of the *jingshen*', many are pericardium points.

- She insists on the fact that the choice of the point is fundamental and that combinations should be accurate and effective.
- She usually uses two to six points at a time.
- The choice is made from about 70 points that are also the most used points in the general clinic.
- She often uses a method of combining points along the same channel, following her family tradition. In cases of *kuang* she frequently selects three points on *Ren Mai*, for example *Jiuwei* Ren-15 (to *Juque* Ren-14), *Shangwan*

---

[3] The verb 'to conduct' is a translation of *yin*. The same term is used with reference to the *daoyin* practices and to radiating pain.

Ren-13 and *Zhongwan* Ren-12 – a combination that is very effective for resolving the phlegm and calming.

- In cases of *dian*, to tonify she often uses two points on the *Du Mai* and a pericardium point, because of the connection between the heart and brain.

- She pays great attention to different techniques of stimulation used in the various phases, adapting them to the individual and to the moment; stronger stimulation is used in the fullness (for example she uses 1.5 *cun* needles for *Renzhong* Du-26, with the lifting–thrusting method until the eyes water) and lighter stimulation in emptiness (often in the *dian* patterns the stimulation is through rotation).

- She often uses the method of 'joining two points with one needle'. She suggests:
  — *dian*: *Yintang* EX-HN-3 (to *Xinqu*),[4] *Neiguan* P-6;
  — *kuang*: *Renzhong* Du-26 (to *Yinjiao* Du-28), *Jianshi* P-5;
  — *diankuang*: peaceful phase: *Yintang* EX-HN-3; agitated phase: *Renzhong* Du-26;
  — depending on the condition and on how the situation evolves one can connect one or two *yuan*, *luo* or *xi* points of the corresponding *zangfu* or *shu* points of the back;
  — if the heart *qi* does not flow and is obstructed: *Tongli* HE-5;
  — if there is excessive liver fire, with anger and swearing manifestations: *Taichong* LIV-3 to drain the channel;
  — if there is insufficient liver *qi*, with fear and terror: *Taixi* KI-3 or *Sanyinjiao* SP-6;
  — if there are dietary disorders, with stomach heat and phlegm: *Fenglong* ST-40;
  — very useful points: *Shenmen* HE-7, *Waiguan* TB-5, *Ligou* LIV-5, *Zusanli* ST-36, *Hegu* LI-4, *Jiuwei* Ren-15 up to *Juque* Ren-14, *Shangwan* Ren-13 and *Zhongwan* Ren-12, *Fengfu* Du-16, *Yamen* Du-15, *Dazhui* Du-14, *Baihui* Du-20, and *Sishencong* EX-HN-1;
  — ear therapy: *Shenmen*, Brain, Subcortex, Forehead, Heart.

- Jin Shubai also makes use of traditional medicines, but she relies mostly on acupuncture. Prescriptions are generally used in the initial *kuang* phases, to treat rapidly, drawing on the energy of the illness to solve it.

---

[4] *Xinqu* is the heart area in the face somatotopic representation, to which face acupuncture, *mianzhen* refers. When the wording 'to…' appears it means that the needle is inserted in one point but it reaches another one, using the method of 'joining two points with one needle' (the same method used by Zhang Mingjiu, see Chapter 19).

Case Study 20.1

Dian[5]

This was a 32-year-old woman, factory worker, 1970. In 1961, because of a heavy emotional strain, she had suffered from suspiciousness, fear and auditory hallucinations. At the hospital psychiatric unit schizophrenia had been diagnosed; after a 3-month hospitalisation she recovered and was discharged. The illness recurred periodically: the patient felt threatened, she thought that everything that happened was related to her, she was in a state of fear and confusion and was never at peace. In the period of the Cultural Revolution her family had been attacked and the symptoms of mental disorder, such as retreat, distrust and auditory hallucinations, had worsened. She was treated for four years with a strong dosage of medicines (chlorpromazine), but her situation did not improve. On the contrary the patient became more and more confused.

Objective examination: she has a tendency to obesity, her mind is unclear, she pays no attention to the surroundings, her affective communication is limited, she does not ask for nor relate anything spontaneously, she is slow in speaking and answering, her movements are apathetic, her memory weak, her ability to count reduced, her mental processes are slowed down, and she is almost without any sense of orientation.

She has had amenorrhoea for the previous 2 years, the tongue coating is white and greasy, the pulse is deep and thready.

Diagnosis
Constraint and knotting of heart and spleen, with phlegm obstructing the heart orifices; schizophrenia.

Therapeutic Principles
Free the constraint, open the orifices, resolve the phlegm.

Treatment
First phase:
- *Sishencong* EX-HN-1, directed towards *Baihui* Du-20;
- *Neiguan* P-6 alternated with *Tongli* HE-5, with rotation.
  We reduce the dosage of the medicines.
  The patient begins to talk and laugh, she is in more lively spirits, she resumes her part-time work, but during the night she still has many dreams, and amenorrhoea.
  Second phase:
- *Yintang* EX-HN-3 (to *Xinqu*);
- *Hegu* LI-4 and *Sanyinjiao* SP-6.

---

[5] Jin Shubai, 1987, p. 9. Cases are described with a double diagnosis: the traditional Chinese one and the conventional, Western one. From this perspective this case is defined as *dian* and *jingshen fenlie* (schizophrenia).

Further reduction of the drug dosage. Menstruation restarts and she becomes pregnant. She has a termination and, after a 2-week rest, regains her normal spirits and starts working full time.

Jin Shubai's comment:

The patient is overweight, there is an accumulation of phlegm caused by a lack of movement in the emotions and by fear and distrust, which cause constraint and knotting of the heart and spleen. Moreover, the prolonged use of sedatives has had the effect of blocking the drainage and resolution of the phlegm, obscuring the pure *yang*, causing hallucinations and distorted thoughts, and progressively dulling and clouding the consciousness like a 'wooden hen'. The pulse corresponds to the symptom described in *Nanjing*, 'double *yin* is *dian*'.

In the first phase of the therapy we used the extra points *sishencong* EX-HN-1 to expel the turbid, raise the pure and open the orifices. When combined, the *luo* point of the pericardium and the *luo* point of the heart have the effect of activating the heart *qi* and allowing it to flow, opening the chest and removing the constraint. The patient consequently became more lively, smiled and was able to communicate spontaneously.

Because of the improvement, in the second phase we chose *Yintang* EX-HN-3 directed towards *Xinqu* to calm the heart and the *shen*, and *Hegu* LI-4 and *Sanyinjiao* SP-6 to regulate the nutritious *qi* and promote the flow of the *qi* in the channels. She also resumed her part-time work.

The treatment lasted for 6 months, with 64 sessions.

The pharmacological therapy was continued with minimum dosage.

The menstrual cycle was again normal; she became pregnant and had an abortion, but recovered without any great problems and was able to return to her work.

Case Study 20.2

Dian[6]

This was a 16-year-old boy, 1972. The family declared that 2 years before he suffered from a cranial trauma sustained in a fight. Since then he has spoken nonsense and wanders about aimlessly. The diagnosis was maniacal psychosis and he was prescribed a pharmacological treatment (chlorpromazine) to calm him.

Five days before the session, while reading *The Little Monkey*, he suffered a relapse.

Objective examination: the lips are dry and cracked, his appearance is untidy, he is anxious and he never stops speaking, he does not cooperate, his tongue is red with

---

[6] Jin Shubai, 1987, p. 35.

a yellow coating, and the pulse is slippery and rapid. He is thirsty, has been constipated for a few days, and cannot sleep.

Diagnosis
The heat pathogen of the *Yang Ming* invades the heart, with loss of clarity of the *shen*.

Maniacal psychosis.

Treatment
Resolve the phlegm, clear *Yang Ming* heat, calm the *shen*, harmonise.
* *Jiuwei* Ren-15 (to *Juque* Ren-14)
* *Shangwan* Ren-13 and *Zhongwan* Ren-12

All the points are treated with strong dispersing manipulation, with the lifting–thrusting technique.

Prescription: *shentieluo* 60 g, *shengshigao* 60 g, *fuling* 12 g, *yuanzhi* 4.5 g, *nanxing* 10 g, fresh *shichangpu* 10 g, for 2 days.

In the second session the spirit is clear, the boy cooperates, his stools are regular, lips and tongue are moister, and the pulse is moderate.

We repeat the same points and the same prescription, but with half the dosage of *shentieluo* and *sheng shigao* (30 g), for 2 days.

In the third session the look, behaviour and spirit are normal and he has gone back to school.

We purify the heart and calm the *shen*, to reinforce the effect: *Yintang* EX-HN-3, *Jianshi* P-5, with light manipulation and we interrupt the prescription.

Jin Shubai's Comment
When the *Nanjing* says 'double *yang kuang*' it means that the *yang* pathogen enters the *yang* channels. The *yang* pathogens in the *kuang* pattern can be *qi*, fire, phlegm and food pathogens. By *yang* channels we particularly refer to gall bladder and stomach, and above all to the stomach channel.

In his text *Zhengzhi zhunsheng* ('Diagnosis and medicine treatment standards'), Wang Ketang says: 'when *Kuang* breaks loose it is violent and crazy like the exploding of the *kuang* of the great fullness of *Yang Ming* in feverish illnesses'. It is always a case of *Yang Ming*, both with an external invasion and with an internal damage; the name is the same but the nature is different: in feverish illnesses the external pathogens transform themselves until they enter the *Yang Ming* in the form of heat and in severe cases there can be loss of the senses. When there is a *Yang Ming* syndrome one insults both relatives and strangers; this is caused by phlegm, fire, *qi* and food pathogens. Similar considerations also emerge in the '*Jingmai*' chapter of the *Lingshu* (Chapter 10) concerning stomach illnesses.

In this case the illness concerns both the channel and the organ *Yang Ming*; the excessive and chaotic speech is a result of the invasion of the heart channel; the untidy look, the yellow coating, the slippery pulse are all caused by the excess of *yang*. The four limbs are the root of all the *yang*, if there is an excess of *yang* the four limbs are full. If these are full they cause disorderly movement and crazy walking. An excess of heat in the body produces the untidy appearance. If the heat disturbs the heart *shen* the speech is muddled and the person cannot sleep at night; there are also symptoms such as thirst, dry and cracked lips, constipation, etc.

In the treatment we have used three anterior points, following the principle of getting to the *yang* through the *yin*, to drain the phlegm and the heart and stomach heat. At the same time we have used a strong dosage of *shentieluo*, which is cold and heavy, to calm and bring the *qi* counterflow downwards, *shigao*, which is spicy, sweet, cold, to purify the heat and drain the fire, and the other components to resolve the phlegm. The overall effect is that of purifying, calming and eliminating the phlegm; if the heart is purified the *shen* is calm.

Case Study 20.3

Diankuang[7]

This was a 25-year-old girl. The family maintained that a deeply deluded love had caused great rage and hatred in the girl: the deep emotional injury, with an accumulation of anguish and constraint, had brought manifestations of folly. This had been going on for 4 years with a diagnosis of schizophrenia and numerous psychiatric hospitalisations.

She had already been exposed to ten electroconvulsive treatments and was under a therapy with chlorpromazine. In the last period, following her parents' suggestion, she had been taking some *Longhuan* pills, which caused vomiting, diarrhoea and severe asthenia, but had left the girl as noisy and messy as before.

The examination reveals a strong body and rude speech. The girl insults everyone violently and does not cooperate; her pulse is deep, slippery and large, and the tongue has a yellow and greasy coating and a red tip.

Diagnosis
Internal constraint of the *Yang Ming* phlegm, disorderly movement of the minister fire of heart and liver; schizophrenia.

Therapeutic Principles
Drain the *yang*, resolve the phlegm, and purify the heart.

Treatment
First phase:
- *Renzhong* Du-26 (to *Yinjiao* Du-28);
- *Jianshi* P-5 (to *Zhigou* TB-6) and *Fenglong* ST-40.

All the points are treated with strong dispersing manipulation, with the lifting–thrusting technique, never leaving the needle in place.

---

[7] Jin Shubai, 1987, p. 59.

After we took the needles out the patient shouted: 'I do not want to be treated with acupuncture, I will come back and take my revenge'. After some days she came back to the practice and tried to hit the doctor; the parents, who did not want to take her back to the study because of her behaviour, having found no other alternatives finally decide to return.

In this first phase of the therapy the girl moves and swears, but the treatment is carried out anyway keeping her still; there were four sessions.

Second phase:

- *Dazhui* Du-14 along the *Du Mai* up to the level of the 12th thoracic vertebra without letting go of the needle.
- *Renzhong* Du-26 up to *Yinjiao* Du-28 until the eyes water, with strong manipulation.

The patient falls asleep for 2 hours with the needle, then she wakes up crying; we take the needle out, she sleeps another half an hour and when she wakes up she has only a vague memory of the acupuncture, yet her consciousness seems clearer.

We treat her in this way for 3 days in a row. Each time she falls asleep for at least 2 hours, but in the evening she is still restless and continues to walk.

After a 1-week break because she is menstruating she undergoes another seven sessions.

At each session the length of the insertion of the needle is reduced, until we go from *Shendao* Du-11, to the level of T5.

The patient now cooperates a little more, but she remains untrusting and still feels constantly threatened. During the night she sleeps and does not wander anymore. During the day she still appears excited and laughs to herself; at times she has a feeling of oppression in the chest and agitation, but these pass spontaneously. She can engage in small tasks.

Third phase:

At first she still has moments when her movements are agitated, she gets angry easily, but the attacks of rage are much shorter and less violent, although her language and thought processes are still confused.

If she sees a young doctor she approaches him in a seductive manner.

The treatment is continued following the principles of purifying the brain, calming the *shen*, clearing the heart, and calming the liver.

- *Renzhong* Du-26 (up to *Yinjiao* Du-28 and horizontally up to *Kouheliao* LI-19);
- *Jianshi* P-5 alternated with *Neiguan* P-6.

If necessary:

- *Anmian* N-HN-54;
- *Fenglong* ST-40;
- *Ligou* LIV-5.

Dispersing manipulation is performed with lifting–thrusting and rotation, leaving the needles in for 30 minutes.

Fourth phase:

The symptomatology has improved by 50%: her responses are adequate, behaviour is harmonious, she can relate to her surroundings, she is not verbally nor physically aggressive, she is punctual when coming to the sessions, she cooperates, is polite to people and speaks calmly, her menstrual cycle is regular, and she spontaneously asks for a certificate to be able to return to work. Her pulse is slippery and small; the tongue is normal.

She has stopped taking chlorpromazine and takes only a small dose of anxiolytic in the evening.

Now we can tonify and disperse, treating the manifestation and root.
- *Fengfu* Du-16 alternated with *Dazhui* Du-14 or with *Renzhong* Du-26;
- *Jianshi* P-5 alternated with *Neiguan* P-6.
  If necessary:
- *Zusanli* ST-36, *Anmian* N-HN-54, *Ganshu* BL-18, *Shenshu* BL-23, etc.
  Fifth phase:
  We continue the treatment, draining the heat and purifying the *shen* to enhance the regulation.
- *Fengfu* Du-16 alternated with *Yintang* EX-HN-3;
- *Jianshi* P-5 alternated with *Neiguan* P-6;
- *Taiyang* EX-HN-9, *Shenmen* HE-7.
  A total of 63 sessions.

Now the girl appears normal, she stops taking anxiolytics and asks to take Chinese medicines. We prescribe *zijuwan* 6 g per day for 2 weeks.

After a period of part time work she starts working full time again and is cured.

Jin Shubai's Comment

This patient initially had phlegm, which transformed into fire and produced *kuang*; inhibition added to this then produced *dian*.

Due to the electroconvulsive treatments, the chlorpromazine and ultimately the *Longhuwan*, the true *qi* was damaged resulting in hallucinations, confusion of thought processes and in the illness reaching a chronic condition.

Longhuwan used in the first phases of the illness can eliminate the phlegm and purify through the purgative and emetic components, but this method is ineffective when, as in this case, the pathology is chronic and the root is deep.

One can drain only by using a constant, slow and correct treatment.

In the 'Nanjing' it is said: 'double *yang* is *kuang*'. Ye Tianshi maintains that *kuang* is a pattern that is connected to the three *yang* that rise up. The Du Mai is the sea of all the *yang*. Consequently one can use the relationship between the *Du Mai* and *Yang Ming* by inserting a large needle (*juzhen*) to disperse strongly from *Dazhui* Du-14 up to the 12th thoracic vertebra.

When *Renzhong* Du-26 is stimulated with a needle that reaches *Yinjiao* Du-28 it eliminates the fire of all the *yang* and enables the correct *yang* to return to the sea while making sure that the pathogen *yang* has nowhere to settle down. This is the reason why the patient sleeps for two hours after the session.

The stimulation with a needle that goes from *Dazhui* Du-14 up to the 12th thoracic vertebra is a method used specifically for chronic *kuang* illness, otherwise *Baihui* Du-20 and *Zhongwan* Ren-12 are enough.

Renzhong Du-26 is one of the 13 *gui* points and it is the meeting point of the hand and foot *Yang Ming* with the *Dumai*. Since ancient times it has been considered of great importance for the treatment of *diankuang* thanks to its ability to open the orifices, eliminate the heat, disperse the *yang*, calm the *shen*.

Yinjiao Du-28 is the meeting point of the *Ren*, *Du* and stomach channels. It can induce *yin* and *yang* to communicate. If it is used in combination with *Renzhong* Du-26, the *yin* rises and the *yang* goes down; if the *yang* goes down *kuang* stops, if the *yin* rises one can sleep; the results are immediate.

Depending on the evolution of the illness, the choice of points shifts from an attacking therapy to a reinforcement treatment.

The pericardium conducts the activities in the place of the heart; this is why we have chosen *Jianshi* P-5 alternated with *Neiguan* P-6: *Jianshi* P-5 purifies the heart fire, and *Neiguan* P-6 helps the heart *qi*.

We have also added *Anmian* N-HN-54 and *Shenmen* HE-7 to calm the heart *shen*, *Fenglong* ST-40 to resolve the phlegm, *Ganshu* BL-18 and *Ligou* LIV-5 to calm the liver, *Taiyang* EX-HN-9 to drain and liberate, *Zusanli* ST-36 to regulate the stomach and sustain the correct *qi*, and *Shenshu* BL-23 to calm the *zhi*.

If *yin* and *yang* are balanced, *qi* and blood stay in place and one can prevent relapses.

In general, in *kuang* syndrome the treatment is short. In this case, however, the pathology was extremely chronic and so we had to adopt a special treatment of the manifestations at the root, in five phases with 63 sessions to regain a normal condition.

YUZHENG

Jin Shubai quotes Ye Tianshi in the chapter 'Yu' [in *Lingzhen zhinan yian*, Guide cases in clinic] to remind us that *yu* means stagnation-*zhi* and lack of flow.

She recalls how in the treatment we use various principles to help the liver, liberate the *qi*, move with the spicy taste, and lower with the bitter, calm the liver, extinguish the wind, purify the heart, drain the fire, reinforce the spleen, harmonise the stomach, move the blood, let the *luo* flow, transform the phlegm, eliminate the fluid chest phlegm, help the *qi*, and nourish the *yin*. But she underlines the importance of 'changing emotions and varying nature'.[8]

Yuzheng principally originates from emotional factors, with constraint and knotting of the liver and gall bladder, which slowly damage the transforming function of the spleen. The heart then fails to be nourished, and all the organs, *yin* and *yang*, and *qi* and blood are disordered.

---

[8] The sentence *yiqing bianxing*, 'changing the emotions-*qing* and varying the nature-*xing*' that is, modifying the internal attitude, recalls the title of the 13th chapter of the *Suwen*, '*Yijing bianqi*', changing the *jing* and varying the *qi*. On this subject see also Chapter 14 on the treatment of emotions in the classics.

In the initial phase the pathogenesis is usually connected to *qi* stagnation, associated with phlegm and dampness, food accumulation, blood stasis, fire transformation – that is, mainly with patterns of fullness. In the chronic phase of pathology, in contrast, there is a shift from full to empty. This means that *yu* is caused internally by the seven emotions and initially attacks the *qi*, then reaches the blood and finally causes breakdown. In any event, since *yin* and *yang* organs, *qi* and blood are affected, in clinical presentations empty and full are usually seen intertwined in the initial phase as well.

In *yu* patterns the blood is usually affected after the *qi*, but sometimes the origin can be an emptiness of the blood followed by damage to the *qi*.

Case Study 20.4

Yuzheng[9]

This was a 38-year-old woman, a journalist, seen in 1970. In the spring of 1965 the patient had gone to the country to teach in the communes. Because of the great effort this involved her sleep had been disturbed for over 20 days, she missed her husband and this had affected her mood greatly (*qingxu*). She had returned to normal after three sessions of electroconvulsive treatment in a hospital in Beijing. In 1967 the same problem emerged for 1 month because of certain family problems. Then she went on holiday with her husband, which distracted her and she got better.

In 1970, after childbirth, she moved to her mother's house to rest and her husband went to see her, but when the holiday was over and he left, the emotional lability recommenced: she feels alone and sad, she is always frightened, anxious, she continuously cries, she stays awake all through the night and has sporadic hallucinations.

She comes to the acupuncture clinic with her husband.

She has a very tidy and clean look, she is polite, her tongue is pale with a white coating, and the pulse is drenched-*ru* and thready-*xi*, her appearance is that of cold, her complexion is dark and dull, her spirit is weak, and when speaking she answers in a correct way, lowering her voice when she talks of her personal problems. She says: 'my husband comes to see me but he bothers about other things, deep inside me I really cannot stand him, I cannot fight against this thought even though I know it is wrong'. Then she cries without stopping. Memory, ability to count, cognitive faculties and neurological examinations are normal.

Diagnosis
Emptiness of the blood after delivery, constraint and knotting of liver and gall bladder, and lack of nutrition of heart *shen*.

---

[9] Jin Shubai, 1987, p. 62.

Therapeutic Principles

Free the constraint, and calm the *shen*.

Treatment

First phase: sessions 1–7
- *Yintang* EX-HN-3 (to *Xinqu*), *Anmian* 1 and 2 alternated, *Neiguan* P-6 + ear acupuncture: Sympathetic point.

All points are treated with light stimulation.

The patient is severely ill, she does not trust acupuncture very much, and she continues to take anxiolytics. After seven sessions of acupuncture there is an improvement in the afternoons, but during the day she is still in a bad mood, sad, and continuously crying.

Second phase: sessions 8–16
- first group of points: as above;
- second group of points: *Xinshu* BL-15, *Ganshu* BL-18, *Pishu* BL-20 + ear acupuncture: Heart point and *Shenmen* point.

All points are treated with the even method and light stimulation.

Jin Shubai went to the patient's house a few times in the evening to treat her before sleeping and she spoke with her very patiently, trying to build up her confidence in the therapy. The patient gave up taking medicines spontaneously. She is now in a better mood, even in the morning, she no longer cries all the time and she accepts the fact that her husband must return to his work at the functionaries' school.

Third phase: sessions 17–30

Vexation in the chest and epigastrium, swollen abdomen, slippery pulse, and tongue with a thick coating.

The doctor notices that the patient uses many tonics, such as milk, pork meat, chicken soup, dragon's eyes (*longyan*, sweet taste, nourishes the blood) and considers this might have an influence on the digestion. She changes the points accordingly:
- *Juque* Ren-14, *Zhongwan* Ren-12, *Jianli* Ren-11, *Neiguan* P-6.

All points are treated with the even method and light stimulation.

The modified *Wendantang* prescription is added.

The patient is cured and she goes back to work. She then writes to Jin Shubai that her mood is much improved and work is going fine.

Jin Shubai's Comment

There is a coexistence of fullness and emptiness: phlegm, accumulation of food and transformation in fire, which affect the *yin*. This means that the root is emptiness and the manifestation is fullness.

The *yu* illness is mainly caused by emotions, but whether or not the emotions affect and conduct to *yu* depends on the constitutional characteristics of the patient. In the *Zabing yuanliu xichu*, chapter *Zhuyu yuanliu* ['The origin of all *yu*'] it is said that: 'All *yu* are illnesses of the *qi* of the organs, their origin is in the excess of thought and apprehension. If they are associated with a weakness of the organ *qi* they generate the illnesses of the six constraints'.

In this case the emptiness of blood following the birth is the internal factor, while the distance of the husband and the miserable emotional condition are the trigger factors. The *Neijing* says: 'If the *shen* is insufficient there is anguish, if the blood is insufficient there is fear'. If there is anguish the *qi* is constricted; if there is fear the *shen* is weak.

The manifestations are an opaque face, depressed mood, lack of courage, apprehension, weeping and insomnia. The liver governs planning, the gall bladder the determination, and the heart the clarity of the *shen*. So in this case we must liberate the constraint and the knotting of the liver and gall bladder and at the same time we must nourish the heart and calm the *shen*.

In the first phase we use *Yintang* EX-HN-3 to *Xinqu*: the *Du Mai* rises to the top of the head and connects to the brain, but with the needle we also reach *Xinqu*, the 'area of the heart'. Because the brain is the palace of the original *shen* and the heart is the home of the spirit, in this way we use the relationship between the brain and the heart; *Anmian* N-HN-54 belongs to the part of *Shao Yang*: it calms the emptiness *yang* and unifies the *yin* to calm the sleep; *Neiguan* P-6 opens the chest and calms the *shen*.[10]

The Sympathetic point of the auricular therapy helps to calm the internal organs. In the second phase, since there is an emptiness of the heart and spleen and a constraint of the liver, we add the *shu* back points of heart, liver and spleen in order to regulate and nourish the heart and spleen, and to free and harmonise the liver *qi*.

In the third phase we regulate the *qi* and harmonise the stomach because during the illness the patient has been eating heavy food that has produced phlegm and dampness. These have impeded the transformation and transport functions, causing tightening and discomfort in the chest, swelling, a thick tongue coating, and slippery pulse. There was a shift from a pattern of emptiness to a pattern of fullness within emptiness.

The *mu* point of the heart *Juque* Ren-14 opens and enhances the flow; the *mu* point of the stomach *Zhongwan* Ren-12 regulates the centre and harmonises the stomach; the points *Jianli* Ren-11 and *Neiguan* P-6 resolve the oppression in the chest.

Moreover the prescription *Wendantang* helps to purify the heart and transform the phlegm, to harmonise the stomach and calm the *shen*.

Slowly the pulse becomes regular, the coating turns thin again, oppression in the chest and swelling of the abdomen are solved and the patient is completely cured.

---

[10] *Xinqu* is the heart area in the face somatotopic representation, and *Anmian* is on the line linking the two points of the channels *Shao Yang Yifeng* TB-17 and *Fengchi* GB-20 (for more details see footnote 19 in Chapter 7 on insomnia).

Case Study 20.5

Zangzao[11]

This was a 35-year-old woman. For 2 years, since giving birth, she has had an excessive menstrual flow, palpitations, anxiousness and fear, anguish and agitation-*fan*, spasms and cramps, insomnia, night sweating, continuous and chaotic dreams, at times oppression of the chest and constraint in breathing, distressed throat, changing mood, and a flushed face.

The tongue is red with a thin coating, and the pulse is thready and wiry.

Diagnosis

Zangzao from emptiness of the blood, and alteration of the heart *shen*.

Therapeutic Principles

Calm the *shen* and regulate the *yin*.

Treatment

- *Baihui* Du-20, backwards direction, insertion of 0.5–1 *cun*.
- *Neiguan* P-6, insertion of 0.5 *cun*, with simultaneous stimulation of the two, dispersion, with lifting–thrusting and rotation technique.
- *Sanyinjiao* SP-6, tonification, with rotation.
- *Yinxi* HE-6, dispersion, with rotation.
- *Fuliu* KI-7, tonification, with rotation.

She is treated every 2 days for 20 sessions, after which she is cured.

Jin Shubai's Comment

After quoting the description by Zhang Zhingjing in the *Jingui yaolue*, Jin Shubai then suggests her own interpretation of the term 'zangzao'. *Zang* refers to the *zizang* uterus; *zao* means an emptiness of the blood. The heart governs the blood, the liver stores the blood, the spleen controls the blood, and the kidney stores the *jing*. Since *jing* and blood share the same origin, the insufficiency of the *qi* of these four organs can cause a lack of nutrition of the heart with the *shen* becoming restless. All the symptoms such as palpitations, insomnia, excessive menstruation, lack of energy, etc. are signs of an emptiness of the blood, which causes *zangzao*.

The treatment must regulate and nourish the heart, liver, spleen and kidney *yin*, but above all the heart, which is the most important. If we regulate all of the *yin* and the heart is nourished, the *shen* has a place to return to and the heart is calm, the *shen* is peaceful: how can there be agitation-*zao*?

We have chosen *Baihui* Du-20, which awakens the brain and calms the *shen*; *Neiguan* P-6 combined with *Sanyinjiao* SP-6 opens the chest, resolves constraint and allows the heart and kidney to communicate. Moreover *Sanyinjiao* SP-6 is the meeting point of the three foot channels and in gynaecology it is a fundamental point

---

[11] Jin Shubai, 1987, p.70.

for the treatment of blood; *Yinxi* HE-6 combined with *Fuliu* KI-7, one with dispersion and the other one with tonification, harmonise water and fire, and allow the heart and kidney to communicate so that the *yin* is stored and the sweating stops.

Case Study 20.6

Bentunqi[12]

This was a 24-year-old girl. Each time the crisis breaks out the patient feels a piece of *qi* of the size of a goose egg rising from the abdomen to the chest and then, when it is very strong, up to the throat. She also feels oppressed in the chest and believes she is going to suffocate and faint.

The attack lasts around 10 minutes; then it disappears and all the symptoms diminish. She has already experienced more than ten episodes of this type. The pulse is wiry and slippery, the coating is white and greasy, and the face is pale.

Diagnosis

Worrying and long-lasting constraints affect the mind-*shenzhi*, the *qi* accumulates in the kidney, and *bentun* breaks out.

Therapeutic Principles

Calm the *shen*, pacify the *zhi*, and regulate the movements of the *qi*.

Treatment

- *Qihai* Ren-6, with the rotation and lifting–thrusting technique; after having obtained the *qi* we first disperse and then tonify.
- *Guanyuan* Ren-4, with the same technique, but only tonifying.
- *Sanyinjiao* SP-6, with the same technique, we first disperse and then tonify.

After the first session the symptoms have improved; after the second one the frequency of the episodes has also decreased and there is further improvement; after the third session there are no more episodes.

The treatment continues with weekly sessions for 2 months to reinforce the results.

Jin Shubai's Comment

The *bentun* pattern is a manifestation of hysteria; it belongs to the *yu* (*yuzheng*) syndromes.

Jin Shubai, after having recalled the *Zhubing yuanhoulun* ('Treatise on the origin and symptoms of illnesses' by Chao Yuanfang, 610), suggests that the pattern can be linked to a lack of regulation of *qi* movements.

---

[12] Jin Shubai, 1987, p. 71.

The constricted *qi* gathers in the lower abdomen, this is why we use *Qihai* Ren-6, sea for the production of *qi* and meeting point of *yuanqi*, to liberate and regulate the movements of the *qi* with a dispersion technique to melt the knotted *qi* and, with a tonifying technique to reinforce the original *yang* so that the *qi* can flow freely.

Guanyuan Ren-4, meeting point of the *Renmai* with the three foot *yin*, is a *yang* point within the *yin*: if combined with *Qihai* Ren-6, it warms the kidney and helps the *yang*; *Sanyinjiao* SP-6, the meeting point of the three foot *yin*, helps the *yin* and tonifies the *yang*, and helps the two above points in the treatment of pathologies with an accumulation of *qi* in the lower *jiao*.

Jin Shubai concludes by saying that this is a well-chosen combination, with a focused and effective action.

Case Study 20.7

Meiheqi[13]

This is a 39-year-old woman. Over the last 10 months she has had a feeling of oppression behind the sternum and in the throat. She feels a blockage as if she had a nut that she cannot swallow. The more she thinks about it the more she feels vexed and has a sensation of blocked throat, while when she does not pay attention it is as if nothing is there.

Other symptoms are dizziness, emotional tension, suspiciousness and emotional lability. The tongue is thin with thin and greasy coating, the left pulse is wiry and the right one is slippery and thready.

Diagnosis

Constraint and knotting of the *qi* and phlegm, and liver-wood invading the stomach.

Therapeutic Principles

Help the liver, free the constraint, harmonise the stomach, and bring down the conversely rising *qi*.

Treatment

Tiantu Ren-22, with the needle inserted for 0.5 *cun* and then directed downwards for a total of 1.5 *cun*, with light manipulation, never letting go of the needle. After the extraction the patient should feel some kind of liberation.

Neiguan P-6, with simultaneous manipulation of the two points, using the lifting–thrusting technique.

---

[13] Jin Shubai, 1987, p. 68.

Zusanli ST-36, first used with dispersion and then tonified when we have obtained an improvement.

Xinjian LIV-2, with dispersion, usually with the lifting–thrusting technique.

Jin Shubai's Comment

After having referred to the *Jingui*, to the *Nanyang huorenshu* and to the *Yizong jin-jian*,[14] Jin Shubai highlights that, since the chest oppression, belching and obstruction of the throat are caused by a constraint of the *qi* – that is by the wood invading the earth – we must resolve the constraint, course the liver, harmonise the stomach, bring down the rising *qi*.

We use *Tiantu* Ren-22, meeting point of the *Yin Wei Mai* and *Ren Mai*, to open the throat to bring the rising *qi* down; *Neiguan* P-6, *luo* point of the pericardium, which goes to the *Sanjiao* channel, meets with the *Yin Wei Mai*, frees the movements of the *qi*, opens the chest and the diaphragm and regulates the centre (the *Yin Wei Mai* is used for heart pain); *Zusanli* ST-36, the *he* point of *Yang Ming* (the *he*-sea points treat *yang* organs illnesses), which reinforces the spleen and harmonises the stomach, and nourishes *qi*, blood and *yin*; and LIV-2, *ying* point of the liver channel: if the liver–wood attacks the stomach we must disperse it through the child point to sedate the liver, resolve the constraint, control the wood and harmonise the centre. If the illness is above, select points from the lower body.

---

[14] Respectively by Zhang Zhongjing, Zhu Hong and Wu Jian; for their quotes see the discussion on *meiheqi* in Chapter 9 on classical syndromes.

Alterations of the *Qi* and their Somatic Manifestations

21

Zhang Shijie

The method presented here stems from the clinical work conducted with Dr Zhang Shijie at the Gulou Hospital of Beijing in August–September 1992 (with Patrizia Adelasco, interpreter Laura Caretto), from the personal teachings twice a week and from the first draft of the text by Zhang Shijie, which was going to be published in Beijing.[1]

The way Zhang Shijie practises acupuncture has the charm of a magical act, i.e. of a simplicity in which the most minute gesture has the greatest effect; his way of observing, describing and interpreting clinical cases is in essence that of finding the basic elements: of *yin* and *yang*, of water and fire, of the movement of the *qi* in the channels; his evaluation of symptomatology from the perspective of the most ancient texts attests to the possibility of finding their current and tangible application.

With consideration to the singularity and pregnancy of Zhang Shijie's discourse, I have been extremely careful to render as faithfully as possible his original descriptions, comments and evaluative processes when referring to theoretical elaborations and clinical cases.

When he was asked about the *shen*, Zhang Shijie would answer: '*Shen* is *wuji* 无极, with no limit, no definition, earth and heaven are not yet separated'.

At first is *hundun* 混沌 (chaos, non-definition). Unseparated *yinyang* is *shen*, unchanging is *shen*, *shen* is the two *jing* reunited. Before it has a shape it is *shen*;

---

[1] From this text I have taken all the quoted passages in this chapter, both for the comments and the clinical cases. The book by Zhang Shijie was later published with the title *Gufa zhengci juou* ('Examples of acupuncture following the antique method'), 1995.

then there is *taiji* 太极, where *yin* and *yang* exist but are not yet separated; *taiji* originates *liangyi* 两义 (the two principles, *yin* and *yang*); *liangyi* generates *sixiang* 四象 (the four shapes); *sixiang* generates the *bagua* 八卦 (the eight trigrams).[2]

And he would add: 'Man depends on the earth, the earth depends on the heaven, the heaven depends on the *dao* 道, *dao* depends on *ziran* 自然. *Ziran* is spontaneous nature; it is like *hundun*; *shen* is like *ziran*, it has no shape, it encompasses all things, it has no internal nor external limit.'

Such an answer recalls texts such as the *Zhuangzi*, where it is said that the *dao* has a reality but does not act and has no shape, it was generated before the heaven and earth and has no time.[3]

We are not used to hearing such discourses from contemporary Chinese doctors: Dr Zhang's whole approach to clinical work and theoretical considerations is most uncommon.

Yet, as confirmation that marginal points of view still have a certain 'official' place, Zhang Shijie, born in 1931, was at the time the director of the acupuncture department of the Gulou Hospital. Formally entitled 'Chief Physician', he was allowed to work in the hospital only three mornings a week, have an internal doctor as a personal pupil, and see his work published.

The article in which I described my work experience with Dr Zhang, giving consideration to the complexity and synthesis of the diagnostic process, opened with this image:

> Even for a Chinese clinic the small room is really full of people: two patients on the cots pushed against the wall, relatives, students, assistants, other patients. And Zhang *laoshi* (master) sits there, with his knowing smile under his Mongolian warrior moustache, reads the paper, smokes, puts some needles here and there, at times lets go of the needles, in other moments he does not, but it looks as if he is using only *Taixi* KI-3.[4]

During the first few days I had to remind myself more than once that masters love to appear under strange forms, again and again I had to prove to him how I could obtain the *qi* (yet, I could not 'hold it'), but some jewel sentences were already popping up such as 'Chinese medicine is undetermined, *mohu* 模糊 (the same term is used in physics to indicate Heisenberg's uncertainty principle), like contemporary theories of knowledge'. At this stage the real work was to begin.

In fact the encounter with Dr Zhang was the result of a 'search for a master' and of an interest in teachings that are slightly different from those given in training centres, to which I nevertheless give all my appreciation, admiration and gratitude.

---

[2] This cosmogenetic discourse refers to the *Yijing*, to which Dr Zhang also referred to in medicine, defining *yin* and *yang* as *taivi*.

[3] *Zhuangzi*, Chapter 6. See the discussion on classical thought in Chapter 1.

[4] E. Rossi, Notes on diagnosis and evaluation of efficacy in TCM, 1993.

Dr Zhang knew how to 'hold' the *qi* and manipulate it, his evaluations could embrace face diagnosis and hand diagnosis, he could always apply the knowledge contained in the classical texts to the cases he was treating so as to bring them to life and turn them into concrete situations in contemporary clinical practice.

At the same time his theoretical reflections were connected to the contemporary discussion on diagnosis in Chinese medicine and to themes ranging across the most recent scientific topics: from the evaluation of traditional medicines to the very issue of the concept of 'scientificity'.

Zhang Shijie's work is presented with the belief that a discussion that is marginal to the TCM *bianzheng* 辩证 method can enrich the comprehension of the movements of the *qi* in highly complex patterns such as those with strong psychic components.

ANALYSIS AND SYNTHESIS IN THE DIAGNOSTIC PROCESS

In Zhang Shijie's work neither the evaluation of the *bianzheng* method for the differentiation of syndromes nor the way he handles the cases correspond to the system predominantly in use in China today. His text discusses the reasons underlying this system that is partially an alternative to the *bianzheng* method.

Zhang Shijie immediately makes clear that the knowledge and interpretation of a case through all the various levels of reference of TCM are the minimum conditions for formulating a diagnosis; the real difficulty is in the next step – that is, when one has to unite all these elements. He identifies this process of synthesis as the *yuanwu bilei* 援 物 比 类 principle, which appears in Chapter 76 of the *Suwen*. Modern comments of the *Suwen* interpret *yuanwu* as 'taking, underlining the thing, the fact', and *bilei* means 'comparing' (比类 is 'analogy'), but also in the sense of tracing the real cause, which does not lie where it manifests.

He begins by saying:

> This text relates 30 clinical cases. It aims at showing that, in acupuncture practice, the eight diagnostic principles, the six couples of *jingluo*, the *zangfu*, *weiqi*, *yingqi*, *xue*, and the three *jiao* are not enough to formulate a differential analysis (*bianzheng*), but that we must also use the *yuanwu bilei* principle, which can be found in the 'Shicong ronglun' chapter of the *Suwen*. This method gives us the possibility of recognising the root of the hundred illnesses and of unifying the therapeutic practice.[5]

---

[5] *Suwen*, Chapter.76. Zha Xiaohu and Paolo Ferrari have also contributed to the translation and the revision of the quotes from the *Neijing*.

Later he specifies: 'If the level of analytical research is not high there can be no high level synthesis, so the more detailed the diagnostic method of the Chinese medicine the more its level of synthesis must be accurate. Otherwise our models will be nothing but mist on the sea.'

These considerations fit in the tradition of the Chinese thought in which, 'with the only exception of the sophists and late Maoists, intelligence corresponds to what Anglo-Saxons call 'common sense' – where what counts is the ability to grasp synthetically the connections between things, over and above the analysis'.[6]

Zhang Shijie recalls how all contemporary scientific domains tend to recognise the complexity of reality and aim at reconstructing models that integrate various interdisciplinary studies. He maintains that 'Chinese medicine is an encounter between numerous disciplines and in practising it one must use objective, dynamic and systemic modalities', meaning that it is necessary to: evaluate pathological processes and results without bias, follow flexible methodologies which take into consideration the continuous movement of reality, and consider the fields of study and intervention as complex systems.

He also reminds us that Chinese medicine grew in a syncretic way, integrating knowledge from other disciplines such as astronomy and astrology, divination of the *Zhouyi*, and *fengshui*-geomancy. This position was expressed early on, in the *Suwen*, in the phase 'one must observe the complexity of the disciplines and submit them to analogical confrontation'.[7]

He also refers to the fact that the term *bianzheng* appeared for the first time in the *Shanghanlun* by Zhang Zhongjing, and to how this method has contributed to the development of Chinese medicine and was honoured by doctors from all schools. But he also highlights that Zhang Zhongjing was drawing from the classical texts *Suwen* and *Nanjing* and was using the knowledge on points and channels, but focusing mostly on prescriptions and pulses.

> Yet *yin* and *yang*, *qi* and blood, the illnesses of the 12 channels, the six *yang* and their related illnesses, the *biaoben* procedure, the *genjie*, the harmonisation and the opening of the *qi* passages, the notion of pivot-*shu* 枢, and the connected pathological transformations are difficult to synthesise with the *bianzheng* method. This is why an acupuncturist cannot work without a method based on comparison and analogy.[8] By using this method one avoids the risk

---

[6] Graham, 1999, p. 348.

[7] *Zhouyi* is the name commonly used in China for *Yijing*. The sentence *languan zaxue jiyu bilei* & 揽 观 杂 学 集 余 比 类 in Chapter 76 of the *Suwen* is explained by some modern comments as an invitation to take into consideration other texts along with the *Neijing*, recalling how the merit of a compiler was precisely in the fact that his work would embrace all previous works.

[8] Here the reference is to the various perspectives in which the illness can be read: the polarity between *yin* and *yang*, its physiological connections, the channels, the layers through which the pathogens enter the body, the recognition of manifestations and roots, the 'root-knot' points, etc. Just as plants have roots that nourish them, channels have points, *gen*-root 0, and points-*jie* 结, meaning 'knot, knotting', but also 'fruits' – it is a moment of condensation, the place where the *qi* collects in the channel. The *gen* points always correspond to the beginning of the channel, while in the most antique texts the *jie* correspond to the peripheral areas of the body.

of not being able to return to a synthesis a differential diagnosis divided into patterns, excessively detailed and subtle. The subtler the analysis the more we need a high level of synthesis. It is the knowledge of the channels which is the foundation of acupuncture; it is based on a 'complete knowledge of the channels', as one can read in the affirmations made in the chapter 'Zhongshi' of the *Lingshu*: 'The principle-*li* of each needling has its origin in the channels' and 'the method of each needle has its conclusion in the *zhongshi*'.[9]

THE IMPORTANCE OF CHANNELS IN THE INTERPRETATION OF PATHOLOGY

The importance of channels is also effectively expressed in the *Suwen*, in the line 'the development of an illness spreads so widely upwards and downwards that it is impossible to seize it only by looking at texts'. Zhang takes as an example the case discussed in the same chapter: 'A person with headache, contraction of the tendons, heaviness of the bones, short breath, belching, swollen abdomen, who is easily threatened and does not like to lie down: by which *zang* is all this caused? The pulse is floating, wiry, as hard as stone; I do not know how to explain all this and I ask myself how it relates to the three *zang* in order to know how to classify it.'[10]

He then comments the passage, maintaining that:

> ... if we analyse this case without using the *bilei* method we can draw three conclusions: 1. The liver channel has its origin in the *Dadun* (LIV-1) point, its *qi* rejoins that of kidney, reaches the top of the head, controls the muscles; if there are headache and muscle problems then the illness depends on the *qi* of the liver channel. 2. The kidney channel has its origin in the *Yongquan* (KI-1) point; it is the source for the production of the *qi* and it controls the bones; if the bones are heavy and there is short breath then the illness depends on the *qi* of the kidney channel. 3. The spleen channel has its origin in the *Yinbai* point; it is connected with the stomach by a vessel; if there are regurgitations, belching, fullness of the stomach, tendency to startlement, and difficulty in lying down, then all disorders come from the *qi* of the spleen channel. In this way we will have a therapy oriented on the three channels. Rather, the answer is: 'What you say ignores the eight winds and the heat accumulations; the five *zang* are consumed and the pathogen-*xie* goes from one to the other. The floating and wiry pulse is the emptiness of the kidney, and the deep and stone-like pulse is

---

[9] *Zhongshi* 终 始 literally: 'end-beginning', is the title of Chapter 9 of the *Lingshu*, which explains how it is necessary to know perfectly the illnesses of the 12 channels. Modern comments specify that the title must be read as 'complete knowledge of the channels'.
[10] 'Suwen', Chapter 76.

the internal block of the kidney *qi*, the jolts and short breath are caused by the blockage of water passages and by the consumption of the shape-*xing* and *qi*, the cough and restlessness depend on the counterflowing-*ni* kidney *qi*. In this person the illness is in one of the *zang*, if you say that it is in three of *zang* you are mistaken.'[11]

And Zhang concludes: 'this shows that it is possible to act only on the kidney and that if we do not proceed with this *bilei* method we would find ourselves looking down at a deep abyss or at floating clouds'.

We cannot work without knowing the keys for the reading of signs and symptoms, nor without a deep knowledge of the dynamics that lie underneath the events and their developments.

The synthesis would emerge as that vision which embraces and explains all the data, unifying them at a higher level (if we think of the theories that have periodically disrupted the world of physics and mathematics, these solutions are usually very simple and elegant).

The concept of *yuanwu bilei* 援 物 比 类 recalls the modes of the Chinese thought: we know that its correlative logic develops through analogies, correspondences and synchronicities, but to subsequently bring this knowledge back to the practice, to use it in the formulation of a diagnosis and in the choice of points, is not always an easy task. The *yuanwu bilei* method – in line with the Chinese tradition – is not expressed in detail. Only scattered remarks suggest the concept.

As we have argued, the most specific aspect in the discussion of the diagnosis seems to be the importance of the physiology and pathology of the channel.

Often one tends to consider as 'channel symptoms' only those that relate to an external development (pain, functional impediments, skin manifestations, etc.) and we do not always pay attention to the overall signs and symptoms 'of the channel'. In contrast, in Zang Shijie's approach the energetic anatomy is considered precisely for its value as *yuanwu bilei* synthesis.

The other aspect that crosses both the clinical practice and the theoretical thought is the reference to the great cosmic movements, so that in evaluating our cases in the microcosm we should continuously take into consideration the relationship between signs or aetiopathogenesis and the elements of the macrocosm.

---

[11] *Suwen*, Chapter 76. The article then quotes a comment by Zhang Jiebin, from the *Leijing*: 'The headache is caused by a lack of water and an abundance of fire; the contractions are caused by the fact that the kidney water cannot nourish the muscles; the heaviness of the bones is connected to the kidney which controls the bones; regurgitation and belching depend on the kidney channel, which crosses the stomach; the fullness of the stomach comes from the perversions of the water, which affects the earth; the jolts appear when one loses *zhi*, which is kept by the kidney; the eyes do not close because of the emptiness of the *yin*: these disorders have their root in the kidney and it is wrong to speak of three *zang* acting at the same level'.

To convey more effectively the flavour of the description, some of the cases presented here have been translated directly from Zang Shijie's text, while of others we have reported the textual comments.

A Case of a 'Typical' Patient

Even if the words and context are different, the description of many of Zhang Shijie's cases reminds us immediately of our patients and of their muddled problems.

A typical situation could be that of a woman in her fifties who has always been working, with grown-up children, who feels depressed and wants only to sleep. At a physical level she says that she feels a weight on the chest, a disorder at the mouth of the stomach, which gets better when she eats something. But at the same time she complains about nausea and says that she has a sensation of perpetually swollen and full stomach.

A similar case is described by Dr Zhang as follows:

Illness of the Kidney Channel

A 56-year-old woman, peasant: 'in the last 6 years, from dawn to sunset, her eyes have refused to open as when one is sleeping, she feels an oppression of the chest, 'suspended' heart, shortness of breath, fullness of the abdomen, languor, and all the symptoms decrease if she eats something, only to reappear shortly after with hunger and nausea but with no desire to eat. The pulse is floating, wiry, and when tested deeply it is slightly slippery. The tongue is pale with white and slightly thick coating'.[12]

The *Yin Qiao Mai* and *Yang Qiao Mai* rejoin and enter one another in the internal corner of the eye; *yin* and *yang* exchange, if the *yin* prevails the eyes close. *Yin Qiao Mai* is a ramification of the kidney channel, if the *yin* is strong and the *yang* is weak the earth is not warmed and there is a feeling of fullness and discomfort in the stomach.

The kidney does not receive the *qi* and this produces shortness of breath and thoracic constraint, when there is an illness of the kidney channel the symptoms are hunger and suspended heart with a desire to eat.

---

[12] 'Suspended heart' is the translation of *xin ruo xuan* 心 若悬, a typical sign of the kidney channel, which is the sensation of having the heart suspended to a thread from above, usually accompanied by languor. 'Languor' is the translation of *caoza* 嘈 杂, which is a strong discomfort in the stomach, a disorder which produces uneasiness and agitation, without any pain or swelling.

We have consequently needled the point *yuan*-source of the kidney, *Taixi* (KI-3). We obtained the *qi* like a fish taking the bite, all symptoms felt immediately relieved. After four sessions the illness had unmistakably improved.

Explanation: 'With the *bianzheng* method using the *zangfu* it would have been difficult to reach a conclusion, whereas by considering it a kidney illness it became quite easy. With an excess of *yin qi* and a lack of *yang qi* it would appear necessary to tonify the *yang*, instead we regulate the water, i.e. we tonify the *yang* from inside the *yin* with the *Taixi* point, which is much better that needling the *Yang Qiao Mai* directly.'[13]

Therefore in this case, needling the *yuan* point of kidney has different functions: it is the root of the *Yin* and *Yang Qiao Mai*; it tonifies the *yang* so as to warm the earth; being an expression of channel pathology it treats other symptoms.

Cases With Strong Psychic Components In Which The *Yang* Is Sustained From Within The *Yin*

Let us briefly relate some cases with strong psychological components, considered from a perspective in which the evaluation is specifically energetic and in which the *yin* prevails on the *yang* and *Taixi* KI-3 is needled in order to reinforce a weak *yang*.

A 50-year-old woman has suffered for the last 20 years from mental numbness, asthenia, difficulty in speaking, continuous yawning, with soft pulse on the surface and choppy in depth, a pale tongue, and white and slightly thick coating. We needle *Taixi* because 'if the *yang* is weak – as in this case, in which the *yin* prevails, forcing the eyes to close during the day – the natural movement of descent goes only half way and the yawning is of help to pull the *yang* downwards'.

A 23-year-old girl, always sad and depressed, continuously cries after an episode where she lost consciousness. In this case we again needle *Taixi* because 'with sadness the heart system *xinxi* becomes urgent-*ji*, the lung no longer distributes, the upper *jiao* is blocked, *zhong qi* and *wei qi* do not distribute, the warm *qi* accumulates in the medium *jiao*, so that the *qi* is reduced, the *yang* becomes weak and the *yin* strong, and there is weeping with sobs'.[14]

This concept of regulating the water-*kan* by conditioning the *yang* within the *yin* is equivalently referred to as 'conditioning the origin of the fire' and it is used also in the case of false heat and true cold, as in the following example.

---

[13] 'Regulating water' is said *tiaokan* 调 坎, where *kan* is the trigram for water, represented by a continuous *yang* line between two open *yin* lines.

[14] *Suwen*, Chapter 39. The term urgent-*ji* 急, which recurs also in the description of *chong mai*, refers to the feeling that there is an emergency. On this issue see also the article by Yu Qingbai, 'The liver suffers from urgency', 1997.

This is a 70-year-old woman, a peasant, whose main symptom is borborygmi (noises in the abdomen), with a sensation of fullness and swelling of the abdomen, scanty urine, irritation of the micturition, and constipated stools.[15] Experimental examinations did not reveal anything specific and various treatments with Western and Chinese medicines were ineffective. Both the pulses are wiry, arrive strong and leave weak, and the tongue is peeled, and deep red.[16] An abdominal palpation reveals the sound of water.

Zhang Shijie quotes a passage which says:

> '... inversion-*jue* and abdominal noises, much cold, borborygmi, difficult stools and urines, one takes *zutaiyin*'[17], and he explains that 'the abdomen is the region where the spleen lives, it is controlled by the spleen, the spleen *qi* is exhausted, this is why there are noises. The spleen controls the *qi* (transformation and transportation), it is the major *yin* (*Tai Yin* 太阴), this is why there are cold and water noises. The earth *qi* turns into clouds when it rises, the heaven *qi* is rain when it comes down; if the earth *qi* does not rise and the heaven *qi* does not come down the tongue has no coating, stools and urines are difficult, the symptoms in this case are of false heat and real cold, there is extreme emptiness, but manifestations of fullness. *Yin* illness is treated with *yang*. We use the method of tonifying the fire origin, we needle *Taixi*, we obtain the *qi* like a fish taking the bite; the noise stops, we do not feel water when palpating.
>
> The method of warming the spleen *yang* is fundamental also for the transformation of dampness and phlegm, for example in the case of asthma. I have used *Taixi* for the kidney, root of the lung, to warm the spleen *yang*, which has the action of transforming so that dampness and phlegm do not accumulate.

Patients With Conversion and *Yin* Emptiness Disorders

The interpretation that Zhang gives of certain symptoms with a psychic origin explicitly recognised by a western contemporary diagnostic classification is quite interesting.

In the following cases the process underlying signs such as weeping, vertigo, convulsions and paralysis is examined and explained. The cases can be classified as Conversion Disorders (DSM-IV), under the first three subtypes: with sensory symptoms (blindness), convulsions, and movement deficit (loss of balance, paralysis, globus hystericus).

---

[15] 'Borborygmi' is the translation of *gugu*: an onomatopoeic term used principally in the classics. Later the expression *lulu* appears, while in modern Chinese the common term is *gulu gulu*.
[16] The pulse has a wave that is strong at first and then weakens, *laisheng qushuai* 来 胜 去 衰, shows that there is a pathologic excess and, at the same time, an initial lack of *zhenqi*.
[17] 'Lingshu', Chapter 26. For the term *jue* 厥 see the Glossary.

Sight Disorders with a Psychic Origin

A 36-year-old woman, factory worker: after having cried all day she loses her sight, with negativity, a slightly red tongue, thin white coating, and deep and choppy pulse.

It is said that: 'the heart regulates the *jing* of all organs. The eyes are its opening [...] if there is fear-*ju* then one cannot see'.[18] And also that: 'the heart is the leader of all the *zangfu*, the eyes are the place where all channels meet, the way of the upper liquids, [...] emotions move the heart, the heart moves, the five *zang* and the six *fu* falter, if they falter all the channels are influenced, the way of the liquids is open, tears run down. The liquids nourish the *jing* and feed the empty orifices. If the ways of the upper liquids are open then the weeping does not stop, the liquids are exhausted, the *jing* cannot be filled, the eyes cannot see, all this is called cringing-*duo* 夺 of the *jing*. We must tonify *Tianzhu*.'[19]

The kidney is water and contains the *jing* of the five *zang*. Above it communicates with heart and lung, it is internal–externally related to bladder; the *jing* of the kidney is the pupil, and if this *jing* is missing one cannot see. Needling *Taixi* her sight immediately returned to normal.

Tetanism with psychic origin

A 30-year-old woman, factory worker: because of anger the body contracts, stiffens and shakes, with tightly closed mouth. She has suffered from similar episodes before. The tongue is impossible to examine. The pulse is deep, weak, rapid.

All sudden and strong stiffenings are due to violent wind: grinding teeth, blowing with closed mouth and clicking teeth are manifestations of *shen* losing control over the body-*xing*; they are fire symptoms. In its movement, the kidney is shivering.

The liver and heart fire is powerful and there is emptiness of *yin*: I needled *Taixi*.

Hysterical paralysis[20]

In the *Suwen* it is said that: 'if the heart *qi* is warm then the lower vessels *qi* rises, the lower vessels become empty, there is atrophy-*wei* of the vessels, the pivots which sustain the body break, the legs cannot carry the body any longer and there is no stability'. And in the *Lingshu*: 'Sadness and misery, worrying and anguish affect the heart; if the heart is affected the five *zang* and the six *fu* are shaken.'[21]

---

[18] 'Suwen', Chapter 81.
[19] 'Lingshu', Chapter 28.
[20] *Yibingxing tanhuang* 癔病性 瘫痪, a modern term.
[21] 'Lingshu', Chapter 8.

So if one is thwarted in his desires and the seven emotions are moved from the inside, there is atrophy-*wei* of the vessels, caused by heat in the heart.'

Cases that Correspond To 'Classical Syndromes'

Now let us see how Zhang Shijie interprets certain cases that belong to the classical description of the *qi* movement.

Bentunqi

A 58-year-old man, a teacher: during the 10 years of the Cultural Revolution an illness caused by fear began, with frequent attacks that appeared repeatedly and without interruption through the years.[22] In 1977 he comes to the clinic complaining about *qi* flowing to the chest from below, restlessness and agitation in the middle of the heart, shortness of breath, and cold limbs. He says that he would like to vomit but cannot and that the distress is more than usual. The two pulses are deep and wiry, the tongue is pale red, and the coating is thin and white.

The diagnosis is *bentunqi*; the two *Taixi* points are needled, the symptoms decreases immediately and there are no more attacks.

The *Jingui yaolue*, chapter 'Illness, pulse, symptoms, prescriptions of the *bentunqi*', says: 'the *bentun* illness, the *qi* begins in the lower abdomen, attacks the throat, the assault is such that one wants to die, it soon stops, all attacks come from fear'.[23] You Zaijing says: 'The kidney is hit by fear, *bentun* is an illness of the kidney, the pig is a water animal, the kidney is a water organ. The kidney is moved from the inside; it assaults the throat like a running piglet; for this reason it is called running piglet; there are also cases in which the source is in a liver illness, because kidney and liver share a common origin in the lower *jiao*, the *qi* of both rises counterflow-*ni*.'[24]

For this reason I needle *Taixi* to treat these illnesses with paroxysmal excesses, obtaining good results.

Meiheqi

A 43-year-old woman, relative of a member of the hospital staff: for the last year she has had the feeling of having something in her throat, and has taken *Banxia houpo tang*, also with modifications, without results.[25] The two pulses

---

[22] Literally: 10 years of disorders, *shinian dongluan* 十 年 动 乱, from 1966 to 1976.

[23] Zhang Zhongjing, *Jinggui Ysaolue* ('Prescriptions of the Golden Chamber'), Chapter 8. See also the discussion in Chapter 9 on classical syndromes.

[24] You Zaijing, *Jingui yaolue xindian* ('Personal selection from the *Jingui yaolue*'). In the correspondence *wuxing* system of the five elements, the pig is connected to water.

[25] A classic prescription that appears for the first time in the *Jingui yaolue*, with *meiheqi* as a specific indication: in the category of formula promoting the qi movement, it helps to transform the phlegm, melt the masses and bring the qi which counterflows downwards.

are deep, slightly wiry, the tongue is slightly red, and the coating is thin and white.

The diagnosis is kidney *qi* rising upwards inverted-*ni*; *Taixi* is needled, the symptoms have decreased by 50% in the first session and have disappeared completely after the second.

Zhang Shijie then recalls how the classics maintain that the *meiheqi* illness derives from a constraint of the *qi* caused by emotions, together with phlegm-*tan*, and how they prescribe *Banxia houpo tang*. On this point he quotes Zhang Zhongjing: 'Women have in their throat something like a piece of roasted meat, the prescription in this case is *Banxia houpo tang*.'[26] And he adds a comment of a later text: 'In the throat they have a piece of roasted meat, in the throat there is phlegm that feels like a piece of roasted meat that cannot be eliminated by coughing nor swallowing, this is like the contemporary *meiheqi* illness.'[27]

He then adds: 'My experience tells me that if there are no symptoms of full chest and hardness under the heart, this prescription is often useless, it is much less effective than another diagnosis of kidney *qi*, in which we needle *Taixi*.

This illness is often caused by constraint and knotting, *yujie* 郁结, from emotions; it is also common in men. The kidney channel travels along the throat, and embraces the tongue. With *Taixi* we can drain the obstruction, bring down the inverted-*ni* flow.'

Cases in Which the Fire Returns to its Origin High Up

Zhang Shijie also uses *Taixi* to reconnect water and fire in cases of constraint of the emotions, with stagnation of the *qi* that transforms into fire and damages the *yin*, resulting in an organic cardiac pathology, or in the cases of emptiness of the fire that disturbs the heart *qi*, for example in case of arrhythmia.[28]

The movement of the fire rising up towards its origin, caused of a lack of *yin*, can also take place through the rise of the kidney *qi* along the *Chong Mai*. The superficial manifestation is consequently in the lung (asthma and oppression of the chest) and in the stomach (nausea and vomit), but the root is in the kidney.

Taixi can also be used in cases in which the rising of the *yang* takes the form of *Shao Yang* pathology. This is because *Shao Yang* is the growing *yang*, born from the water.

---

[26] Zhang Zhongjing, *Jingui yaolue*, Chapter 22.
[27] Wu Jian, *Yizong jinjian* (Golden mirror of the principles of medicine), chapter 'Zhiqi zhifa' (Method for the treatment of qi stagnations).
[28] *Zhengzhong* is 'true' arrhythmia, which appears without any connection to an external cause, whereas palpitations, called *xinji* or *jingj*, are a consequence for example of fright-*jing*, and are therefore less serious.

A classical example is the case of headache from liver stagnation with an emotional origin: the liver loses its function of expansion and is the origin of fire that ascends and disturbs the clear orifices. The fire damages the *yin* so the kidney does not nourish and does not contain the wood; the *yang* rises and there is pain.

There are also many cases of phlegm-heat in which it is necessary to act on the water. Phlegm and heat gather and obstruct the channels, as in the case of a patient with sequelae of a cerebrovascular accident in which after a cerebral thrombosis there were still amimia, dysphasia, loss of saliva from the right side, uncontrolled weeping and laughter, a floating, wiry, rapid pulse, and a bright red tongue with greasy yellow coating.

> If there is a constitutional *yin* emptiness in which the water does not contain the liver, then the *yang* rises upwards, the liver invades the spleen, the dampness condenses in phlegm-heat, and the water does not control the fire, which burns too strongly. The obstruction impairs the swallowing action. The kidney channel crosses the earth–centre, it connects with heart and lung, and it reaches the root of the tongue. We also needle *Yifeng* TB-17 and *Wangu* SI-4 because *Shao Yang* is a pivot, *Tai Yang* is opening, and *Yang Ming* is closing.

Hyperactivity and Attention Deficit Disorder

22

Julian Scott

This chapter has been reproduced from a previous book by Julian Scott entitled *Acupuncture in the Treatment of Children.*

INTRODUCTION

Hyperactivity is almost unknown in China, whereas it is now well recognised in the West as a major problem. The term 'hyperactive' is used to describe a whole spectrum of behaviour in children ranging from very energetic to disruptive and rude and to positively violent.

From a Chinese point of view the categories are very clear, and although there may be slight overlaps, the main problem is usually easily identified. This is one of the great strengths of Chinese medicine and is part of the reason that hyperactivity can be treated so well with acupuncture. To be able to identify the cause, and to treat the condition, we can cure the child.

This is in stark contrast to conventional medicine, where the cause is unknown, and there are few tools with which to help these children other than drugs – which do not always work – and possibly some dietary advice.

Having a child who is hyperactive is exhausting for parents. These children can completely disrupt the whole family with their screaming, shouting, throwing tantrums, breaking things, fighting, and so on. Even when they are comparatively 'quiet' they don't sit still, are unable to concentrate, and demand constant attention. The problem usually extends to school, and the parents often receive letters telling them of their child's behaviour; in extreme cases, the child may be asked to leave.

Two of the most exasperating things for parents are that there seems to be no rhyme or reason for their child being like this, and there is little in the way of reliable treatment. Child psychiatry may help in some cases, but not always, and the drugs prescribed are of limited use. In some cases diet helps, but often these children crave the very thing that makes them worse (sugar, food colouring) and find ways to get hold of the stuff. It is partly because there is so little in the way of help that we see a lot of hyperactive children in the clinic – and also because word soon gets around that acupuncture is very effective in helping these children.

Although it can be very stressful treating such children – they upset other patients, make a lot of noise, kick, scream, bite, wreck the clinic – they are, in some ways, the most rewarding cases to treat. They do not want to be like this; they are often desperate to stop their behaviour, and are miserable because of it. With your treatment you can actually 'bring them back' to their parents and family. They can turn from aggressive, difficult children into happy, lively, and contented kids who are a joy to be with.

From the perspective of traditional Chinese medicine, there are four patterns. The first two are the most commonly seen and are 'true' forms of hyperactivity. The third is almost identical to the hyperactive Spleen *qi* deficiency pattern described in Chapter 3, and is usually seen in older children. The fourth pattern stems from deficiency and is therefore not 'true' hyperactivity. The four patterns are:

- heat;
- heat plus phlegm (mania);
- weakness in the middle burner;
- kidney deficiency.

Heat

These children are hot! They have red faces or lips, get angry, throw tantrums, and cannot sit still. They tend to be clingy children. Their sleep is disturbed, as they are restless and tend to wake up early. They are the ones that run about the clinic shouting, screaming, and disturbing all the other practitioners. The cause of the heat is varied. Among the common sources are immunisations, hot-type foods, food flavourings, food colourings, or heat transferred from the mother during pregnancy.

Heat and Phlegm

These children are hot too, but they are also full of phlegm and seem to be more aggressive and violent than the pure heat types. Most have red faces (some do not) and have the same irritability, tantrums, and insomnia, but in addition have signs of phlegm and tend to be wilfully destructive, and even cruel, to other children. They may also have genital or anal fixations. These children make comments about your privates and try to grab hold of them during treatment. They also delight in destroying your clinic, tearing up clean paper and throwing it all over the floor, pulling the arms and legs off the cuddly toys, and hitting and kicking you during treatment.

Weakness in the Middle Burner

This is a manifestation of hyperactive spleen *qi* deficiency. The basis of the pattern is deficiency, even though the child appears to have lots of energy. As with hyperactive spleen *qi* deficiency, the parents are often exhausted, while the children are manipulative, and tend to have poor appetites and other signs of spleen deficiency. However, there are some aspects that are slightly different and put these children into the hyperactive bracket. They tend to be full of 'hate'. They are the ones that love to play video games with names like 'Doom', 'Mega-Kill', 'Death', and other such pleasantries. They can be really destructive and nasty, but it is cold and calculating. Unlike the previous two patterns where the child is boiling up with rage, these children are pale or grey in the face, and possibly even cold in energy. But inside there is this terrible hatred. You would expect hatred to be linked with anger, which stagnates the liver *qi* and transforms into heat, but this does not seem to happen. (For example, LIV-2 (*Xingjian*) does nothing for these children.) Theirs is a cold hatred; one can find oneself quite shocked by them, almost frightened, and they can be very difficult to help.

Kidney Deficiency

This is not a true type of hyperactivity. These children are tall and beautiful, and tend to be frail, and often ill. They have weak kidney energy, and so become hyperactive when they are tired or excited: the kidneys cannot hold down the energy, and it rises up to the head. Typically, they do not like to go to bed; even though they are tired they can keep themselves up for ages. They get 'hyper' when they are excited–perhaps hysterical–running around, unable to be controlled, although they do not become violent as a rule. By contrast, during the daytime they may be quite weak and floppy.

AETIOLOGY AND PATHOGENESIS

Heat

The heat in the body rises up to affect the Heart, which houses the spirit and is easily affected by heat. The spirit becomes disturbed, causing irritability and restlessness. Common causes include:

- Food: some foods create heat in the system; curries, spicy foods, and shellfish are all hot in energy.

- Food additives: including colourings and flavourings.
- Womb heat: if the mother has a very hot nature, or if she eats a lot of oranges during pregnancy, heat can transfer across the placenta to the child and it is born hot.
- Lingering pathogenic factor (LPF) from an immunisation: a lingering pathogenic factor can be hot in nature – measles and HIB immunisations, in particular, tend to leave heat in the body.
- After a febrile disease: if a hot pathogenic factor is not properly cleared from the body; for example, if antibiotics are used to cool a fever, the heat can remain locked inside the body as a lingering pathogenic factor.
- Accumulation disorder: this can be the cause of heat in young children.

Heat and Phlegm (Mania)

Heat and phlegm rise up and affect the Heart, disturb the spirit, and lead to anger and wilful acts of aggression that are characteristic of this type of hyperactivity. The presence of phlegm causes 'misting' or clouding of the mind, which can lead children to do things they know to be wrong. Their morals get blotted out. Among the causes of this type of hyperactivity are the following:

- Lingering pathogenic factor (LPF): a lingering pathogenic factor that is hot in nature and causes the formation of a lot of phlegm in the body. Typical examples are LPFs from measles and HIB immunisations.
- Food: a diet that is rich in phlegm-producing foods (dairy products, refined sugar, wheat). In young children the diet can cause accumulation disorder – producing heat and phlegm – and in older children the food itself can be both hot and phlegm producing. It is common for these children to have a gluten allergy; because gluten produces dampness, when they eat wheat a nasty thick goo develops. If taken off wheat, there is often a dramatic improvement.
- Accumulation disorder: diet and regularity of feeding in young children can cause accumulation disorder, which produces heat and phlegm in the body.

Weakness of Middle Burner

Hyperactive spleen *qi* deficient children must draw their middle burner energy from people around them. Usually parents can prevent this by setting up boundaries, thereby forcing the child to get energy for itself – from food. Where there are no such boundaries, the child can help itself to all it wants, commonly from parents, who are nearest at hand. The parents become exhausted and then cannot establish boundaries. This situation seems to promote in the child a sort of greedy, grabbing mentality – selfishness, which then develops into cruelty and hatred. The child becomes demanding out of all proportion (i.e. hyperactive), and furious when it can't get what it wants. This hyperactivity is especially noticeable when the child does not get what it wants and the parents withhold their energy.

The pathology of this condition is complex. It seems that the spleen energy is weak and that the child draws *qi* from those around it. When *qi* is withheld for some reason, the child gets angry, probably because it is frightened by the sudden loss of energy. The *qi* becomes temporarily deficient and the blood does not circulate properly, withholding nourishment from the Heart. The child then gets anxious, restless, fidgety, and cannot sit still. Common causes include:

- Spleen *qi* deficiency: this can arise from many causes – immunisations, lengthy childbirth, anesthetics in childbirth, and long-term accumulation disorder, to name but a few. It can also stem from drinking too much fruit juice.
- No boundaries: these children seem to be able to manipulate their parents mercilessly. They manage to get their way in most things. In addition, they draw on their parents' energy, who in turn become more and more exhausted, and thus less able to stand up to their child.

Kidney Deficiency

The *yuan qi* (basal *qi*) kidney energy is weak, and rises up to affect the heart and the mind, resulting in hyperactive behaviour. It is more obvious when the child is tired or overstimulated. Causes of kidney deficiency include:

- constitutional kidney weakness: the kidney energy can be weak from birth, usually from weakness in the parents, genetic disorders, or severe illness during pregnancy;
- long-term illness: if a child has been ill over the years, the kidney energy can be weakened;
- severe illness: a very severe illness, such as a long febrile disease or meningitis, can deplete the kidney energy.

PATTERNS AND SYMPTOMS

Heat

- In younger children there may be accumulation disorder.
- Very active.
- Restless.
- Talkative.
- May destroy things.
- Insomnia: wakes up early (5 a.m.) or may be awake for an hour or two in the middle of the night.
- Red lips.

- Possibly whole face red.
- Tongue: red.
- Pulse: rapid, but hard to take.

Heat and Phlegm

- In younger children there may be accumulation disorder.
- Irritability.
- Restlessness.
- Shouts.
- Tantrums.
- Insomnia: wakes early, restless while sleeping.
- Violent.
- Wilfully destructive.
- May be sexually premature.
- Possible anal or genital fixation.
- Cannot concentrate.
- Tongue: red, possibly with yellow coating.
- Pulse: rapid, slippery, but hard to take.

Weakness of Middle Burner

- Grey or pale face.
- Dull or resentful eyes.
- Lips may be dull.
- Appetite poor.
- Manipulative.
- Sleep is poor, or only needs little sleep.
- Often has great thirst and drinks a lot of fruit juice.
- Loves to play destructive games: video games, or aggressive games with guns.
- May be cruel to brothers or sisters, and rude to parents.
- Tongue: pale, possibly with a red tip.
- Pulse: possibly weak, or wiry.

Kidney Deficiency

- Thin, tall, beautiful.
- Pale face.
- Frail body.
- Often ill.
- Eyes are too bright, glittering.
- When overexcited the face may become red.
- Hyperactive at the end of the day, when tired.
- Hyperactive when overstimulated (e.g., at a party).
- Hyperactive after watching television.

- Often terrified of needles.
- Tongue: may be pale, or red.
- Pulse: fine, floating.

One way to distinguish a child with 'false' hyperactivity from one with a 'true' type is to feel the back of the child. If it feels weak and is curved, then it is likely that the child is of the kidney-deficient pattern. If the bone structure is good, and the back straight and strong, then it is more likely to be another type of hyperactivity, if indeed it is pathological at all. The child may just be inquisitive and a bit annoying.

Case History

Master G, aged eight, was brought to the clinic because he was behaving badly at school. He had always been demanding, but now was completely out of hand – never sitting still, always wanting attention, and being very difficult if he didn't get it. His mother was very upset. She felt as if she were 'losing' her son. They had always been very close, but now he was becoming more and more distant and rude toward her.

Master G fell into the category of weak middle burner – very choosy about food, pale grey face, and manipulative. When it came to treating him he would scream 'NO, NO!' at full volume and curl up in a ball on the floor. When I did manage to get a needle in him, he would break out into a big smile! However, the next point was the same – screams and protestations, then a smile when the needle was in. Things were slightly easier if the mother left the room, but still hard.

This ritual was infuriating as it would take a good 45 minutes to treat him, which is a problem if your clinic is full and you are already running late. One student observing in the clinic was so fed up with him one day that he bribed him: ten pence per point. Master G was not impressed and negotiated twenty pence! After this, provided the rate was agreed beforehand, I was allowed to treat him. After about ten treatments he was noticeably different and we did not even need a bribe. Eventually, we reached the end and he did not have to come anymore. He was always going to be strong-minded, but he was not nearly as rude, and could control his temper much better. His mother was delighted; she felt as if she had 'found her son again'. I thought Master G himself would be delighted: no more torture! But on the last day he came up to me with a sad look and gave me a very loving hug and a 'thank you'.

TREATMENT

Treating a child with hyperactivity is no easy task. They can start off by wrecking the clinic, disturbing other patients and practitioners, and then irritating you. During treatment they hit, kick, scream, and make life difficult, to say the least. However, do persevere: the results can be quite astonishing – perhaps not immediate – but gradually the child will calm down.

Taking the pulse: with some children this can be virtually impossible, but hopefully it will not matter, as you should have a pretty good idea of what is going on by having read through the case history.

Advice about advice: try to be realistic about your advice to parents. A long list of 'don'ts' is daunting and often unworkable within the structure of the family. Try to provide alternatives so that parents don't have to think too much themselves – they are often exhausted!

Heat

Treatment principle: clear the heat and calm the spirit
   Main points:

- HE-7 (*Shenmen*) – calms the spirit;
- LIV-2 (*Xingjian*) – calms the spirit, clears the heat, subdues the manic behaviour;
- ST-44 (*Neiting*) – clears heat from the Stomach.

If the main points don't seem to be working, try substituting HE-8 (*Shaofu*) in place of HE-7 (*Shenmen*). This point calms the spirit and clears heat from the heart. Other points might include:

- LI-4 (*Hegu*) – clears heat;
- LIV-3 (*Taichong*) – calms the spirit, clears heat, and regulates the circulation of *qi*.

Method: use a strong reducing technique.
If there is accumulation disorder, use *Sifeng* (M-UE-9).

Reaction to Treatment

There are two common reactions during treatment with these children. On the one hand they tend to react strongly: they howl and scream, quite often just for effect. On the other hand they do not feel the needles at all, especially if there is a great deal of heat. (The interior heat disrupts the flow of *qi* to hands and feet, dulling sensation.) Thus, you can tell the child is improving when the drama of the treatment diminishes; and improvement in the condition brings increased response – and screams – to the needles.

In all children with this type of hyperactivity, they can go wild after treatment, as some heat is released. Do warn the parents of this. If you tell them, they can prepare themselves, and they will have faith that you actually know what you are doing!

Prognosis

Generally, 10 to 15 treatments are needed, depending on the severity and the amount of heat. If less severe, perhaps things will improve sooner. There should be gradual improvement in all cases.

Advice

As a matter of course, the child should be taken off all food colourings, additives, dairy products, oranges, orange juice, and sugar. There should be no coloured soda pop or junk food. Regular meals, with a well-cooked and a well-balanced diet, are essential. The child should be encouraged to exercise, watch less television, and play fewer video games and the like. If the child has accumulation disorder, advise appropriately.

Phlegm and Heat (Mania)

Treatment principle: clear heat, resolve phlegm, and calm the spirit
   Points:

- HE-7 (*Shenmen*) – calms the spirit;
- HE-8 (*Shaofu*) – calms the spirit and clears heat from the heart;
- LIV-2 (*Xingjian*) – clears heat, calms the spirit, and subdues the manic behaviour;
- ST-40 (*Fenglong*) – transforms the phlegm;
- GB-34 (*Yanglingquan*) – transforms the phlegm;
- P-5 (*Jianshi*) – calms the spirit and clears the phlegm surrounding the heart.

   Method: use a strong reducing technique

Reaction to Treatment

There will, over the course of treatment, be a discharge of phlegm – usually through the bowels and the nose, but it may be vomited. The stools may be loose for 1 to 2 months depending on the amount of phlegm present. This is a surprisingly long time, but it seems to be all right. A productive cough may also develop. As with the previous pattern, following treatment, the child may get very angry as heat is released. The reaction during treatment is likewise similar to that in the previous pattern.

Prognosis

Ten to thirty treatments may be required, depending on the severity of the condition. Once all the phlegm and heat has been cleared you may well find an underlying Spleen dysfunction that may need treatment.

Advice

Similar to the previous pattern, and no peanuts or peanut butter.

Weakness in the Middle Burner

Treatment principle: strengthen the middle burner, tonify the spleen. Encourage the parents to establish boundaries.

Points:

- SP-6 (*Sanyinjiao*) – tonifies the spleen;
- ST-36 (*Zusanli*) – tonifies the stomach and spleen;
- LIV-3 (*Taichong*) – calms the spirit and regulates the circulation of *qi*;
- HE-7 (*Shenmen*) – calms the spirit;
- Ren-12 (*Zhongwan*) – use moxa.

Reaction to Treatment

These children will often scream blue murder! They will cry crocodile tears and make such a noise that even your colleagues will look at you with a 'What were you doing to that poor child?' expression. It is somewhat infuriating as you know that it doesn't hurt that much: the child is just being difficult and manipulating its parents! It can reach such a pitch that the parents will begin to doubt you, and may give in and stop bringing the child.

One way around this is to get the parents to leave the room, if the child is old enough. In this way the child cannot play up to them so much, and cannot draw so much *qi* from them. When we have done this, far from being a trauma, the child often becomes very calm.

Prognosis

Quite variable – possibly 10 treatments, and up to 30. A lot depends on the home situation.

Advice

The main advice is to the parents: they must set boundaries. This is often very difficult because the first few weeks can be hell for the family as the child gets very upset at being told what to do and having all his free energy withheld. Keep off fruit juice and limit consumption of liquids. Also important for these children is to stop them from watching television and playing video games. Also – as with the other patterns – diet, exercise, and a regular lifestyle are important.

Kidney Deficiency

Treatment principle: tonify the kidney energy, calm the spirit

These children are usually genuinely afraid of needles, so don't use them. Using needles is actually counterproductive as their fear weakens the kidney energy further. Herbal medicine is often useful, although they may find it too disgusting to take.

Points:

- BL-23 (*Shenshu*);
- KI-1 (*Yongquan*);
- LU-8 (*Ququan*);
- SP-6 (*Sanyinjiao*).

Method: use moxa at all points. You may also advise that they drink teas like limeflower or passiflora.

Reaction to Treatment

If you just use moxa the child should be happy, but if you try to use needles the child may really freak out. You can tell the difference between these children and those with the previous pattern by looking at their eyes and feeling the lower back. If the eyes are bright and glittery and the back is weak, then they fall into this category. If the eyes are intense and the back is reasonably strong, then it is likely they are of the hyperactive weak middle burner type. It is not always easy to tell though.

Prognosis

It takes time for these children to recover. Depending on the severity of the kidney weakness, you may need to treat them for many months.

Advice

The child must be encouraged to rest, early nights, no television or any form of stimulation for a couple of hours before bedtime. They must also avoid sugar, and should take gentle exercise. Suggest something like artistic acting.

NOTES

Some children are labelled hyperactive and put on drugs when actually they are simply bored with school. Often they are strong, wilful, and intelligent children who simply do not want to sit still for long periods, and are easily bored with simple schoolwork. Identifying these children can be hard, but important, especially if they are going to be put on drugs, which simply dampens their enthusiasm for life. Moreover, the drug Ritalin, a derivative of speed that is commonly prescribed for hyperactivity in children, is very damaging to the spleen. Long-term use inevitably leads to spleen *qi* or yang deficiency.

Anxiety Disorder: Protocol Applied in a Public Health Unit

23

The aim of the project is to evaluate an acupuncture protocol as a treatment of anxiety disorders.

Anxiety disorders induce widespread consumption of anxiolytics, with abuse and addiction. They are particularly frequently used by people suffering from addiction/abuse of alcohol; their consumption during a period of abstinence is one of the primary causes of relapse.

The Alcohol Unit (Nucleo Operativo Alcologia, NOA) is a specialised structure with institutional duties for the prevention, diagnosis, treatment and rehabilitation of alcohol addiction and alcohol-related problems. The NOA in Vimercate carries out the following activities:

- projects for prevention and public awareness both for the general population and for specific targets;
- individual and couple psychotherapy;
- psychotherapy groups;
- non-therapeutic groups (multi family self-help);
- systemic relational therapy (family therapy);
- evaluation of the patient with relation to the state of alcohol addiction;
- home visits and detoxifications;
- mobile clinic medicine detoxifications;
- Acudetox mobile clinic, for detoxification with ear acupuncture and treatment of postacute abstinence symptoms;
- somatic acupuncture mobile clinic for the treatment of problems related to weaning and/or reinforcement of abstinence state;
- prevention and treatment of alcohol-related pathologies;
- visits and support in hospital;
- coordination of the intervention between medical staff (GP, specialists, nurses);

- supporting families with problems linked to detoxification therapies;
- vaccinations;
- introduction in protected workplaces;
- introduction in a therapeutic community;
- counselling for professional retraining.

TRADITIONAL CHINESE MEDICINE IN THE TREATMENT OF GENERALISED ANXIETY DISORDERS

Protocol applied in the Alcohology Operative Unit (Nucleo Operativo Alcologia, NOA) Vimercate, Milano.

Project by Roberto Cipollina MD.
Supervisor: Elisa Rossi MD.

Aim of the Project

The aim of the project is to evaluate an acupuncture protocol as a treatment of generalised anxiety.

Project Motivation

At some point in life, 5% of the population suffers from problems linked to generalised anxiety disorders.

The course is chronic, it usually worsens during stressful periods, produces an attitude that creates behaviours which tend to interfere with one's normal social, emotional and working life, and often causes high consumption of anxiolytics with abuse and addiction phenomena.

Anxiety disorders appear frequently in people suffering from addiction/abuse of alcoholic substances; anxiolytics consumed during a period of abstinence are one of the primary causes of relapse.

Criteria for Admission in the Project

Inclusion Criteria

The protocol may include all patients who have a Generalised Anxiety Disorder as defined in the DSM-IV, even if under pharmacological or psychotherapeutic treatment.

Although pre-existing therapy does not constitute a criterion for exclusion it will be submitted to a specific evaluation in terms of greater or lesser effectiveness.

Exclusion Criteria

- Anxiety disorder induced by the use of substances.
- Anxiety disorder from general medical condition.
- Anxiety disorder with manifestations only during mood alterations.
- Anxiety disorder related to psychosis.
- Patients who are already being treated with acupuncture for other reasons.

Patients are admitted in the study on the basis of the following:

- anamnestic interview;
- inclusion criteria as in the DSM-IV;
- objective evaluation using STAI;
- self-evaluation questionnaire IPAT-ASQ;
- evaluation of the impairment produced by the anxiety state in the social, working and affective life;
- evaluation of current medication.[1]

Method and timing of the therapy

Standard Therapeutic Method

- Fifteen persons will be considered by the study. They will be patients using the service and with a period of abstinence of over 3 months.
- The patients are treated in sessions twice a week for 6 weeks; the sessions will last 20 minutes; during the sessions the patients will be left alone in a relaxing environment.
- The study will be carried out over a period of 2 years.
- Patients will be evaluated using Traditional Chinese Medicine diagnosis in order to define the pathological patterns and to consequently select among the points listed below.

Protocol for the Treatment With Acupuncture

The protocol includes seven or eight points:

- a couple of fixed points;
- a group of three or four points, chosen among two groups on the basis of a TCM differential diagnosis;
- one or two points chosen from among seven points.

Fixed Points

- *Yintang* M-HN-3 + *Juque* Ren-14

---

[1] American Psychiatric Association: DSM-IV, *Diagnostic and Statistical Manual of Mental Disorders*, 1994; Consulting Psychologists Press, STAI, *State-trait anxiety inventory – Forma Y*, Palo Alto, 1983; S. E. Krug, I. H. Scheier, R. B. Cattel, IPAT-ASQ, 1976.

Group of Three or Four Points According to a TCM Basic Diagnosis (Emptiness or Fullness)

Fullness – *shi* (Three Points):

'Plethoric' pattern: red face, feeling of heat, agitation, thirst, bitter mouth, abundant urine, red tongue or tongue with red spots, yellow coating, full, rapid pulse. We alternate between:

- *Neiguan* P-6 + *Gongsun* SP-4 + *Qihai* Ren-6;
- *Tongli* HE-5 + *Dazhong* KI-4 + *Qihai* Ren-6.

Emptiness-*xu* (Four Points):

'Deficiency' pattern: asthenia, easily tired, pale face, spontaneous sweating, anxiousness, shortness of breath, pale tongue, difficulty in speaking, a weak, thready, empty pulse.

- *Shenmen* HE-7 + *Taixi* KI-3 + *Zusanli* ST-36 + *Guanyuan* Ren-4.

One or Two Points To Be Chosen From Among The Seven Points

These include:

- *Baihui* Du-20 if there is phlegm blocking the pure orifices;
  – feelings of unreality, depersonalisation, significant signs of affective/ cognitive alterations (e.g. hypomania, depression, obsessions).
- *Fengchi* GB-20 if there is wind and *yang* ascending:
  – headache, dizziness, blurred vision, cervical tension or pain.
- *Shanzhong* Ren-17 if there is an obstruction in the circulation of the *qi* to the upper *jiao*:
  – feelings of oppression in the chest, tachycardia, shortness of breath.
- *Taichong* LIV-3 if there is liver *qi* stagnation:
  – globus hystericus, unsteady mood, muscle tensions or contractions, premenstrual syndrome, dysmenorrhoea, irregular cycle, irritable bowel syndrome.
- *Neiting* ST-44 if there is stomach fire:
  – postprandial vomiting, heartburn and pain, 'violent' hunger, thirst for cold drinks, nausea, acid regurgitations, irritated mouth.
- *Xingjian* LIV-2 if there is liver fire:
  – irritability, constipation or dry stools, pain at the hypochondria, dreams that disturb the sleep, bitter mouth, thirst.
- *Taibai* SP-3 if there is spleen *qi* deficiency:
  – easily tired, lack of appetite, loose stools, pale, swollen or tooth-marked tongue, weak pulse.

Patients are required to leave the study if they miss two consecutive sessions.

During the treatment patients must not start any new specific therapy (psychotherapy, AA groups, pharmacological therapies).

Patients who have started drinking again will also be excluded.

The therapy will be suspended if there is a worsening of the anxiety.

Monitoring and Evaluation of the Study

At the end of the treatment we will evaluate the state of the patient through a re-submission of the tests (STAI and ASQ) and a re-evaluation of the data related to the initial state (specific symptoms, behaviours interfering with daily life, usage of medication).

The *follow-up* will be conducted with the same methodology (interview, STAI and ASQ) and it will take place after two weeks and after three months from the end of the therapy.

COLLECTING THE INITIAL DATA

Here we present the initial data from the protocol that was devised and applied in the Alcohol Operative Unit in Vimercate, Milano.

The patients all suffer from a Generalised Anxiety Disorder, following the criteria of the DSM-IV and a diagnosis based on TCM; the treatment is supplied twice a week for 6 weeks; the level of anxiety is calculated with specific tests at the beginning of the therapy, at the end and 15 days after it has finished.

Case 23.1

46-year-old woman, married with two children, housewife.

Under medication with Seroxat ½ cp/day, prescribed by a psychiatrist for a dysthymic disorder.

- She suffers from heat; during the night she feels hot and she sweats.
- She is never thirsty, except during the menstrual period.
- Sometimes she feels heat in her face and ears.
- Regular menstruation both in duration and flow, no pain, sometimes accompanied by moderate premenstrual headache in the right front–temporal region.
- Disturbed sleep: she falls asleep easily but wakes up often during the night; she has many dreams.
- She has no problems with digestion or pain or stomach distress except when she is stressed; in the evening she feels a slight abdominal distension, regular normal stools, clear urine.
- Palpitations in the evening when she lies down to rest.
- She has no vertigo but she sometimes feels empty headed when walking.

- Pain starting behind the neck on the right and spreading down to the back and the arm to the elbow following *San Jiao*
- Tongue: slightly thin, with upturned edges, red spots on the tip; red purplish body colour; coating almost absent at the front, dry surface.
- Pulse: normal frequency, thready on the left, slightly slippery on the right.

Diagnosis
Emptiness of heart (and kidney) *yin*.

Points
- *Yintang* EX-HN-3, *Juque* Ren-14, *Guanyuan* Ren-4, *Shenmen* HE-7, *Taixi* KI-3, *Zusanli* ST-36.

Evaluation of the Level of Anxiety
Baseline Questionnaires: 08.02.01
- STAI form Y: State 63 (T = 53) – Trait 74 (T = 56). She did not fill in the ASQ test.

End Questionnaires: 15.03.01
- STAI form Y; State 63 (T = 53) – Trait 75 (T = 57).

Follow-up Questionnaires 15 Days After the End of the Treatment: 29.03.01
- STAI form Y: State 10 (T = 36) – Trait 81 (T = 59).

In this case there is a noticeable difference between the state test (conditions at the moment of the test) and the trait test (anxiousness as a relatively stable trait of the personality).

The former value (10) is widely below average (41, 30), the latter (81) is among one of the highest values. Such a discrepancy between values means that the conditions for the test were relatively good (neutral).

In this case the wide divergence can be ascribed to the patient's psychological condition following a severe accident 9 days earlier in which her son had been involved.

Interview: 03.09.01
The patient feels very well, with a distinct improvement in her relationship with the family. The trauma deriving from the son's accident seems to have passed rapidly; the patient has obtained greater autonomy within the family, something that had never happened before. The medication remains unchanged.

Case 23.2

45-year-old woman, single, living with her parents, a teacher.

She is referred from the psychiatric unit. For 7 years she has been suffering from a generalised state of anxiety, she is now taking Anafranil 3 cp/day and Tavor, which have noticeably reduced the symptoms; she takes Tegretol following an intervention for double cerebral aneurysm in February 2000.

- Continuous palpitations during day and night (she feels the heart beating in the head).
- Constant fear.
- Regular sleep with many dreams.
- Disturbed sight (like dazzling sun on water).
- Vertigo and feelings of heat in the head.
- Regular menstruation, light red with some clots, at times mammary strain.
- Abundant urine, stools usually constipated.
- Feeling of fullness of the chest, sighing.
- Asthenia.
- Desire to drink hot drinks.
- Tongue: slightly pale, dry, thin and white coating, red tip with small dark red spots, visible congestion of the sublingual vessels.
- Pulse: rapid, thready and deep on the right.

Diagnosis

Emptiness of heart and liver blood.

Points

- *Yintang* EX-HN-3, *Fengchi* GB-20, *Juque* Ren-14, *Guanyuan* Ren-4, *Shenmen* HE-7, *Taixi* KI-3, *Zusanli* ST-36

Evaluation of the Level of Anxiety
Baseline Questionnaires: 20.09.01

- ASQ: score 10.
- STAI form Y: State 83 (T = 59) – Trait 91 (T = 64).
  Very high level of anxiety, in the ASQ a score of 10 is found only in 1 person out of 20 since it corresponds to a 99 percentile range.

End Questionnaires: 05.11.01

- STAI form Y: State 22 (T = 40) – Trait 45 (T = 48).
- ASQ: score 7.
  The two tests reveal a strong reduction of the level of anxiety, which is now in the average range.

Follow-up Questionnaires 15 Days After the End of the Treatment: 19.11.01

- STAI form Y: State 4 (T = 36) – Trait 4 (T = 34).
- ASQ: score 6.
  Standard level of anxiety (percentile range 50).

Notes

Following the suggestion of a psychiatrist the woman has reduced the dosage of Anafranil from 3 to 2 pills and no longer takes Tavor. In mid December the psychiatric visit confirms the resolution of anxiety, the suspension of the anxiolytic and also considers the suspension of the antidepressant.

Interview: 20.12.01

The patient reports a disappearance of the anxiety. She defines the result as 'amazing'.

Case 23.3

42-year-old woman, married, one son, housewife.
Under medication: Valium gtt. for anxiety state.
- Lack of appetite, heaviness in the stomach and bad digestion.
- Drinks a lot, preferably cold drinks.
- Often has cold hands, feet and nose but says that she warms up very quickly.
- Constipated stools with dry stools.
- In the last month noticeable asthenia.
- Pale constitution.
- Scanty and white leucorrhoea without smell.
- Regular sleep.
- Palpitations even when resting.
- Regular menstruation in amount, frequency, colour and duration.
- Swollen stomach especially after having eaten.
- Feelings of oppression in the chest, sighs, yawns, sometimes a feeling of not being able to breathe.
- Frequent migraines that start in the right frontal region and then extend to the temporal region involving the whole head.
- Tongue: indented, central crack that reaches the tip, small red spots on the tip, small purple marks in the middle region. 'Geographic' tongue: coating with no root and peeled patches.
- Pulse: empty, slightly slippery.

Diagnosis

Emptiness of spleen *qi* and heart *yin*.

Points

- *Yintang* EX-HN-3, *Juque* Ren-14, *Guanyuan* Ren-4, *Shenmen* HE-7, *Taixi* KI-3, *Zusanli* ST-36, *Taibai* SP-3

Evaluation of the Level of Anxiety

Baseline Questionnaires: 28.02.01

- STAI form Y: State 75 (T56) – Trait 81 (T59).
- ASQ: score 9.

High levels of anxiety, corresponding to the percentile range 90, high levels of general frustration and instability.

End Questionnaires: 03.05.01

- STAI form Y: State 8 (T37) – Trait 26 (T42).
- ASQ: score 5.

Notes

The patient is no longer under any specific therapy.

We did not undertake the follow-up evaluation after 15 days because the patient, feeling better, had returned for a couple of months to her place of birth in Eastern Europe.

Interview: 16.1.02

After a long period of well-being the patient started drinking alcohol again, more or less one month ago. She is now abstinent and will start a second cycle of the treatment in 2 months.

Case 23.4

51-year-old man, married, one son, traffic warden.

Anxiety lasting for many years, under medication with anxiolytics.

- Insomnia, the patient wakes up at 3 a.m.
- Bitter mouth.
- Hypoacusis.
- Problems of loss of memory.
- Asthenia.
- Abundant urine with a normal colour, regular stools.
- Hypertension.
- Tendency in suffering from heat.
- Anxiousness, restlessness, rage attacks.
- Tongue: normal colour, purple on the left side, very thin coating.
- Pulse: wiry.

Diagnosis

Liver *yang* ascending.

Points

- *Yintang* EX-HN-3, *Juque* Ren-14, *Qihai* Ren-6, *Taichong* LIV-3, *Neiguan* P-6 and *Gongsun* SP-4 alternated with *Tongli* HE-5 and *Dazhong* KI-4.

Evaluation of the Level of Anxiety

Baseline Questionnaires: 20.09.01

- STAI: State 84 (T60) – Trait 80 (T58).
- ASQ: score 7.

The levels of anxiety of both State and Trait are widely above the average (39.68 and 43.85 respectively).

In the ASQ the score (7) corresponds to the percentile range 77, meaning that in the general population three-quarters of the men have smaller scores than that of the patient and one-quarter have higher ones.

End Questionnaires: 05.11.01

- STAI: State 34 (T44) – Trait 57 (T48).
- ASQ: score 6.

The results show that the level of the State of anxiousness is normal, while the level of Trait anxiety has improved but still remains above the average range.

ASQ: the level of anxiety is average, percentile range 60.

Follow-up Questionnaires 15 Days After the End of the Treatment: 20.11.01

- STAI: State 70 (T54) – Trait 87 (T62).
- ASQ: score 8.

There has been a new rise of the level of anxiety, especially in the Trait scale.

ASQ: the patient has a high level of anxiety, percentile range 90 (found in 10% of the population).

Notes

After the Twin Towers tragedy in New York on 11 September 2001, the patient decided to look after his savings, and his anxiety started again.

18.12.01

The patient was tested again after approximately 1 month. He revealed high levels of anxiety.

- STAI: State 83 (T59) – Trait 92 (T64).

SECTION V

APPENDICES

Appendix A

THE PULSE

Since emotional illnesses result from a great variety of patterns, it is possible to find all kinds of pulses. We have thus chosen to present all 28 pulses with descriptions borrowed from classical texts, using their pictures and their analogies. We have also recalled in a few words their clinical interpretation, which must always be integrated with the four methods of diagnosis.[1]

The classical quotes are borrowed from the article by Laura Caretto 'I polsi nei classici' ('Pulses in the classics').[2]

FU 浮-Floating

Classic Description

'The *fu* pulse under the fingers presents immediately a floating shape, when we press it weakens but is never empty; when searching in the centre it feels fluent and flowing.'[3]

'Taken on the surface it is in excess, taken in depth it is insufficient.'[4]

'If we take the *fu* pulse with a light hand it is like a piece of wood floating in water'; 'like a gentle wind puffing up the back feathers of a bird.'[5]

Diagnosis

- Attack from external pathogens:
  —wind-heat: floating and rapid;
  —wind-cold: floating and wiry.
- Emptiness of *yin* and *yang*; floating, large and weak.

Notes

In the first case the defensive *qi* becomes superficial to rejects the pathogens. In the second case it stays on the surface only because of its weakness.

In the *Neijing* it is also called *mao* (hair).

CHEN 沉-Deep

Classic Description

'Taken on the surface it is insufficient, taken in depth it is in excess.'[6]

'It is like a stone thrown into the water, it must reach the bottom.'[7]

---

[1] Among the references in English are: Beijing Medical College, *Common Terms of Traditional Chinese Medicine in English*, Beijing, 1980; Liu Gongwang, Akira Hyodo eds, 1994; Zhao Xin, Fu Jianping eds, 1994; Wiseman N., Feng Ye, *A Practical Dictionary of Chinese Medicine*, 1998; the Blue Poppy edn translations of the classical texts: Li Shi Zhen, *The Lakeside Master's Study of the Pulse*, 1998; Wang Shu-he, *The Pulse Classic*, 1997.

[2] In MediCina, summer 1996. The introduction by G. Rotolo reads: 'The first step is to describe the tactile feeling, i.e. to define what we feel under our fingers. Once this has been memorised it constitutes a useful guide for future observations. We feel the pulse looking for the images that we have memorised and which allow us to place it in a category with a diagnostic value. But the description of the pulse is not immediate nor direct, it must be filtered by language, in this case the language of a culture which is distant from us both in time and space.'

[3] *Zhenzongsanmei* (Three secrets of diagnosis).

[4] *Maijing* (Classic of the pulses).

[5] *Maique* (Definition of the pulse).

[6] *Maijing* (Classic of the pulses).

[7] *Binghu maixue* (The science of the pulse by Binghu).

'It flows in depth between the tendons and the bones, like a stone sunk in water.'[8]

The *chen*-deep pulse flows between the tendons, the *fu*-hidden pulse flows above the bones.'[9]

The *chen* pulse is felt only under strong pressure... while the *fu*-hidden pulse can not be perceived even if we press down to the tendons and bones; to feel it we must open the tendons by pushing with the fingers.'[10]

Diagnosis

- Accumulation of pathogens on the inside: deep and strong:
  — cold: deep and slow;
  — heat: deep and rapid;
  — phlegm: deep and slippery or wiry.
- Emptiness of *qi* and *yang*: deep and weak.

Notes

In the first case the accumulation of pathogens causes an obstruction of the *qi* and blood and takes the *qi* in depth. In the second case the weakness of the *qi* prevents it from rising to the surface.

In the *Neijing* it is also called *shi*, 'stone'.

CHI 迟 -Slow

Classic Description

'*Chi* means it does not arrive on time.'[11]

The *chi* pulse arrives every three breathings, it comes and goes very slowly.'[12]

The *chi* pulse governs the illnesses of the organs, *yang qi* is concealed, if it is strong it indicates pain, if it is weak it implies cold emptiness.'[13]

Diagnosis

- Accumulation of cold with pain:
  — cold from external pathogens: slow and floating;
  — accumulation of cold on the inside: slow and deep;
  — cold from emptiness: slow and weak.
- Accumulation of heat (rarer): slow and strong.

Notes

Usually it is cold that stops the circulation of *qi*, but heat may also obstruct the blood circulation, for example in the *yangming* syndrome.

NB: The pulse can be normally slow (athletes).

SHUO 数 -Rapid

Classic Description

'In the time of one breath it arrives six or seven times.'[14]

'*Shuo* governs the heart, it arrives five times or more.'[15]

Diagnosis

- Heat:
  — full heat: rapid and strong;
  — heat from emptiness of *yin* or blood: rapid and weak.
- Floating *yang* because in emptiness (rarer): rapid, large and empty.

Notes

The heat accelerates the movement of the *qi* and blood. But the rapid pulse can also be a sign of false heat originated by an emptiness of *yin* and consequent floating of the remaining *yang*.[16]

---

[8] *Maijue qiwu* (Awakening of the consciousness in distinguishing the pulse).
[9] *Binghu maixue* (The science of the pulse by Binghu).
[10] *Maijue kanwu* (Correction of mistakes in the definition of the pulse).
[11] *Zhenjia shuyao* (Fundamental elements of the diagnosis).
[12] *Maijing* (Classic of the pulses).
[13] *Siyan juyao* (Brief fundamentals).
[14] *Maijing* (Classic of the pulses).
[15] *Yixue shiziyi* (Simple medicine).
[16] See also Chapter 6 on restlessness and agitation, in which *fanzao* is explained by Sun Simiao as a sign of false heat and true cold from floating of the *yang*.

JI 急-Urgent

Classic Description

'We say *ji* when it is faster than *shuo*, that is, seven or eight times during one breath.'[17]

Diagnosis

• Excess of *yang* and exhaustion of *yin*.

Notes

The movement is accelerated by the heat originate by the consumption of *yin*, and it precedes an exhaustion of the true *qi*, *zhen qi*.

XUAN 弦-Wiry

Classic Description

'Its shape is like the string of a bow, if we press it does not move.'[18]

'The *xuan* pulse is as strait as the string of a bow, if we press it feels like the string of a violin; its shape is that of a kite string passing right in the centre, neat under the fingers.'[19]

Diagnosis

• Stagnation of liver and gall bladder *qi*.
• Accumulation of phlegm, pain.
• Exhaustion of the *qi* of the middle *jiao*, dominated by the liver.

Notes

The lack of regulation of the *qi* on the side of the liver prevents a flowing circulation, which worsens with the appearance of other pathological patterns.

In modern Chinese the character 玄, 'string of a musical instrument, string of the bow, clock spring', is read *xian*, but when it refers to the pulse the pronunciation *xuan* is still frequently used.

JIN 紧-Tense

Classic Description

'The *jin* pulse has strength, needles the fingers on the left and right, it is like touching a tense and vibrant rope.'[20]

Diagnosis

• Cold, with pain:
  — in the external layers: tense and floating;
  — internally: tense and deep.

Notes

The conflict between cold pathogen and correct *qi* and the obstruction of the latter causes a contraction of the pulse.

HUA 滑-Slippery

Classic Description

'*Hua* is the opposite of *se* (choppy); it comes and goes in a flowing manner just like the marbles on the abacus which slide, round and smooth.'[21]

Diagnosis

• Accumulation of phlegm.
• Stagnation of food.
• Damp-heat.

Notes

It can be a sign of abundance of *qi* and blood, for example during pregnancy.

XU 虚 -Empty

Classic Description

---

[17] *Zhenjia shuyao* (Fundamental elements of the diagnosis).
[18] *Shanghanlun* (Treatise on feverish illnesses).
[19] *Binghu maixue* (The science of the pulse by Binghu).
[20] *Zhenjia zhengyan* (The correct eye of the diagnosis).
[21] *Zhenjia shuyao* (Fundamental elements of the diagnosis).

'The pulse is slow, large and soft, if taken in depth it is insufficient, if taken on the surface it feels empty as an open valley.'[22]

'Under the fingers it is empty, large and soft, the feeling is that of stroking the feathers of a chicken, both in the centre and in depth it is weak and with no strength.'[23]

Diagnosis

• Emptiness of *qi* and/or blood.

Notes

The beats have no strength owing to a lack of *qi*, which does not move the blood, and the feeling of emptiness under pressure is caused by a lack of blood.

XI 细-Thready

Classic Description

'It is slightly larger than the *wei*-minute pulse, it is more constant, it is only thready.'[24]

'It is thready because its shape is as thin as a silk thread.'[25]

'It is more evident than the *wei*-minute pulse.'[26]

Diagnosis

• Emptiness of *yin* and *yang*, of blood and *qi* (mainly of *yin* and blood).
• Dampness (rarer).
• Heat invading the nutritious and blood layer (rarer): thready and rapid.

Notes

Qi and blood are insufficient to fill the pulse or there is dampness, which compresses the vessels.

It is also known as *xiao* (small).

WEI 微-Minute

Classic Description

'The *wei* pulse is unperceivable as the layer of fat which forms on the surface of the soup, thin as the thread of the silkworm.'[27]

'It is extremely thready and limp, it gives the impression of exhaustion as if it was and was not there.'[28]

'The *wei*, *ru*-drenched and *ruo*-weak pulses belong to the same category: *ru* is very limp, superficial and thready; *ruo* is very limp but deep and thready; *wei* is very limp and thready with no difference between surface and depth.'[29]

Diagnosis

• Emptiness of *yin*, *yang*, *qi* and blood:
  — exhaustion of *yang*: if not very visible under light pressure;
  — consumption of *yin*: if not very visible under strong pressure.

Notes

The collapse of *yang* in acute illnesses and the exhaustion of *zhengqi* in chronic illnesses do not supply sufficient *qi*.

RUO 弱 -Weak

Classic Description

'The *ruo* pulse is limp, small and thready, it can be found in depth, brushing the surface one does not find it, it is only found by pressing in depth.'[30]

Diagnosis

• Emptiness of *qi* and blood.

---

[22] *Maijing* (Classic of the pulses).
[23] *Zhenzong sanmei* (Three secrets of the diagnosis).
[24] *Maijing* (Classic of the pulses).
[25] *Yixue shiziyi* (Simple medicine).
[26] *Zhenjia zhengyan* (The correct eye of the diagnosis).
[27] *Shanghanlun* (Treatise on feverish illnesses).
[28] *Maijing* (Classic of the pulses).
[29] *Maijue kanwu* (Correction of mistakes in the definition of the pulse).
[30] *Zhenjia zhengyan* (The correct eye of the diagnosis).

Notes

The emptiness of the blood does not fill the vessels; the emptiness of the *qi* gives no strength to the beat.

RU 濡-Drenched

Classic Description

'The *ru* pulse is very limp but superficial and thin like a piece of silk in water; it can be perceived with a gentle hand. It is not there if we press in depth, like a drenched cloth floating on water.'[31]

Diagnosis

• Severe emptiness of blood and *jing*.
• Dampness, mainly from spleen deficiency.

Notes

Blood and *jing* are insufficient and do not nourish the pulse, the dampness obstructs and compresses the vessels.

SE 涩 -Choppy

Classic Description

'The *se* pulse is thready and slow, it proceeds with difficulty, it can be either short or scattered, at times it can suffer some interruption; it does not have a regular frequency and it can come three or five times, it is like a small knife scratching bamboo, like rain wetting the sand, like an ill silkworm nibbling a mulberry leaf.'[32]

Diagnosis

• Blood stasis.
• Choppy, weak and thready: blood stasis in conditions of emptiness of *qi* and blood.
• Choppy and full: blood stasis in conditions of fullness.

• Emptiness of blood or *jing*
• Accumulation of dampness or food, *qi* stagnation.

Notes

The blood or *jing* deficiency prevents a good circulation, which can also be disturbed by stasis or accumulations.

SHI 实-Full

Classic Description

'The *shi* pulse has strength, it is long, large and firm; it responds to the touch with determination and is such at all levels.'[33]

Diagnosis

• Fullness of pathogens on the inside.

Notes

The fullness is caused by the conflict between *qi* and pathogens, both strong.

HONG 洪-Flooding

Classic Description

'The *hong* pulse is extremely large under the fingers, it arrives strong and leaves weaker, it arrives large and leaves long.'[34]
'The *hong* pulse is superficial but also large and has strength; this is why it fills the three positions at all levels. Its strength is like the flooding of the water, the rise of the waves, the pulse arrives large and bulging.'[35]

Diagnosis

• Heat and fire hit the *qi*.
• Pathogens that overtake the *qi* (consumptive illnesses, haemorrhages, chronic diarrhoea).

---

[31] *Binghu maixue* (The science of the pulse by Binghu).
[32] *Binghu maixue* (The science of the pulse by Binghu).
[33] *Zhenjia zhengyan* (The correct eye of the diagnosis).
[34] *Binghu maixue* (The science of the pulse by Binghu).
[35] *Maishuo* (Sayings on the pulse).

Notes

The heat fills and expands *qi* and blood of the pulse, both in the fullness and in the emptiness.

In the *Neijing* it is also called *gou* ('hook') because it arrives strong and leaves weaker.

CHANG 长-Long

Classic Description

'The *chang* pulse is long (far, distant), the head and tail are well apart, it is straight above and below, at the top it reaches *Yuji* (LU-10), at the bottom it overtakes its own position, it is like touching a long reed.'[36]

Diagnosis

* Heat on the inside.
* Liver or wind *yang*.

Notes

If the *chang* pulse is not hard and tense but harmonious, it is a sign of a good condition of the *qi* and blood.

HUAN 缓-Moderate or Slackened

Classic Description

'It comes and goes slowly but a bit quicker than the *chi*-slow pulse. During one breath it arrives four times, it responds to the finger in a gentle and peaceful way, it comes and goes uniformly [...] it reminds one of weeping willows dancing in the wind at the beginning of the spring, when their tops gently sway in the breeze.'[37]

Diagnosis

* Dampness, stomach and spleen *qi* deficiency: slackened and superficial.

Notes

If calm and regular and with no other pathological characteristics it is a sign of good health.

DUAN 短-Short

Classic Description

'The *duan* pulse does not reach its position, it touches the finger and goes back, it is not able to fill the position.'[38]

'The two ends sink, only the middle floats-*fu*.'[39]

Diagnosis

* Emptiness of *qi*. short and weak.
* Stagnation of *qi*: short and full.
* Accumulation of dampness or phlegm or blood stasis (rarer): short and slippery.

Notes

The *qi* deficiency does not allow a good circulation while its stagnation or other accumulations prevent it.

SAN 散-Scattered

Classic Description

'The *san* pulse is like scattered leaves.'[40]

'It is large but scattered, the surface has no inside, scattered and un-gathered. It has no government nor discipline, it has no restrictions; its frequency is not regular, it is messy like the flowers of the poplar tree.'[41]

Diagnosis

* Exhaustion of *yuan qi*.

Notes

The *qi* is so scarce that it cannot maintain the continuity and route of the pulse.

---

[36] *Zhenjia zhengyan* (The correct eye of the diagnosis).
[37] *Binghu maixue* (The science of the pulse by Binghu).
[38] *Binghu maixue* (The science of the pulse by Binghu).
[39] *Zhenjia zhengyan* (The correct eye of the diagnosis).
[40] *Neijing*
[41] *Binghu maixue* (The science of the pulse by Binghu).

KOU 芤-Hollow

Classic Description

'The kou pulse is floating and large but limp, when we press the centre it is empty while the sides are full.'[42]
'Kou is the name of a herb, its leaf is similar to that of an onion, in the middle it is empty.'[43]

Diagnosis

- Internal emptiness caused by haemorrhages produced by fire pathogens.

Notes

The deficiency of nutritious qi and blood produce emptiness at the centre of the pulse, with the yang rising to the surface.

GE 革-Like a Drum Skin

Classic Description

'Ge means skin, it is floating, wiry, large but empty. It is like pressing on a drum skin: it is tense on the outside but empty on the inside.'[44]

Diagnosis

- Emptiness of blood.
- Emptiness of jing.

Notes

The emptiness of dense qi prevents the qi from consolidating and the yang floats towards the outside.

DAI 代 -Intermittent

Classic Description

'The dai pulse is interrupted during the movement, it is as though it is unable to recover alone, that is why it returns after a while (the pause is long).'[45]

'The pauses of the pulse dai are regular, they do not fail.'[46]

Diagnosis

- Emptiness of qi, particularly heart qi (from fear and fright, pain, trauma).
- During pregnancy: yuan qi deficiency.

Notes

The emptiness of the qi causes irregularity in the pulse.

JIE 结-Knotted

Classic Description

'The jie pulse arrives huan-moderate, sometimes it pauses and then comes back; pauses are irregular.'[47]

Diagnosis

- Stagnation of qi caused by excessive yin.
- Blood stasis.
- Cold phlegm.

Notes

Severe: the prevalence of the yin is such that it sometimes stops the pulse.

LAO 牢-Imprisoned or Firm

Classic Description

'The lao pulse has the characteristics of the deep and hidden pulse; it is full, large and long, slightly wiry.'[48]

'Lao has two meanings, one is that of firm, compact, the other is that it is found inside or at depth. That is why trees are firm-lao when they have deep roots that penetrate deeply. When we say that it is deep and hidden we speak of

[42] Maijing (Classic of the pulses).
[43] Maijue kanwu (Correction of mistakes in the definition of the pulse).
[44] Gejin yitong (Past and present medicine).
[45] Binghu maixue (The science of the pulse by Binghu).
[46] Maijue kanwu (Correction of mistakes in the definition of the pulse).
[47] Shanghanlun (Treatise on feverish illnesses).
[48] Binghu maixue (The science of the pulse by Binghu).

lao in relation to the position; by saying that it is full, large, wiry, long it is *lao* in relation to the shape, consistency.'[49]

Diagnosis

- Fullness of cold on the inside.

Notes

Severe: the accumulation of cold on the inside corresponds to an exhaustion of *yang* that causes a lack of *qi* on the surface of the pulse.

CU 促-Hurried

Classic Description

'The *cu* pulse comes and goes quickly, sometimes it stops and then comes back as if it had tripped; its speed is inconstant.'[50]

Diagnosis

- Heat and fire penetrating in the three *jiao* or in the organs.
- *Qi*, blood and phlegm stasis.

Notes

Severe: The fire has produced a deep disorder of *yin* and *yang*.

DONG 动-jumping

Classic Description

'The *dong* pulse can be perceived in the middle-*guan* position, it has no head nor tail, it is as big as a soya bean and it moves as though it was rolling.'[51]

Diagnosis

- Disordered *yin* and *yang* following fear or fright.

Notes

Severe: the disorder of the *yin* and *yang* and of the rising and descending *qi* movements prevents the flow of the pulse, which appears to be jumping or quivering.

FU 浮-Hidden

Classic Description

'*Fu* means hidden, covert, the *fu* pulse is even lower than the *chen*-deep pulse, we can only feel it by separating the tendons and reaching the bones.'[52]

Diagnosis

- Pathogens hidden on the inside, *jue* (syncope–inversion of the *qi*).

Notes

Severe: the pathogens persist in depth, obstruct the *qi* and can result in *jue*.

SHI GUAIMAI 'the ten Strange Pulses' 十怪脉

There are another seven pulses, which indicate approaching death: *quezhuo* 雀啄 (pecking sparrow), *yuxiang* 鱼翔 (swaying fish), *xiayou* 虾游 (darting lobster), *fufei* 釜沸 (boiling pot), *wulou* 屋漏 (leaking roof), *tanshi* 弹石 (clacking stones), *jiesuo* 解索 (shredded rope); and three others: *yandao* 偃刀 (blade turned upwards), *zhuandou* 转豆 (rotating bean) and *macu* 麻促 (hurried sesame seed).

---

[49] *Zhenjia zhengyan* (The correct eye of the diagnosis).
[50] *Binghu maixue* (The science of the pulse by Binghu).
[51] *Maijing* (Classic of the pulses).
[52] *Zhenjia zhengyan* (The correct eye of the diagnosis).

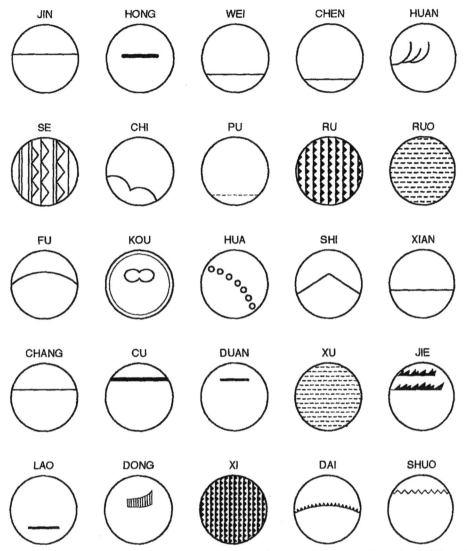

Figure A.1 Classic representations of the pulses, from the article by Laura Caretto, *I polsi nei classici* ('The pulses in the classics'), *MediCina*, summer 1996.

Appendix B

NOTES ON DIAGNOSTIC FRAMING IN CONVENTIONAL PSYCHIATRY

The patients treated in general medicine present a vast majority of depression, anxiety and somatoform disorders that can be greatly disabling.[1]

The most common symptomatology includes symptoms such as easily tired, gastroenterological disorders, headaches, dysmenorrhoea, feelings of instability, of thoracic constraint, of abdominal swelling, pain or muscle contraction, and insomnia, with no internal or neurological problems.

In Chinese medicine the procedure is different and in the clinical practice the superimposition of different symptomatological clusters is quite common.[2] Yet, since the most widespread psychiatric classification (DSM-IV) distinguishes these three categories, we have decided to report here the diagnostic criteria of a number of patterns which are most common in the practice of acupuncturists; those to which we have referred in the text; those that will be useful to the orientation of the reader in the region of mental illnesses.

Anxiety, Depression, Neurosis and Psychosis

This passage does not deal with the terminology and nosological questions that still exist in institutional psychiatry. It is a space where we remember a basic terminology that is more directly connected with the themes discussed in this text.

The current English term is *anxiety*, the German one is *Angst*; they are linked to the terms anxiousness and anguish.[3] 'Anguish' is a term that is now less used in psychiatry, but it is sometimes preferred when there are exceptionally spectacular somatic manifestations.

In states of anxiety there are worrying, apprehension, and restlessness which are scarcely controllable, too often they are accompanied by muscle tension, difficulty in concentrating, or disturbed sleep.

Depression was once called melancholia. It consists of a dysthymic disorder, a shift of the mood towards a deep sadness with a reduction of self-esteem, sense of

---

[1] A OMS study has examined 25 000 patients in 15 general medicine ambulatories of 14 different nations: among the 5500 who were submitted to further psychiatric tests, 25% suffered from a mental disorder (depression in 10%, anxiety in 8% of the cases). In: Sartorius, N. et al, Depression comorbid with Anxiety: Results from the WHO Study on Psychological Disorders in Primary Care, *British Journal of Psychiatry*, 168, 1996.

[2] The meta-studies show a strong association between anxiety and depression: from 33% to 85% of cases. In: Maser, J.D., Cloninger C.R., eds, *Comorbidity of Mood and Anxiety Disorders*, American Psychiatric Press, 1990.

[3] 'Anguish is a philosophical term introduced by Kirkegaard to designate the condition of the world. While Fear is always something definite, Anguish does not refer to any precise object. Instead it designates the emotional state of the human existence which is not reality but *possibility*, in the sense that humans become what they are on the basis of their choices and of the possibilities which they accomplish.' Translation from: Galimberti, 1992.

Freud gives a psychogenetic definition, as opposed to the previous psychiatric one, which would consider it as an alteration of the vegetative system.

guilt and need for self-punishment. It produces somatic and neurovegetative disorders such as insomnia, lack of appetite, diminishing of sexual interest, hepatobiliary dysfunction ('melancholia' originally meant 'black spleen'), alterations of the affections, with feelings full of a deep and persistent sadness, insensibility under external stimulations; loss of interest in life, with apathy in the behaviour and inhibition of thought processes.

In neurosis the function of reality is preserved, the subject maintains a critical consciousness so that he/she is aware of the absurdity of certain fantasies or anxieties; its social adaptation is usually acceptable. In the Freudian model, neurosis is a dysfunctional expression of the displacement of individual and instinctive requests in the frame of the conflict between the former and the social rules of coexistence.[4]

In contrast, in psychosis there is a deep alteration in the evaluation of reality; breakdown at deep levels of the personality; excess or flattening of imagination and feelings; loss of boundaries between the body and the external world and a consequent sense of inviolability of one's thoughts; alteration of the logical thought, hallucinations and delusions; and social disarrangement. The psychosis corresponds to a fracture between the self and the external reality caused by the pressure of instinctive requests on the self, which then tends to build an individual reality in its delirium.

The DSM: Diagnostic and Statistic Manual of Mental Disorders

Here are the specific reports of the diagnostic criteria of certain patterns according to the definitions of the DSM-IV. 'The DSM-IV is a classification of mental disorders that was designed to be used in clinical, didactic and research areas.'[5]

The DSM is a non-theoretical and descriptive text, with a nosology of a categorial type: it defines the classes of disorders using inclusion and exclusion criteria, specifying possible subtypes and developments, and attributing a series of codes which allow the computerisation of the data. The approach adopted follows a descriptive methodology, with a structure that does not include any reflection on the mechanisms of origin and development of the illness, nor any interpretation hypothesis or reference to their conceptual frames.

The first edition of the DSM-I is dated 1952, and is a variation of the classification set by the World Health Organisation ICD-6 (International Classification of Diseases, WHO). The DSM-III was published in 1980 and presented different methodological innovations such as the definition of explicit criteria for diagnosis, a multiaxial system, and a descriptive approach free of aetiological theories. The version DSM-IV-R, compatible with the ICD-10, was compiled using the new data obtained from research on diagnosis and it takes into consideration certain cultural differences and particularly the Culturally Characterised Syndromes.

Generalised Anxiety Disorder

A. Excessive anxiety and worry (apprehensive expectation) occurring more days than not for at least 6 months, about a number of events or activities (such as work or school performance).

B. The person finds it difficult to control the worry.

C. The anxiety and worry are associated with three (or more) of the following six symptoms (with at least some symptoms present for more days than not for the past 6 months):
   1. restlessness or feeling keyed up or on edge;
   2. being easily fatigued;
   3. difficulty concentrating or mind going blank;
   4. irritability;
   5. muscle tension;
   6. sleep disturbance (difficulty falling or staying asleep, or restless unsatisfied sleep).

D. The focus of the anxiety and worry is not confined to features of an Axis I disorder [...].

E. The anxiety, worry, or physical symptoms cause clinically significant distress or impairment in social, occupational, or other important areas of functioning.

---

[4] For example see: Sigmund Freud, *Neurosis and Psychosis*, 1923.
[5] DSM-IV, 1994, p. xxiii.

F. The disturbance is not due to the direct physiological effects of a substance (e.g. a drug abuse, a medication) or a general medical condition (e.g. Hyperthyroidism) and does not occur exclusively during a Mood Disorder, a Psychotic Disorder, or a Pervasive Developmental Disorder.

Panic Attack

It consists of an episode of great fear or discomfort in which at least 4 out of the 13 somatic symptoms listed below reaches its peak within 10 minutes.

1. palpitations, pounding heart, accelerated heart rate;
2. sweating;
3. trembling or shaking;
4. sensations of shortness of breath or smothering;
5. feeling of choking;
6. chest pain or discomfort;
7. nausea or abdominal distress;
8. feeling dizzy, unsteady, lightheaded, or fainting;
9. derealisation (feelings of unreality) or depersonalisation (being detached from oneself);
10. fear of losing control or going crazy;
11. fear of dying;
12. paresthesiae (numbness or tingling sensations);
13. chills or hot flushes.

The Panic Attack Disorder tends to become chronic. In those cases in which the disorder can be reduced by avoiding certain situations, patients tend to construct a behaviour that interferes with their normal social life.
The PAD poses some problems for differential diagnosis with pathologies that are both intrinsic and psychiatric and this often causes a delay in the diagnosis or the impossibility of recognising a specific pathology. On the contrary for the patient it is extremely important to have a diagnosis. In fact the belief of having a severe and unrecognised illness, organic or psychiatric, can lead to a state of continuous anxiety, demoralisation and depression, and to an anticipatory fear, all of which are elements that often involve the abuse of medicines and alcohol and the evolving of the disorder into a chronic state.

Dysthymic Disorder

A. Depressed mood for most of the day, for more days than not, as indicated either by subjective account or observation by others, for at least 2 years.
B. Presence, while depressed, of two (or more) of the following:
    1. poor appetite or overeating;
    2. insomnia or hypersomnia;
    3. low energy or fatigue;
    4. low self-esteem;
    5. poor concentration or difficulty in making decisions;
    6. feelings of hopelessness.
C. During the 2-year period (1 year for children or adolescents) of the disturbance, the person has never been without the symptoms in criteria A and B for more than 2 months at a time.
D. During the first 2 years there were no episodes of Major Depressive Disorder.

We must also exclude a Manic or Hypomanic or Cyclothymic Episode or Chronic Psychotic Disorder, the effects of substances or a general medical condition. The symptoms must cause a significant clinical distress or impairment of social, occupational, or other important areas of functioning.

Major Depressive Episode

A. Five (or more) of the following symptoms have been present during the same 2-week period and represent a change from the previous functioning; at least one of the symptoms is either 1) depressed mood or 2) loss of interest and pleasure:
    1. depressed mood most of the day, nearly every day, as indicated by either subjective report (e.g. feels sad or empty) or observation made by others (e.g. appears tearful);
    2. markedly diminished interest or pleasure in all, or almost all, activities most of the day, nearly every day (as indicated by either subjective report or observation made by others);
    3. significant weight loss when not dieting or weight gain (e.g. a significant change of more than 5% of body weight in a month), or decrease or increase in appetite nearly every day;

4. insomnia or hypersomnia nearly every day;

5. psychomotor agitation or retardation nearly every day (observable by others, not merely subjective feelings of restlessness or being slowed down);

6. fatigue or loss of energy nearly every day;

7. feelings of worthlessness or excessive or inappropriate guilt (which may be delusional) nearly every day (not merely self-reproach or guilt about being sick);

8. diminished ability to think or concentrate, or indecisiveness, nearly every day (either by subjective account or as observed by others);

9. recurrent thoughts without specific plan, or a suicide attempt or a specific plan for committing suicide.

B. The symptoms do not meet the criteria for a Mixed Episode.

C. The symptoms cause clinically significant distress or impairment in social, occupational, or other important areas of functioning.

D. The symptoms are not due to the direct physiological effects of a substance (e.g. drug abuse, a medication), or a general medical condition (e.g. hypothyroidism).

E. The symptoms are not better accounted for by bereavement, i.e. after the loss of a loved one, the symptoms persist for longer than 2 months or are characterised by marked functional impairment, morbid worrying with worthlessness, suicidal ideation, psychotic symptoms, or psychomotor retardation.

Manic Episode

A. A distinct period of abnormally and persistently elevated, expansive, or irritable mood, lasting at least 1 week (or any duration if hospitalisation is necessary).

B. During the period of mood disturbance, three (or more) of the following symptoms have persisted (four if the mood is only irritable) and have been present to a significant degree:

1. inflated self-esteem or grandiosity;

2. decreased need for sleep (e.g. feels rested after only 3 hours of sleep);

3. more talkative than usual or pressure to keep talking;

4. flight of ideas or subjective experience that thoughts are racing;

5. distractibility (i.e. attention too easily drawn to unimportant or irrelevant external stimuli);

6. increase in goal directed activity (either socially, at work or school, or sexually) or psychomotor agitation;

7. excessive involvement in pleasurable activities that have a high potential for painful consequences (e.g. engaging in unrestrained buying sprees, sexual indiscretions, or foolish business investments).

Moreover: the symptoms do not satisfy the criteria for other disorders, they are sufficiently severe to cause a noticeable impairment, they are not caused by the direct effect of a substance or a general medical condition.

The diagnosis of Hypomanic Episode follows similar criteria. The main difference is in the fact that, even though changes in the behaviour and action may be noticed by others, the episode is not severe enough to cause a major impairment in social or occupational areas nor to call for hospitalisation, and there are no psychotic manifestations.

Somatisation Disorder

A. A history of many physical complaints beginning before age 30 years that occur over a period of several years and result in treatment being sought or significant impairment in social, occupational, or other important areas of functioning.

B. Each of the following criteria must have been met, with individual symptoms occurring at any time during the course of disturbance:

1. *four pain symptoms*: a history of pain related to at least four different sites of functions (e.g. head, abdomen, back, joints, extremities, chest, rectum, during menstruation, during sexual intercourse, or during urination);

2. *two gastrointestinal symptoms*: a history of at least two gastrointestinal symptoms other than pain (e.g. nausea, bloating, vomiting other than during pregnancy, diarrhoea, or intolerance of several different foods);

3. *one sexual symptom*: a history of at least one sexual or reproductive symptom other than pain (e.g. sexual indifference, erectile or ejaculatory

dysfunction, irregular menses, excessive menstrual bleeding, vomiting throughout pregnancy);

4. *one pseudoneurological symptom*: a history of at least one symptom or deficit suggesting a neurological condition not limited to pain (conversion symptoms such as impaired coordination or balance, paralysis or localised weakness, difficulty in swallowing or a feeling of a lump in the throat, aphonia, urinary retention, hallucinations, loss of touch or pain sensation, double vision, blindness, deafness, seizures; dissociative symptoms such as amnesia; or loss of consciousness other than fainting).

C. Either 1) or 2):

1. after appropriate investigation, each of the symptoms in Criterion B cannot be fully explained by a known general medical condition or the direct effects of a substance (e.g. a drug of abuse, a medication);

2. when there is a related general medical condition, the physical complaints or resulting social or occupational impairment are in excess of what would be expected from the history, physical examination, or laboratory findings.

D. The symptoms are not intentionally produced or feigned (as in Factitious Disorder or Malingering).

The Undifferentiated Somatoform Disorder includes one or more physical complaints (e.g. tiredness, lack of appetite, gastrointestinal or urinary disorders) and a clinically significant distress, but the only time criterion is a duration of the symptom of at least 6 months. Criteria C and D of the Somatisation Disorder must also be respected.

Appendix C

TCM ON THE INTERNET

These brief annotations are not designed to offer a complete picture of the websites linked to TCM and its specific applications; this is impossible owing to the vastness of the field and to the speed of evolution on the web, which prevents the production of complete and precise information.

We have selected the sites that are the most involved with research and with the deepening and widening of the study of TCM. We have excluded those sites whose primary aim is to promote courses, sell material or propose therapies, avoiding any judgement on the significance of their work. The data have been gathered with the collaboration of Monica Curioni.

World Wide Web

We refer mainly to the English-speaking area but we remember that other linguistic areas such as France have a long tradition of acupuncture. A way to obtain an overview of the existing websites is, for example, to search for 'acupuncture' in Yahoo.france or other search engines specifying the nation in which one is interested.

The panorama of English-language websites is vast, there are thousands. Among the most well organised, which are also interactive, are the following:

http://www.acubriefs.com/newsletter is a newsletter that can be read and to which you can send comments and papers.

http://www.acupuncture.com offers a section for 'Treatment Testimonials', comments from patients; a 'Forum Message Board' where it is possible to share opinions; a rich and up to date 'News' section; the directory 'Aculinks – Oriental Medicine across the Web' proposing a vast choice of websites.

http://www.acupuncturetoday.com has a well-frequented discussion forum, open to both therapists and patients. It has a rich and up to date 'Archives' section, which includes the work on the treatment of anxiety with auriculotherapy (acupuncturetoday.com/archives2001/may/05anxiety.html).

http://www.bluepoppy.com is the website of the Blue Poppy Enterprises: well organised, it focuses on the distribution of books published by Blue Poppy press. It is notable because it covers a vast TCM horizon, including subjects in the psychological area. In the website there is also an online review to which you can subscribe and to which articles can be sent (bob@bluepoppy.com).

http://www.ejom.co.uk, edited by the British Council of Acupuncture, is connected with 'The European Journal of Oriental Medicine', a review that gives particular attention to matters that relate to Chinese medicine in its totality. Under subscription the website offers the possibility of accessing the published articles.

http://www.jcm.co.uk/ is the website of 'The Journal of Chinese Medicine', one of the main publications for clinical and theoretical reference. It is possible to send clinical cases and read the most recent contributions (http://www.jcm.co.uk/SampleArticles.html). There is an updated 'News' section (http://www.jcm.co.uk/News.html) and the bookshop catalogue is rich and up to date.

http://www.medicalacupuncture.org/aama_marf/journal/index.html is an American acupuncture review in which one can find articles, poster presentations and case reports.

http://www.paradigm-pubs.com is the website of Paradigm Publications press, presenting in its catalogue the book 'Soothing the Troubled Mind' on clinical studies of schizophrenia treated with moxa and acupuncture. Connected to this text there is the possibility of accessing various clinical histories in the psychiatric/psychological area (http://www.paradigm-pubs.com/paradigm/refs/soothingcases).

http://www.TCMcentral.com is a space with open forums, for patients and therapists. It has a TCM chatroom: it gives the impression of being slightly disorganised but interesting.

Italy

An online discussion at a national level is still under construction. There are more than 700 sites in which the word 'acupuncture' appears: from schools to rest homes, from unconventional medicine sites to the institutional site of the Chinese Popular Republic.

The sites that focus more on the construction of discussion areas are the following:

http://www.agopuntura-fisa.it is the website of the FISA – Federazione Italiana Società Agopuntura (Italian Federation of Acupuncture Societies), useful for all that relates to schools and acupuncture doctors. It has a 'Questions and answers' section, which unfortunately is still under construction, but which is a good project to start a debate among an audience with clinical abilities and needs.

http://www.agopuntura.org gives access to an open forum, which unfortunately tends to be dispersive because it deals with all types of unconventional medicine (http://www.promiseleland.it/forum/).

http://www.fondazionericci.it is the website of the Matteo Ricci Foundation. It offers an up to date 'News Area'; an active discussion forum; the index of the articles published on the 'Rivista Italiana di MTC' (rivitmtc@tin.it). It also has a good section of links, many of which are addresses of Chinese TCM Universities.

http://www.planet.it/freewww/ass.medicin is the website of the Association MediCina. In addition to the presentation of courses and seminaries it has the intention of functioning as a cultural meeting place: every 2 months it proposes new articles on different subjects of TCM and reports the results of certain research works.

Appendix D

BASIC CHRONOLOGY

Zhou Period (c.1040–22BC)

Qin Period (221–207BC)

Western Han Period (202BC–AD24)

Eastern Han Period (AD24–220)

Three Kingdoms Period (AD220–265)

Jin Period (AD265–420)

Northern and Southern Dynasties Period (AD420–589) (Six Dynasties)

Sui Period (AD589–618)

Tang Period (AD618–907)

Five Dynasties Period (AD907–960)

Song Period (AD960–1279)

Yuan Period (Mongolians) (AD1279–1368)

Ming Period (AD1368–1644)

Qing Period (AD1644–1911)

First Republic of China (AD1911–1949)

People's Republic of China

Appendix E

GLOSSARY

Agitation-*zao* 躁. Often used together with restlessness-*fan* 烦. See the pertinent chapter (Chapter 6).

Anger-*nu* 怒. See the chapter on emotions (Chapter 2).

Anguish-*you* 忧. Term that often appears in the discussion on emotions (Chapter 2).

Apprehension-*lü* 虑. Term that appears often in the discussion on emotions (Chapter 2). It also means 'reflection', as in Chapter 8 of the *Lingshu*.

Calm-*an* 安. 'Calming, peace'. The term is similar to *jing* 精 and *ning* 宁. *An* is often used in relation to the heart *qi*.

Communicating-*jiao* 交. 'To unite, to cross; reciprocal' (the character shows a person with crossed legs). It usually refers to the relation between heart and kidney, water and fire (see also Chapter 22).

Conducting-*dao* 导. This refers to *qi*. See also the discussion on the internal practices of *daoyin* (Chapter1) and on needle stimulation techniques (Chapter12).

Confusion-*huo* 惑. A classical term, it usually refers to serious disorders of the *shen* but also of the appetite, sleep and sight.

Conscience-*shi* 识. Term that belongs essentially to philosophical discourse.

Constraint-*yu* 郁. See the pertinent chapter (Chapter 4).

Correct *qi-zhengqi* 正气. 'Upright'. Sometimes it is translated as 'antipathogenic *qi*', it opposes to the pathogen *qi* 邪气 *xieqi*, deviated, evil, irregular qi.

Damaging-*sun* 损. 'Damage, loss'. It is serious because it refers to the consumption of substance.

Easiness-*shang* 伤, 'Disposition', for example to fear or to excessive dreaming.

Emotions-*qing zhi* 情志. See the pertinent chapter (Chapter 2) and the terminology discussion in the introduction.

Euphoria-*xi* 喜. See the chapter on emotions (Chapter 2) and the terminology discussion in the introduction.

Exhaustion-*lao* 劳. 'Heavy physical work; fatigue'. It is mainly connected with the *qi* but it can also be used with a general sense.

Fear-*kong* 恐. See the chapter on emotions (Chapter 2).

Fright-*jing* 精. See the chapter on emotions (Chapter 2).

Fullness-*shi* 识 **and emptiness-*xu*** 虚.[1]

Ghosts and spirits-*guishen* 鬼神. See the discussion on the *gui*-ghost (Chapter 3).

Happiness-*le* 乐. See the chapter on emotions (Chapter 2) and the terminology discussion in the introduction.

Harmonising-*he* 和. This refers to the emotions and to the *qi* in its various forms, including blood.

---

[1] The other two couples with a similar meaning are: *youyu* 忧郁 'to have in excess' and *buzu* 不足 'insufficient'; *sheng* 盛 'strong, flourishing, in excess' and *shuai* 衰 'weak'.

Heart-*xin* 心. A term used also as a synonym of *shen*. For its use in many modern terms see the terminology discussion in the introduction.

Heart orifices-*xinqiao* 心 窍. Openings of the heart, in relation with *shen* and conscience. See also the chapter on madness-*diankuang* (Chapter 8) and the chapter on clinic (Chapter 10).[2]

Hitting-*shang* 伤. 'To wound, to damage' (the antique form of the character contained an arrow).

Inversion-*jue* 厥. This means loss of consciousness both in the classical language and in the modern use, but it also implies a coldness rising from the extremity towards the centre.[3]

Counterflow-*qini* 气 逆. 'Rebel *qi*, upstream *qi*', which rises oppositely to the physiological movement of the *qi*.[4]

Knotting-*jie* 结. Also means 'to knot', 'knotted' and it usually refers to the *qi* and phlegm.

Mess-*luan* 乱. In this context it refers to the movements of the *qi*. See also the discussion on needle stimulation techniques (Chapter 12).

Nourishing life-*yangsheng* 养 生. See the chapter on internal practices and *qigong* (Chapter 1).

Nutritious *qi-yingqi* 营 气. In the classical texts it is also called *rongqi*. It often appears in relation to the defensive *qi-weiqi* 卫 气 to define more internal or external areas.

Original *qi-yuanqi* 原 气. In close relationship with the anterior heaven – *xiantian* 先 天, also referred to as *yuanshen* 原 神.

Pathogenic *qi-xieqi* 邪 气. 'Deviated *qi*', translated in contemporary texts as 'external pathogen factors', or as 'perverse energies'.[5]

Phlegm-*tan* 痰. Also translated as 'mucus, catarrh'. See also the chapter on constraint-*yu* (Chapter 4) and the chapter on clinic (Chapter 10).

Regulating-*tiao* 调. Generally used in acupuncture with reference to the regulation of the *qi* and blood, *tiao qi xue* 调 气 血.[6]

Responding-*ying* 应. 'Reacting', it is combined with *gan* 感 'awaken, stimulate, influence'. It indicates the spontaneous and immediate relations that precede thought. See also the discussion on Chinese thought (Chapter 1).[7]

Restlessness-*fan* 烦. See the chapter on *fanzao* (Chapter 6).

Sadness-*bei* 悲. See the chapter on emotions (Chapter 2).

Shape-*xing* 形. Term also used commonly in the classics to define that which can be seen, i.e. the body, as opposed to *qi* or *shen*.

Shifting-*dong* 动. The term appears in the classics with reference to the emotions, to the 'centre'.[8]

Sorrow-*ai* 哀. Term that often appears in the discussion on emotions (Chapter 2).

---

[2] Whereas *qingqiao* 清 窍 are the 'pure-clear orifices', generally corresponding to the sensory organs. Verbs related to *xinqiao* 心 窍 are: *mi*-cloud 迷 , *kai*-aprire 开 , *zu*-obstruct 组 , *meng*-blunt 蒙 and *qing*-purify 清 .

[3] This is a serious sign, which derives from a severe disorder of the movement of the *qi*, an inversion of the circulation of yin and yang. It mostly shows itself in the four limbs, with rise of the cold because *qi* and *yang* cannot reach the extremities, or in the head, *jueni* 厥 逆 with syncope. The character has a radical 'cliff' and the phonetic part consists of *ni* 'inversion, obstruction', and *qian* 'yawn, lack'. It also means 'exhaustion', as in *jueyin* 厥 阴 , the state in which the *yin* exhausts and transforms into its opposite. Wiseman translates it as *reversal* and explains it as 1.fainting or syncope; 2. cold which expands in an opposite direction from the extremities upwards.

[4] Wiseman translates it as *qi counterflow*. Originally it was composed of the only radical 'person' *da* written backwards. If it hits the lung it produces cough, asthma, thoracic oppression, if it hits the stomach it produces hiccups, nausea, vomit, and if it rises to the head it produces migraine, vertigo and disorders in the sensory orifices.

[5] Wiseman translates it as *evil* and defines it as 'any entity that threatens the health from the outside or from the inside'. He includes the six excesses, heat, and the various types of toxins.

[6] On the contrary to regulate the *qi* or blood with prescriptions *li* 理 is more commonly used. In general one can also say *tiao li* 调 理.

[7] This concept of a response without mediation of the thought can also be found in philosophical treaties such as the *Zhuangzi* or the *Yijing*, but also in medical texts like the *Neijing*.

[8] It means 'to move, movement' but, since it if often used to describe a pathological action (*shi dong* 是 动 is the term that unites all the channels in the description of the pathology, for example in Chapter 10 of the *Lingshu*), we have chosen to distinguish the translation. Also used to describe a characteristic of the pulse.

Spreading and draining-*shuxie* 疏泄. A term commonly used in relation to the liver. See the specific discussion in the chapter on constraint-*yu* (Chapter 4).

Stabilising-*ding* 定. Usually used in relation to *zhi* 志. As 'concentrate' *zhuan* 专 it can be found in the discussion on *jing, shen, yangsheng*. See also the discussion on *zhi* (Chapter 3).

Stagnation-*zhi* 滞. This is generally referred to *qi*, whereas for the blood we use stasis-*yu* 郁

Thought-*si* 思. See the chapter on emotions (Chapter 2) and the terminology discussion in the Introduction.

Trepidation-*ju* 惧. See the chapter on emotions (Chapter 2).

True *qi-zhenqi* 真气. 'Authentic, genuine', it indicates all the *qi*, including *yuanqi* 原气.

Urgent-*ji* 积. This refers to a feeling of urgency.[9]

Worrying-*chou* 愁. Term that often appears in the discussion on emotions (Chapter 2).

For the terms *shen* 神, *hun* 魂, *po* 魄, *yi* 意 and *zhi* 志 see the specific discussion (Chapter 3).

Ai, sorrow

An, calm

Bei, sadness

Chou, worrying

Dao, conducting

Ding, stabilising

Dong, shifting

Fan, restlessness

Guishen, ghosts and spirits

He, harmonising

Huo, confusion

Ji, urgent

Jiao, communicating

Jie, knotting

Jing, fright

Ju, trepidation

Jue, inversion

Kong, fear

Lao, exhaustion

Le, joy

Lü, apprehension

Luan, mess

Nu, anger

Qingzhi, emotions

Qini, counterflowing *qi*

Shang, easiness

Shang, hitting

Shi, fullness

Shi, conscience

Shuxie, spreading and draining

Si, thought

Sun, damaging

Tan, phlegm

Tiao, regulating

Xi, euphoria

Xieqi, pathogenic *qi*

Xin, heart

Xing, shape

Xingqiao, ear orifices

Xu, emptiness

Yangshen, nourishing life

Ying, responding

Yingqi, nutritious *qi*

You, anguish

Yu, constraint

Yuanqi, original *qi*

Zao, agitation

Zhenqi, true *qi*

Zhi, stagnation

---

[9] It recurs in cases in which there is an acute symptom to which one feels the need of putting an end urgently, it can be related to heart, liver, *Chong Mai* 冲脉, abdomen, anus, or stomach. Also used to describe a characteristic of the pulse.

Appendix F

BIBLIOGRAPHY

Classical Sources

Cao Xiaozhong et al., *Shenji zonglu*, (Imperial medicine encyclopaedia, 1117). Cheng Yunlai (ed.), *Shenji zonglu zuanyao* (Selection from the Imperial medicine encyclopaedia), in Cao Bingzhang (ed.), *Zhongguo yixue dacheng,* vol L.

Chao Yuanfang, *Zhubing yuanhoulun* (Treatise on the origin and symptoms of illnesses, 610). Ding Guangdi (ed.), Zhongyi guji chubanshe, Beijing, 1991.

Chen Menglei et al., *Gujin tushu jicheng, yibu quanlu* (Collection of images and ancient and modern books, complete register of works on medicine, 1725). Renmin weisheng chubanshe, Beijing, 1988, 12 vols.

Chen Shiduo, *Shishi milu* (Secret notes on the stone chamber, 1751). In: Qiu Peiran (ed.), *Zhongguo yixue dacheng sanbian*, vol.IX.

Chen Wuze, *Sanyin jiyi bingzheng fanglun* (Treatise on the three categories of illness causes, 1174), Renmin weisheng chubanshe, Beijing, 1983.

Cheng Guopeng (Cheng Zhongling), *Yixue xinwu* (Medicine revelations, 1732). In: Cao Bingzhang (ed.), *Zhongguo yixue dacheng*, vol. XLVI, Shanghai kexue jishu chubanshe, Shanghai, 1990.

Dai Sigong (1324–1405), *Zhengzhi yaojue* (Essential elements of diagnosis and therapy).

Dou Hanqin (Dou Jie), *Zhenjing zhinan* (Guide to the classics of acupuncture, 1295). It contains: 'Biaoyoufu' (Ode to reveal the mysteries) and 'Tongxuan zhiyaofu' (Ode to understand the basic principles of the depths). In: He Puren, *Zhenjiu geshu lingchuan yingyong* (Clinical use of odes on acupuncture and moxibustion), Kexue jishu wenxian chubanshe, Beijing, 1992.

Gao Wu, *Zhenjiu juying* (Glorious collection of acupuncture and moxibustion, 1529), Renmin weisheng chubanshe, Beijing, 1995. It contains: 'Yulongfu' (Ode for the jade dragon), 'Xuqiufu guibing shisanxuege' (Chant of the thirteen points of the *gui* illnesses by master Xu), 'Baizhenfu' (Ode of the hundred symptoms), 'Zabing shiyixuege' (Chant of the method of the point in various illnesses).

Ge Hong (281–341), *Baopuzi* (The master who embraces simplicity, ca.330). In: Qiu Peiran (ed.), *Zhongguo yixue dacheng sanbian* vol.II.

Gong Tingxian, *Shoushi baoyuan* (Reaching longevity preserving the source, 1615). Beijing, Renmin weisheng chubanshe, 1993.

Gong Xin, *Jingui yuhanjing* (Hidden treasures of the Jingui) and *Gujin yijian* (Ancient and modern medicine reflections,1589).

He Mengyao, *Yibian* (Elements of medicine, 1751). Shanghai kexue jishu chubanshe, Shanghai, 1982.

Hua Tuo, *Huashi zhongzangjing* (Classic of the organ of the centre), attributed to Huatuo but more likely a work from the period of the Six Dynasties, 317–618). In: Qiu Peiran (ed.), *Zhongguo yixue dacheng sanbian,* vol.I.

Huainanzi, Liu Wendian (ed.), Huainan honglie jijie, Shanghai, 1926.

Huangdi neijing (Medicine internal classic of the yellow emperor). Guo Aichun (ed.), 'Huangdi neijing lingshu jiaozhu yuyi' (Commented and translated critical edn of the *Huangdi neijing lingshu*), Tianjin kexue jishu chubanshi, Tianjin 1989; Guo Aichun (ed.), *Huangdi neijing suwen jiaozhu* (Commented critical edn of the *Huangdi neijing suwen*), Renmin weisheng chubanshi, Beijing 1992.

Huangfu Mi, *Zhenjiu jiayijing* (The systematic classic of acupuncture and moxibustion, 259). In: Xu Guoren (ed), *Jiayijing jiaozhu*, Renmin weisheng chubanshe, Beijing, 1996.

Kong Yingda (574–648), *Wujing zhengyi* (The correct meaning of the five classics).

Kou Zongshi, *Bencao yanyi* (Development of the meaning of the Bencao, 1116).

Li Chan (Li Jianzhai), *Yixue rumen* (Introduction to medicine, 1575).

Li Dongyuan, *Lanshi mizang* (The secrets of the orchid chamber, 1336). In Ye Chuan (ed.) *Jinyuan sida yixuejia mingzhu jicheng*, Zhongguo zhongyiyao chubanshe, Beijing, 1995.

Li Dongyuan, *Neiwai shangge bianhuolun* (Treatise on the differentiation in the confusion on the damages from internal and external causes, 1231). In: Ye Chuan (ed.) *Jinyuan sida yixuejia mingzhu jicheng*, Zhongguo zhongyiyao chubanshe, Beijing, 1995.

Li Dongyuan, *Piwei lun* (Treatise on spleen and stomach, 1249). In: Ye Chuan (ed.) *Jinyuan sida yixuejia mingzhu jicheng*, Zhongguo zhongyiyao chubanshe, Beijing, 1995.

Li Zhongzi, *Yizong bidu* (Essential readings of the medical tradition, 1637). Zou Gaoqi (ed.), Renmin weisheng chubanshe, Beijing, 1995.

Liu Wansu (or Liu Hejian), *Suwen xuanji yuanbingshi* (Exam of the original patterns of the illness of the mysterious mechanisms of the Suwen, 1182). In Ye Chuan (ed.), *Jinyuan sida yixuejia mingzhu jicheng*, Zhongguo zhongyiyao chubanshe, Beijing, 1995.

Luo Tianyi, *Weisheng baojian* (Precious mirror for the defence of life, 1281), Renmin weisheng chubanshe, Beijing, 1987.

Lushi chunqiu (Annuals of spring and autumn), In Xu Weiyu (ed.), *Lushi chunqiu jishi, Shangwu yinshuguan*, Beijing, 1955.

Ma Shi, *Huangdi neijing suwen zhuzheng fawei* (Study and comment of the *Huangdi neijing suwen*) and *Huangdi neijing lingshu zhuzheng fawei* (Study and comment of the *Huangdi neijing lingshu*, 1586).

Mengzi, Yang Boyun (ed.), Zhonghua Shizhu, Beijing, 1960.

Nanjing (Classic of difficulties, 1st century BC), Renmin weisheng chubanshe, Beijing, 1989.

Qi Shi, *Lixu yuanjian* (Mirror of the treatment of emptiness of the origin, 1771). In Cao Bingzhang (ed.), *Zhongguo yixue dacheng*, vol. XIX.

Qin Bowei, *Lunganbing Qin Bowei yiwenji* (Collection of medical writings on liver illnesses by Qin Bowei), 1928.

Shi Dinan (Shoutang), *Yiyuan* (The origin of medicine), 1861. In Cao Bingzhang (ed.), *Zhongguo yixue dacheng*, 1990, vol XXI.

Sun Simiao, *Beiji qianjin yaofang* (or *Qianjin yaofang*) (Remedies worth a thousand golden pieces for urgencies, 625), Renmin weisheng chubanshe, Beijing, 1955. It contains: 'Sun zhenren shisan guixuege' (Chant of the thirteen *gui* points by Sun Zhenren).

Sun Simiao, *Qianjin yifang* (Supplement to the thousand golden remedies, 682).

Sun Yikui, *Chishui xuanzhu* (The mystical pearl of the purple water, 1573). Renmin weisheng chubanshe, Beijing, 1988.

Tang Zonghai (or Tang Rongchuan), *Jingui yaolue qianzhu buzheng* (Comment and correction of the Jingui yaolue, 1893).

Tang Zonghai (or Tang Rongchuan), *Xuezhenglun* (Treatise on the illnesses of the blood, 1884), Pei Zhengxue (ed.), Renmin weisheng chubanshe, Beijing, 1979.

Tang Zonghai (or Tang Rongchuan), *Zhongxiyi huitong yijing jingyi* (Essential meaning of the classics in the connection between Chinese and Western medicine, 1892).

Wang Bing, *Zhu Huangdi suwen* (Commentary to the *Huangdi suwen*, 762)

Wang Guorui, *Bianque shenying zhenjiu yulong jing* (Spiritual classic of the jade dragon by Bianque, 1329). In Qiu Peiran (ed.), *Zhongguo yixue dacheng sanbian*, vol.IX. It contains: 'Yulongge' (Chant of the jade dragon) and 'Ma danyang tianxing shierxue bingzhi zabingge' (Chant by Ma Danyang of the twelve star points for the treatment of various illnesses).

Wang Huaiyin, *Taiping shenghui fang* (Wise prescriptions from the Taiping period, 992).

Wang Ketang, *Zhengzhi zhunsheng* (Clinical patterns and treatments,1602). Shanghai guji chubanshe, Shanghai, 1991.

Wang Kuang *Quansheng zhimi fang* (Secrets for the preservation of the integrity of life, ca.1150). In Qiu Peiran (ed.), *Zhongguo yixue dacheng sanbian,* vol. IV.

Wang Qingren, *Yilin gaicuo* (Correction of the mistakes in medicine works, 1830). Zhongguo zhongyiyao chubanshe, Beijing,1995.

Wang Shuhe, *Maijing* (Classic of the pulse, 316), Renmin weisheng chubanshe, Beijing,1988.

Wang Tao, *Waitai miyao* (Secret remedies of a functionary, 752). Beijing, Huaxia chubanshe, 1993.

Wang Weiyi, *Tongren shuxue zhenjiu tujing* (Illustrated classic of the points of the bronze statue, 1027). In Qiu Peiran (ed.) *Zhongguo yixue dacheng sanbian*, vol. X.

Wei Zhixiu, *Xu mingyi leian* (Continuation of the Clinical cases of famous doctors, 1770). In Qiu Peiran (ed.) *Zhongguo yixue dacheng sanbian*, vol.XI.

Wu Jian, *Yizong jinjian* (The golden mirror of medicine, 1742). Renmin weisheng chubanshi, Beijing,1992 (1st edn 1963).

Wu Kun, *Yifang kao* (Studies of medical prescriptions, 1584). In Cao Bingzhang (ed.), *Zhongguo yixue dacheng*, vol.XLIX.

Wu Shangxian (Wu Shiji), *Liyue pianwen* (Rimed discourse on new therapies, 1864), Renmin weisheng chubanshe, Beijing, 1984.

Xu Chunpu, *Gujin yitong dacheng* (Great compendium of ancient and modern medicine 1556). Cui Zhongping (ed.), Renmin weisheng chubanshe, Beijing, 1991.

Xu Dachun, *Yixue yuanliu lun* (Treatise on the origins of medicine, 1704). In: *Zhongguo yixue dacheng*, Shanghai, Shanghai kexue jishu chubanshe, 1990, vol. XLV.

Xu Feng, *Zhenjiu daquan* (Complete work of acupuncture and moxibustion, 1439). It contains: 'Tianxing shixuege' (Chant of the eleven star points) and 'Xihongfu' (Ode by Xi Hong) and 'Lingguangfu' (Ode of the splendour of the spirit).

Xu Xun (Korean), *Dongyi baojian* (The precious mirror of medicine, 1611).

Yang Jizhou, *Zhenjiu dacheng* (Great compendium of acupuncture and moxibustion, 1601), Renmin weisheng chubanshe, Beijing, 1984. It contains: 'Shenyuge' (Chant that wins the dragon).

Yang Shangshan, *Huangdi neijing taisu* (Comprehensive annotations to the *Huangdi neijing*, ca. 610), Beijing, Renmin weisheng chubanshi, 1983 (1st edn 1965).

Ye Tianshi, *Lingzhen zhinan yian* (Guide cases in clinic, 1766). Shanghai kexue jishu chubanshe, Shanghai, 1993 (1st edn 1959).

You Yi (You Zaijing), *Jingui yaolue xindian* (Personal selection from the *Jingui yaolue*, 1732).

Yu Chang (or Yu Jianyan), *Yimen falu* (Principles and prohibitions of the medical practice, 1658). Shanghai kexue jishu chubanshe, Shanghai, 1983.

Yu Tuan (Yu Tianmin), *Yixue zheng chuan* (The real tradition of medicine,1515). Renmin weisheng chubanshe, Beijing,1981.

Zhang Jiebin (Zhang Jingyue), *Jingyue quanshu* (The complete works of Jingyue, 1640), Zhongyi guji chubanshe, Beijing, 1991.

Zhang Jiebin (Zhang Jingyue), *Leijing tuyi* (Illustrated supplement to the classic of cathegories,1624). Renmin weisheng chubanshe, Beijing, 1982.

Zhang Jiebin (Zhang Jingyue), *Leijing* (The classic of categories, 1624). Renmin weisheng chubanshe, Beijing, 1995 (1st edn 1965).

Zhang Lu (Zhang Shiwan), *Zhangshi yitong* (General medicine according to master Zhang, 1695). Shanghai kexue jishu chubanshe, Shanghai, 1990 (1st edn 1963).

Zhang Mingjiu, *Toupizhen zhiliao huanjue 296 lide jingyan* (Craniopuntura in 296 casi di schizofrenia con allucinazioni), Zhongyi zazhi 6:52, 1987.

Zhang Xichun, *Yixue zhongzhong canxilu* (Notes on medicine based on tradition and taking into account the Western world, 1924). Hebei kexue jishu chubanshe, Shjiazhuang, 1985.

Zhang Yuansu (Zhang Jiegu), *Yixue qiyuan* (The origin of medical science,1186).

Zhang Zhicong (Zhang Yinan), *Huangdi neijing lingshu ju jizhu* (Collection of comments to the Lingshu, 1672). In Cao Bingzhang (ed.), *Zhongguo yixue dacheng*, 1990, vol.II

Zhang Zhicong (Zhang Yinan), *Huangdi neijing suwen jizhu* (Collection of comments to the Suwen, 1670). Shanghai kexue jishu chubanshe, Shanghai, 1980.

Zhang Zhongjing, *Jingui yaolue* (Prescriptions in the golden chamber , ca. AD220). In: Liu Duzhou (ed.), *Jingui yaolüe quanjie*, Tianjin kexue jishu chubanshe, Tianjin, 1984.

Zhang Zhongjing, *Shanghanlun* (Treatise on feverish illnesses, ca. AD200). In: Nanjing zhongyi xueyuan (ed.), *Shanghanlun yishi* (Translation and explanation of the Shanghanlun), Shanghai kexue jishu chubanshe, Shanghai, 1992 (1st edn 1959).

Zhang Zihe (Zhang Congzheng), *Rumen shiqin* (Confucian responsibilities towards family and parents, 1228). In: Ye Chuan (ed.), *Jinyuan sida yixuejia mingzhu jicheng*, Zhongguo zhongyiyao chubanshe, Beijing, 1995.

Zhao Xianke, *Yiguan* (Deep knowledge of medicine, 1647). In: Qiu Peiran (ed.), *Zhongguo yixue dacheng sanbian*, vol.XI.

Zhou Xuehai, *Duji suibi* (Notes from medicine readings, 1898), Jiangsu keji chubanshe, Nanjing, 1985.

Zhu Danxi (pupils of), *Danxi xinfa* (Teachings of [the master] Danxi, 1481). In: *Danxi yiji*, Renmin weisheng chubanshe, Beijing, 1993.

Zhu Danxi (or Zhu Zhenheng), *Gezhi yulun* (Extra treatises based on the research of things, 1347). *Jinyuan sida yixuejia mingzhu jicheng*, Zhongguo zhongyiyao chubanshe, Beijing, 1995.

Zhu Danxi *Jingui gouxuan* (The mysteries of the Jingui, unknown date, attributed from some to Zhu Danxi). In Ye Chuan (ed.), *Jinyuan sida yixuejia mingzhu jicheng* (Collection of famous works by the four great), Zhongguo zhongyiyao chubanshe, Beijing, 1995.

Zhu Hong, *Nanyang huorenshu* (Nanyang's book to save the life, 1111).

Zhu Xi, *Zhuzi yulei* (Updated collection of the sayings of master Zhu, 1270). Zhonghua shuju, Beijing, 1986.

Zhuangzi zishi, Guo Qingfan (ed.), Zhonghua shuju chuban, Beijing, 1979.

Contemporary Texts in Chinese

Cao Bingzhang (ed.), *Zhongguo yixue dacheng* (Great compendium of Chinese medicine) Shanghai kexue jishu chubanshe, Shanghai, 1990, 50 vols.

Fang Chunyang (ed.), *Zhongguo qigong dacheng* (Great compendium of Chinese Qigong), Jilin kexue jishu chubanshe, Changchun, 1989.

Gao Lishan, *Zhenjiu xinfei* (Notes oh heart of acupuncture and moxibustion), Xueyuan chubanshe, Beijing, 1997.

Guo Aichun (ed.), *Huangdi neijing cidian* (Dictionary of the *Huangdi neijing*), Tianjin kexue jishu chubanshi, Tianjin, 1991.

He Puren, *Zhenjiu gefu linchuan yingyong* (Clinical use of the odes on acupuncture and moxibustion), Kexue jishu wenxian chubanshi, Beijing, 1992.

He Yuming, *Zhongguo chuantong jingshen binglixue* (Mental illness pathology in Chinese medicine), Shanghai kexue puji chubanshi, Shanghai, 1995.

Jin Shubai, *Zhenjiu zhiliao jingshenbing* (Acupuncture and moxibustion in the treatment of mental illnesses), Shanghai zhongyi xueyuan chubanshi, Shanghai, 1987.

Kang Yin, *Wenzi yanliu qianhuo* (Essay on the origins of Chinese writing), Rongbaozhai, Beijing, 1979.

Li Junchuan, *Qingzhi yixue* (Medicine of the emotions), Beijing guji chubanshi, Beijing, 1994.

Li Qingfu and Liu Duzhou, *Zhongyi jingshen bingxue* (Psychiatry in Chinese medicine), Tianjing kexue jishu chubanshi, 1989.

Nie Shimao, *Huangdi neijing xinlixue gaiyao* (Elements of psychology in the *Huangdi neijing*), Chongqing, Kexue jishu chubanshi, Chongqing, 1986.

Niu Yunduo, *Jinzhen zaichuan* (Transmission of the experience of Wang Leting 'golden needle'), Kexue jishu chubanshi, Beijing, 1994.

Qiu Peiran (ed.), *Zhongguo yixue dacheng sanbian* (New compilation of the great compendium of Chinese medicine), Yueli shushe, Shanghai, 1994, 12 vols.

Qiu Peiran, *Zhongyi mingjia xueshuo* (Theories of famous doctors in Chinese medicine), Renmin weisheng chubanshi, Beijing, 1992.

Wang Keqin, *Zhongyi shenzhu xueshuo* (Theory of the *shen* in Chinese medicine), Zhongyi guji chubanshi, Beijing, 1988.

Wang Ling (ed.), *Zhenjiu gefu jizhu* (Collection and comment to the odes on acupuncture and moxibustion), Zhongguo yixue keji chubanshi, Beijing, 1998.

Wang Miqu et al., *Zhongyi xinlixue* (Psychology in Chinese medicine), Hubei kexue jishu chubanshi, Tianjing, 1985

Wang Miqu, *Zhongguo gudai yixue xinlixue* (Ancient Chinese medical psychology), Guizhou renmin chubanshi, Guiyang, 1988.

Wang Zhanxi, *Neike zhenjiu peixue xinbian* (Revision of the combination of points in the internal medicine in agomoxa), Kexue jishu wenxian chubanshi, Beijing, 1993.

Yang Jiasan (ed.), *Zhenjiu xue* (Treatise of acupuncture), Renmin weisheng chubanshi, Beijing, 1989.

Yang Jiasan (ed.), *Zhongguo zhenjiu dacidian* (Great dictionary of Chinese acupuncture), Renmin weisheng chubanshi, Beijing 1988.

Zhang Shijie, *Gufa zhengci juou* (Examples of acupuncture following the ancient method), Huaxue gongye chubanshe, Beijing, 1995.

Zhong Meiquan, *Zhenjiu linzheng zhinan* (Clinical guide of acupuncture and moxibustion), Hu Ximing (ed.), Renmin weisheng chubanshe, Beijing, 1991.

Zhou Youguang (ed.), *Hanyu pinyin zhengcifa weiyuanhui de gongzuo qingkuang* (State of the works of the committee for a correct orthography in pinyin of the words of the Chinese language). In: *Hanyu pinyin zhengcifa lunwen xuan*. Editor for the reformation of writing, 1985.

Zhu Wenfeng, *Zhongyi xinlixue yuanzhi* (Principles of psychology in Chinese medicine), Hunan kexue jishu chubanshi, Changsha, 1987.

Reference Texts for the Chinese Language

Ciyuan (Origin of the words), Shangwu yinshuguan, Beijing, 1991 (1st edn 1915) 2 vols.

Gu hanyu changyongzi zidian (Dictionary of the most used characters in ancient Chinese), Shangwu yinshu guan, Beijing,1986.

Gudai hanyu cidian (Dictionary of ancient Chinese characters), Zhang Shuangdi et altri (eds.), Beijing daxue chubanshe, 1998.

Hanying cidian, *A Chinese–English Dictionary*, Beijing waiguoyu daxue, Waiyu jiaoxue yu yanjiu chubanshe, 1997.

Hanying cidian, *A Chinese–English Dictionary*, Shangwu yinshu guan, Beijing, 1988.

Kalgren, B., 'Grammatica serica, script and phonetics in Chinese and Sino Japanese', *Bulletin of the Museum of Far Eastern Antiquities*, 12, 1–471, 1940.

Viotti-Bonfanti, *Chinese–Italian and Italian–Chinese Dictionary*, Le Lettere, Firenze, 1991.

Wenlin Software for Learning Chinese, Version 2.1, Wenlin Institute, 1999.

Wieger, L.S., *Chinese Characters*, New York, Dover, 1915.

Xiandai hanyu cidian, *Dictionary of Modern Chinese*, Shangwu yinshu guan, Beijing, 1985.

Xie Guan (ed.), *Zhongguo yixue dacidian*, (Great dictionary of Chinese, 1921), Zhongguo shudian, Beijing, 1988.

Xu Shen, *Shuowen jiezi* (Explanation of characters and words, AD121). Zhonghua shuju, Beijing, 1963.

Western Language References

American Psychiatric Association: *DSM-IV, Diagnostic and Statistical Manual of Mental Disorders*, American Psychiatric Association, Arlington VA, 1994.

Balint, M., *The Doctor, his Patient, and the Illness*, Churchill Livingstone, Edinburgh, 1957.

Beijing Medical College, *Common Terms of Traditional Chinese Medicine in English*, Beijing, 1980.

Bensky, D., Barolet, R., *Chinese Herbal Medicine Formulas and Strategies*, Eastland Press, Seattle, 1990.

Bi Yongsheng et al., *Chinese Qigong*, Publishing House of Shanghai College of TCM, Shanghai, 1990.

Bian Zhizhong, *Daoist Health Preservation Exercises*, China Reconstruct Press, Beijing, 1987.

Bion, W. R., *Attention and Interpretation*. Aronson, London, 1970.

Bleuler, E., *Trattato di Psichiatria* (Psychiatry treatise), Handbuch der psychiatrie, Leipzig, 1911.

Boschi, G., *La Radice e i Fiori* (The root and the flowers), Erga, Genova, 1997.

Chen Ping (ed.), *History and Development of Traditional Chinese Medicine*, Beijing, 1999.

Cheng, A., *Histoire de la Pensée Chinoise* (History of Chinese thought), Paris, 1997, (trad.it. Einaudi 2000).

Corradin, M., Di Stanislao, C., *Lo Psichismo in Pedicina Energetica* (Psychism in energetic medicine), Associazione Medica per lo Studio dell'Agopuntura, L'Aquila, 1995.

Deadman, P., Al Khafaji, M., *A Manual of Acupuncture*, Journal of Chinese Medicine, Hove, 1998.

Despeaux, C., *Immortelles de la Chine Ancienne. Taoisme et Alchimie Feminine* (The immortals of ancient China. Taoism and female alchemy), Pardès, Puiseax, 1990.

Despeaux, C., *Phisiologie et Alchimie Taoiste* (Taoist physiology and alchemy). Le Weisheng shenglixue mingzhi, Les Deux Océans, Paris, 1979.

Dey, T., (ed.), *Soothing the Troubled Mind*, Paradigm Publications, Brookline, 2000.

Esposito, M., *L'alchimia del Soffio* (The alchemy of the breath), Ubaldini, Roma, 1997.

Eyssalet, J.M., *Le Secret de la Maison des Ancetres* (The secrets of the house of the ancient), Guy Tredaniel, Paris, 1990.

Farquhar, J., *Knowing Practice: The Clinical Encounter of Chinese Medicine*, Blue Poppy Press, Boulder,1994.

Faubert, A., *Initiation a l'Agopuncture Traditionelle*, Pierre Belfond, Paris, 1974.

Fingarette, H., *Confucius: The Secular as Sacred*, Harper Torchbooks, New York, 1972.

Flaws, B., Lake, J., *Chinese Medical Psychiatry*, Blue Poppy Press, Boulder 2001.

Freud, S., *Dynamics of Transference, Complete Psychological Works of Sigmund Freud*, vol.6, 1912 (republished Hogarth Press and the Institute of Psycho-analysis, London , 1999)

Galimberti, U., *Dizionario di Psicologia* (Dictionary of psychology), UTET, Torino, 1992.

Giberti, F., Rossi, R., *Manuale di Psichiatria,* Piccin, Padova, 1983.

Graham, A.C., *Disputers of the Tao. Philosophical Argument in Ancient China*, Open Court, La Salle,1989; Italian edn Neri Pozza 1999.

Granet, M., *La Pensée Chinoise* (Chinese thought), Albin Michel, Paris, 1934.

Hammer, L., *Contemporary Pulse Diagnosis,* Eastland Press, Seattle, 2001.

Hammer, L., *Dragon Rises, Red Bird Flies*, Station Hill Press, New York, 1990.

Hinsie L.E., Campbell R.J., *Dizionario di Psichiatria* (Dictionary of psychiatry), Astrolabio, Roma, 1979.

Hou Jinglun (ed.), *Traditional Chinese Treatment for Psychogenic and Neurological Diseases*, Academy Press, Beijing, 1996.

Huang Jinwei, *Muscle Region Therapy*, Traditional Chinese Medicine Publishing House, vol. 91,1996.

Inglese, S., Peccarisi, C., *Psichiatria Oltre Frontiera. Viaggio Intorno Alle Sindromi Culturalmente Ordinate* (Psychiatry across the border. A voyage among culturally ordered illnesses), UTET, Milano, 1997.

Jarrett, L.S., *Nourishing Destiny. The Inner Tradition of Chinese Medicine*, Spirit Path Press, Massachusetts, 1998.

Jullien, F., *Eloge de la Fadeur*, Editions Philippe Picquier, 1991.

Jung, C. G., *Praxis der Psychotherapie* (The practice of psychotherapy), vol.16, 1958. In: *The Collected Works of C. G. Jung*, London, 2nd edn Bollingen, Princeton, 1966.

Karcher, S., Ritsema, R., (ed.), *I Ching*, Element, Shaftesbury, 1994.

Kernberg, O., *Severe Personality Disorders*, London, 1984, paperback edn Yale University Press, New Haven, 1993.

Kirschbaum, B., *Atlas und Lehrbuch der Chinesischen Zungendiagnostik*, 1998.

Kleinman, A., *Social Origins of Distress and Disease. Depression, Neurasthenia, and Pain in Modern China*, Yale Press, New York, 1988.

Knoblock, J., *Xunzi: A Translation and Study of the Complete Works*, vol.I, Stanford, Stanford University Press, 1988.

Kohn, L. (ed.), *Taoist Meditation and Longevity Techniques*, Center for Chinese Studies: University of Michigan, 1989.

Kraepelin E., *Trattato di Psichiatria* (Psychiatry treatise), 1883, Milan, 1907.

Laplanche, J, Pontalis, J.B., *Enciclopedie de la Psychanalyse* (The encyclopaedia of psychoanalysis), Laterza, Bari, 1967.

Larre, C., Rochat de la Vallée, E., *Les Mouvements du Coeur*, Institut Ricci, Paris, 1992.

Larre, C., Rochat de la Vallée, E., *The Seven Emotions*, Monkey Press, Cambridge, 1996.

Lau, D.C., *Mencius*, Penguin, Harmondsworth, 1970.

Li Shi Zhen, *The Lakeside Master's Study of the Pulse*, trans. Bob Flaws, Blue Poppy Press, Boulder, 1998.

Liu Gongwang (ed.), *Clinical Acupuncture and Moxibustion*, Tianjin Science and Technology Translation and Publishing Corporation, Tianjin, 1996.

Liu Gongwang (ed.), *Techniques of Acupuncture and Moxibustion*, Tianjin, 1998.

Liu Gongwang, Akira Hyodo (ed.), *Fundamentals of Acupuncture and Moxibustion*, Tianjin, 1994.

Maciocia, G., *The Practice of Chinese Medicine*, Churchill Livingstone, Edinburgh, 1994.

Martucci C., Rotolo G., *Qigong*, Li Shizhen, Milano, 1991.

Maspero, H., *Le Taoisme et les Religions Chinoises* (Daoism and the Chinese religions), Paris, 1971.

Needham, J., *Celestial Lancets*, Cambridge University Press, Cambridge, 1980, reprinted RoutledgeCurzon, London, 2002; Italian edn Saggiatorre, Milan 1982.

Nielsen, A., *Guasha: A Traditional Technique for Modern Practice*, Churchill Livingstone, Edinburgh, 1995.

Onians, N.B., *The Origins of European Thought*, Cambridge University Press, Cambridge, 1998.

Pieri, P., *Dizionario Junghiano* (Jungian dictionary), Boringhieri, Torino, 1998.

Porkert, M., *The Theoretical Foundations of Chinese Medicine*, M.I.T. Press, Cambridge Mass., 1974.

Pregadio, F., *Ko Hung: Le Medicine della Grande Purezza* (The medicines of the great pureness), Edn Mediterranee, Roma, 1987.

Robinet I., *Histoire du Taoisme des Origines au XIV Siècle* (History of Daoism from the origins to the XIV century), Cerf, Paris, 1991; Italian edn Ubaldini, Rome 1993.

Sabattini M., Santangelo P., *Storia della Cina* (History of China), Laterza, Bari, 1985.

Santangelo, P., *Emozioni e Desideri in Cina* (Emotions and desires in China), Laterza, Bari, 1992.

Scott, J., Barlow, T., *Acupuncture in the Treatment of Children*, Eastland Press, Seattle, 1999.

Selye, H., Stress senza paura (Stress without fear), 1971.

Shao Nianfang (ed.), *The Treatment of Knotty Diseases*, Shandong Science and Technology Press, Jinan, 1990.

Shen, J., *Chinese Medicine*, Educational Solutions, New York 1980.

Sivin N., *Science and Medicine in Chinese History*, Brookfield, Variorum, 1995.

Unschuld P., *Medicine in China*, University of California Press, Berkeley, 1985.

Unschuld, P., *Introductory Readings in Classical Chinese Medicine*, Kluver Academic Publisher, Dordrecht/Boston/London, 1988.

Unschuld, P., *Medicine in China: a History of Ideas*, University of California Press, Berkeley, 1985.

Unschuld, P., *Nan-ching, The Classic of Difficult Issues*, University of California Press, Berkeley, 1986.

Watson, B., *Records of the Historian*, Columbia University Press, New York, 1969.

WHO, *A Proposed Standard International Acupuncture Nomenclature*, WHO, Geneva, 1991.

Wilhelm, R., *Das Geheimnis der Goldenen Blute* (Secret of the Golden Flower): *Ein Chinesisches Lebensbuch*, 1929. Con il commento di C.G.Jung. Trans. English 1931.

Winnicott, D.W., *Through Paediatrics to Psycho-Analysis*, Tavistock Publications, London 1958.

Wiseman N., Feng Ye, *A Practical Dictionary of Chinese Medicine*, Paradigm Publications, Brookline, 1998.

Zhang Mingwu, *Chinese Qigong Therapy*, Shandong Science and Technology Press, Jinan, 1985.

Zhao Xin, Fu Jianping (ed.), *A Guide-book to the Proficiency Examination for International Acupuncture and Moxibustion Professionals*, China Medico-Pharmaceutical Science and Technology Publishing House. Beijing, 1994.

Zingarelli N., *Vocabolario della Lingua Italiana* (Dictionary of the Italian language), Zanichelli, Bologna, 1994.

Articles

Al-Khafaji M., Running Piglet Qi, *The Journal of Chinese Medicine*, 30, 1989.

Angelini C., Considerazioni su alcuni punti ad azione psichica (Considerations on certain points with psychic action), *Comunicazione IV Congresso Mazionale SIA*, Luino 1985.

Barnes, L., The psychologising of Chinese healing practices in the United States, *Culture, Medicine and Psychiatry*, 22, Kluwer Academic Publishers, Netherlands, 1998.

Chase C., Ghosts in the Machine, *European Journal of Oriental Medicine*, vol.1(1), 1993.

Deadman P., A reply to Bob Flaws, *The Journal of Chinese Medicine*, 38, 1992.

Deadman P., Al-Khafaji M., Treatment of psycho-emotional disturbance by acupuncture with particular reference to the Du Mai. *The Journal of Chinese Medicine*, 47, 1995.

Deporte P., Le terme gui dans les noms des points d'acupuncture, *Médecine Chinoise & Médecine Orientales*, 1, 1992.

Di Stanislao C., Le sindromi ansioso-depressive (yuzheng) in agopuntura e medicina cinese (The anxiety-depressive syndrome (yuzheng) in acupuncture and Chinese medicine). *Yi Dao Za Zhi*, 11, 1999.

Diebschlag F., Ants and acorns, *European Journal of Oriental Medicine*, 2, p. 25–30, 1996.

Flaws, B., The importance of spirit in prognosis: what this means in clinical practice. *Australian Journal of Acupuncture*, 18, 1992.

Flaws, B., Thoughts on acupuncture, internal medicine, and TCM in the West, *The Journal of Chinese Medicine*, 38, 1992.

Garvey M., Theory and practice, *European Journal of Oriental Medicine*, 2(1), 1996.

Garvey, M., Qu, L., The liver's *shuxie* function, *European Journal of Oriental Medicine*, 3(5), 2001.

Goldberg, D., Epidemiology of mental disorders in primary care settings, *Epidemiology Review*, 17, 1995.

Groves, J., Taking care of the hateful patient. *New England Journal of Medicine*, 298, 1978.

Gu Yuehua, *Baihe* syndrome, *The Journal of Chinese Medicine*, 40, 1992.

Gu Yuehua, Le sindrome *baihe* (*baihe* syndrome). *Médecine Chinoise & Médecine Orientales*, 6, 1993.

Hammer, L., Integrated acupuncture therapy for body and mind, *American Journal of Acupuncture*, vol.8, 2, 1980, pp163–169.

Hsu, E., Spirit (*shen*): styles of knowing and authority in contemporary Chinese medicine. *Culture Medicine and Psychiatry*, 24, 2000.

Huang Xing Yi, Tom Dey (eds), Hysterical diseases, *European Journal of Oriental Medicine*, 2(2), 1996.

Idelman Simon, Stress ed agopuntura (Stress and acupuncture). *Rivista Italiana di Medicina Tradizionale Cinese*, 2, 1991.

Kaptchuk, T., Maciocia G., Moir F., Deadman P., Acupuncture in the West, *The Journal of Chinese Medicine*, 17, 1985.

Kleinman, A., Kleinman J., Somatization: The interconnections in Chinese society among culture, depressive experiences, and the meaning of pain, In: Kleinman A,. Good B. (eds). *Culture and Depression*, University of California Press, Berkeley 1985.

Low, C., Perfectly organized chaos, *European Journal of Oriental Medicine*, vol.2, 1, 1996.

Maciocia, G., The psyche in Chinese medicine, *European Journal of Oriental Medicine*, 1, 1993.

Morandotti, R., Viggiani B., Le depressioni (Depressions). *Rivista Italiana di Agopuntura*, 78, 1993.

Morelli, G., Rossi E., L'Attacco di Panico: *zhen*, il drago dal profondo si lancia verso il cielo (Panic attack: the dragon rises from the depths to the heaven), *MediCina*, autumn 1995.

Qi Jinping, Shui Hai He, Trattamento delle sindromi depressive con agopuntura (Treatment of depressive syndromes with acupuncture). *Orientamenti MTC*, 2, 1996.

Qiao Wenlei, Clinical experience: the treatment of stress syndromes by acupuncture, *The Journal of Chinese Medicine*, 61, 1999.

Rossi, E., Il corpo, la mente e noi (The body, the mind and ourselves), *MediCina*, autumn 1994.

Rossi, E., Note di diagnosi e valutazione di efficacia nella medicina tradizionale cinese (Notes on diagnosis and evaluation of efficacy in TCM), *MediCina*, spring 1993 (English translation in: *European Journal of Oriental Medicine* vol.1, 5, 1995).

Rossi, E., The space shared between patient and acupuncturist, *European Journal of Oriental Medicine*, vol.3, 2, 2000.

Rotolo, G., *Diankuang*: follia calma e follia agitata (*Diankuang*: calm madness and agitated madness). *Rivista Italiana di Agopuntura*, 56, 1986.

Scheid, V., Bensky D., Medicine as signification, *European Journal of Oriental Medicine*, vol.2, 6, 1998/99.

Scheid, V., Orientalism revisited, *European Journal of Oriental Medicine*, 1(2), 1993.

Stone, J., Ethics and the therapeutic relationship, *European Journal of Oriental Medicine*, 2, 1996.

Wagner, E., La moxibustione nella clinica HIV+ (Moxibustion in the HIV+ clinic), *MediCina*, inverno 1996.

Wang Chenhui, '*Fure* calore nascosto' (Fire, hidden heat), ed. E. Rossi, *MediCina*, estate 1994.

Yu Qingbai, 'Il Fegato soffre di urgenza' (The liver suffers from urgency), *MediCina*, autumn 1997.

Yu Yongxi, Il modello delle catastrofi a cuspide ('The cusp catastrophe model'), *MediCina*, spring 1996.

Zhao Yanling et al., 'Needling *yanglingquan* G.B.-34 for relieving spasm and its influence on gamma-aminobutyric acid in cerebrospinal fluid', *Chinese Acupuncture and Moxibustion*, 9, 1998.

Zhang Mingjiu, 'Thoupizhen zhiliao huanjue 296 lide jingyan' (Craniopuncture in 296 cases of schizophrenia with hallucinations), *Zhongyi Zazhi*, 6(52), 1987.

Zheng Yan-Ping et el., Comparative study of diagnostic systems: Chinese classification of mental disorders – 2nd edn versus DSM-III-R, Comprehensive Psychiatry, 35(6), 1994.

Appendix G

LIST OF POINTS MENTIONED

BL-17 *Geshu*
BL-42 *Pohu*
BL-43 *Gaohuangshu*
Du-4 *Mingmen*
Du-8 *Jinsuo*
Du-11 *Shendao*
Du-14 *Dazhui*
Du-16 *Fengfu*
Du-20 *Baihui*
Du-24 *Shenting*
Du-26 *Renzhong*
EX-HN-3 *Yintang*
GB-20 *Fengchi*
GB-34 *Yanglinquan*
HE-3 *Shaohai*
HE-4 *Lingdao*
HE-5 *Tongli*
HE-6 *Yinxi*

HE-7 *Shenmen*
HE-8 *Shaofu*
HE-9 *Shaochong*
KI-3 *Taixi*
KI-4 *Dazhong*
KI-6 *Zhaohai*
LI-4 *Hegu*
LIV-2 *Xingjian*
LIV-3 *Taichong*
LU-3 *Tianfu*
LU-7 *Lieque*
P-3 *Quze*
P-4 *Ximen*
P-5 *Jianshi*
P-6 *Neiguan*
P-7 *Daling*
P-8 *Laogong*
P-9 *Zhongchong*

Ren-4 *Guanyuan*
Ren-6 *Qihai*
Ren-12 *Zhongwan*
Ren-14 *Juque*
Ren-15 *Jiuwei*
Ren-17 *Shanzhong*
Ren-22 *Tiantu*
SI-7 *Zhizheng*
SP-3 *Taibai*
SP-4 *Gongsun*
SP-6 *Sanyinjiao*
SP-10 *Xuehai*
ST-21 *Liangmen*
ST-36 *Zusanli*
ST-40 *Fenglong*
ST-44 *Neiting*
TB-3 *Waiguan*

Index

A

affectivity, 342–343
aggression, 343
agitation, 97
    acupuncture effects, 293–294
    case studies, 91–95, 101–102
    sleep disturbance, 103, 108
    yin, 98–100
    see also anxiety; hyperactivity
alarm reaction, 316
alcohol abuse, case study, 244–245
Alcohol Unit (Nucleo Operativo Alcologia, NOA), Milano, 397–398
    case studies, 401–406
    data collection, 401
    evaluation, 401
    treatment protocol, 399–401
amnesias, 346
anger-*nu*, 30–31, 34–35
    case study, 42–43
    liver and, 76
    obsessive, 268–269
    see also emotions
anorexia, case study, 224–227
anxiety, 297–298, 343, 397–406, 419
    case studies, 229–232, 401–406
    Nucleo Operativo Alcologia (NOA)
        project, 397–406
        case studies, 401–406
        data collection, 401
        evaluation, 401
        treatment protocol, 399–401
    see also agitation
appearance, 339
appetite, 174
attention disorders, 344
    see also hyperactivity

B

back *shu* points, 255
baihebing, 151–154
    aetiology, 152–153
    case study, 161–163
    clinical notes, 153–154
behavioural disorders, 340–341
bentunqi, 145–151
    aetiology, 146–150
    case studies, 158–161, 367–368, 381
    clinical notes, 150–151
BL-1 *Jingming*, 109, 122
BL-3 *Meichong*, 333, 342, 349
BL-4 *Shentang*:
    for psychiatric pathology, 334, 336, 340, 342–346
    for *yin* deficiency, 119
BL-5 *Wuchu*, 138
    for psychiatric pathology, 334, 339–340, 342–346, 349
BL-6 *Chengguang*, 341, 347
BL-7 *Tongtian*, 338, 341–343, 347
BL-8 *Luoque*, 337, 340, 344, 346
BL-10 *Tianzhu*, 346
BL-13 *Feishu*:
    baihebing treatment, 162
    for emptiness, 220
    for phlegm, 189
    for *qi* stagnation, 178
    moxibustion and, 235
BL-15 *Xinshu*:
    for blood stasis, 193
    for chronic disease, 303
    for emptiness, 211, 222
    for fire, 185
    insomnia treatment, 109, 111, 112, 113, 119
    moxibustion and, 235
    yuzheng treatment, 364
BL-17 *Geshu*, 191–192
    for blood stasis, 191–192, 193
    for emptiness, 215
    for fire, 185
    for *qi* stagnation, 178
    hiccups treatment, 43
    principal actions, 192
BL-18 *Ganshu*:
    baihebing treatment, 162

diankuang treatment, 361, 362
    for blood stasis, 193
    for chronic disease, 303
    for emptiness, 215, 222, 224
    for *qi* stagnation, 179, 224
    insomnia treatment, 109, 111
    moxibustion and, 235
    stress treatment, 319
    whiplash injury treatment, 329
    yuzheng treatment, 364
BL-19 *Danshu*:
    for emptiness, 214, 224
    for *qi* stagnation, 179, 224
    stress treatment, 319, 320
BL-20 *Pishu*:
    for blood stasis, 193
    for chronic disease, 303
    for emptiness, 212, 222, 291
    for phlegm, 189
    for psychiatric pathology, 339
    for *qi* stagnation, 178, 194
    moxibustion and, 235
    yuzheng treatment, 364
BL-21 *Feishu*:
    for emptiness, 212
    for phlegm, 189
    for *qi* stagnation, 178, 194
    stress treatment, 320
BL-23 *Shenshu*:
    diankuang treatment, 361, 362
    for blood stasis, 193
    for emptiness, 214, 219, 222, 224
    for *qi* stagnation, 224
    hyperactivity treatment, 395
    insomnia treatment, 111, 112, 113, 119
    moxibustion and, 235
    stress treatment, 320
    whiplash injury treatment, 329
BL-31 *Shangliao*, 164
BL-32 *Ciliao*, 164
BL-40 *Weizhong*, 185, 321
BL-42 *Pohu*, 162, 255
    for lung *yin* emptiness, 220
    insomnia treatment, 111

BL-43 *Gaohuangshu*, 220–221, 235
BL-44 *Shentang*, 255
  for blood stasis, 193
  for emptiness, 211, 222
  for fire, 185
  insomnia treatment, 109
BL-47 *Hunmen*, 255
  baihebing treatment, 162
  for emptiness, 222
  insomnia treatment, 109, 111
BL-49 *Yishe*, 255
BL-52 *Zhishi*, 255
  for emptiness, 214, 219
  insomnia treatment, 119
BL-58 *Feiyang*, 342, 346, 348, 349
BL-60 *Kunlun*, 164
BL-62 *Shenmai*:
  diankuang treatment, 136
  insomnia treatment, 109, 111, 122
BL-67 *Zhiyin*, 334
bleeding-*Sanlengzhen Liaofa*, 236, 238
  insomnia treatment, 110
  stress treatment, 321
  whiplash injury treatment, 326
blood:
  emptiness, 205, 214–215, 348
    case study, 221–223
    insomnia, 105, 107, 116
    zanzao, 143
  stasis, 80, 189–193, 349
    aetiology, 189
    case study, 43–45
    clinical manifestations, 190
    clinical notes, 190–191
    development, 189
    treatment, 191–193
breathing, 10, 15
  fetal, 15

C

channels, 375–377
  illness of the kidney channel, 377–378
chronic disease case study, 301–302
confabulation, 346
Confucius, 5, 19
confusion, 333, 334
consciousness, 333–334
  confusion of, 333
constraint-*yu*, 73–74, 76–79, 89–90,
  108, 172
  case studies, 196–199, 224–229,
    356–357
  in *meiheqi*, 155
  see also stagnation
conversion disorders, 379–381

convoluted thought, 335
cranial acupuncture-*Touzhen*, 241–243
  insomnia treatment, 110
  see also scalp acupuncture
cupping-*Baguan Liaofa*, 236–237

D

dantian, 12–13, 247–248
dao (way), 5–8, 41
daoyin practices, 10–11, 15
de power, 5–7, 9
delirium, 334
delusions, 336–338
dementia, 345
depression, 297–298, 419–420
  case studies, 196–199, 244–245
  major depressive episode, 421–422
  manic *see diankuang*
desires, 19–20
determination, 40–41
diagnosis, 373–375
  in conventional psychiatry, 419–423
  tongue diagnosis, 307–311
diankuang, 125–140, 352–362
  aetiology, 129–134, 352–353
    emotions and heat, 131–132
    phlegm, 132–134
    yin and *yang*, 129–131
  case studies, 137–140, 356–362
  description, 127–129, 353–354
  treatment, 134–137, 354–355
    gui points, 136
doctor–patient relationship *see*
  therapeutic relationship
dreams, 56
dryness, in *zangzao*, 143–144
DSM:Diagnostic and Statistic Manual of
  Mental Disorders, 420–423
Du Mai, 247–248, 251–254
Du-1 *Changqiang*, 135
Du-3 *Yaoyangguan*, 164
Du-4 *Mingmen*, 251–252
  for emptiness, 214, 219, 222
  for psychiatric pathology, 344
  moxibustion and, 236
  principal actions, 251
Du-8 *Jinsuo*, 252
  principal actions, 252
Du-11 *Shendao*, 252
  for emptiness, 211, 222
  for psychiatric pathology, 339
    diankuang, 360
  insomnia treatment, 109, 119
  principal actions, 252
Du-12 *Shenzhu*, 137, 339

Du-14 *Dazhui*, 252
  bleeding, 238, 321
  for chronic disease, 302
  for fire, 200
  for psychiatric pathology, 339, 344,
    345
    diankuang, 355, 360, 361
  for *qi* stagnation, 81
  insomnia treatment, 116
  meiheqi treatment, 164, 165
  moxibustion and, 236
  principal actions, 252
  stress treatment, 321
Du-15 *Yamen*, 355
Du-16 *Fengfu*, 253
  diankuang treatment, 136, 355, 361
  for fire, 200
  for *qi* stagnation, 81
  meiheqi treatment, 164
  principal actions, 253
Du-18 *Qiangjian*, 335, 338
Du-19 *Qianding*, 345, 346
Du-20 *Baihui*, 248, 253
  agitation treatment, 94
  anxiety treatment, 400
  bleeding, 238, 321
  for emptiness, 212, 219, 222
  for fire, 200
  for psychiatric pathology, 334–335,
    338, 340–341, 343,
    345–346, 349
    diankuang, 138, 355, 361
  insomnia treatment, 111, 116
  moxibustion and, 236
  principal actions, 253
  stress treatment, 321, 323, 324
  whiplash injury treatment,
    326, 327
  zangzao treatment, 366
Du-21 *Qianding*, 343, 345, 349
Du-22 *Xinhui*, 335, 344, 346
Du-23 *Shangxing*:
  diankuang treatment, 136
  for severe psychiatric pathology, 333,
    335, 339, 344–346, 348
Du-24 *Shenting*, 253–254
  agitation treatment, 93
  bleeding, 238, 321
  diankuang treatment, 136, 138
  for emptiness, 211, 219, 222
  for *qi* stagnation, 210
  for severe psychiatric pathology,
    333–334, 339, 344–346,
    348–349
  insomnia treatment, 111, 117
  principal actions, 253
  stress treatment, 321, 324
Du-25 *Suliao*, 334, 335, 342

Du-26 *Renzhong*, 254
  agitation treatment, 93
  for psychiatric pathology, 339, 343
    diankuang, 136, 137, 355, 359,
      360, 361–362
  principal actions, 254
Du-28 *Yinjiao*, 362
dysthymic disorder, 421

E

E-HN-37 *Haiquan*, 136
E-HN-54 *Anmian/Yiming*, 109
ear acupuncture therapy-*Erzhen*,
  238–240
  anxiety, 230, 231
  bentunqi, 159
  diankuang, 355
  insomnia, 109–110, 115, 120, 122
  primary points, 239, 240
  qi stagnation and emptiness, 224, 225
  stress, 321
  yuzheng, 364
earth, 30, 36–37
  heaven and, 53–54
  see also elements
earth point, 257–258
eccentricity, 340
echolalia, 338
echopraxia, 338
electrostimulation-*Dianzhen*, 243–244
  for liver *qi* stagnation, 194
elements, 18
  relationships with emotions, 30–31,
    34–39
emotional instability, 342
emotions, 4, 17–18, 32–33
  as causes of illness, 20–23, 78–79,
    90–91
    pathogenic processes, 28–30
  classical thought and, 19–20
  control of, 266–268
  diankuang and, 131–132
  fire and, 85–86
  movement of *qi* and, 23–26, 34
  obsessive, 268–269
  organs and, 30–31, 34–39
  perceptions of, 33–34
  relationships with elements, 30–31,
    34–39
  treatment of, 3
  treatment with, 261–268
    going around the obstacle, 264–266
    physician as guide, 262–263
  yu and, 76–77

zhi as, 68–69
  see also anger; euphoria; fear;
    sadness; thought
empathy, 286
emptiness-*xu*, 107, 203
  aetiology, 204
  anxiety and, 400, 401–405
  case studies, 221–227, 291–292,
    323–324, 401–405
  clinical manifestations, 204
  clinical notes, 204–205
  in psychiatric pathology, 334, 335,
    336, 338
  jing, 218–219
  stress and, 317–318, 320
  treatment, 205–211
  see also blood; *specific organs*; *yang yin*
euphoria-*xi*, 30–31, 35–36, 343
  see also emotions
EX-BW-35 *Huatuojiaji*, 255
EX-HN-1 *Sishencong*, 200
  agitation treatment, 93
  for emptiness, 219
  for psychiatric pathology, 335, 339,
    345
    diankuang, 355, 356, 357
EX-HN-3 *Yintang*, 248, 254
  agitation treatment, 92, 93, 94
  anxiety treatment, 230, 231, 402–405
  bentunqi treatment, 159, 160
  diankuang treatment, 355, 356–357,
    358, 361
  for emptiness, 211, 219
  for fire, 200
  for *qi* stagnation/constraint, 201,
    228, 229
  for severe psychiatric pathology, 334,
    339, 340
  insomnia treatment, 109, 111, 116,
    117, 119
  meiheqi treatment, 164
  principal actions, 254
  yuzheng treatment, 364, 365
  zangzao treatment, 156, 157
EX-HN-6, 319, 320
EX-HN-9 *Taiyang*, 224, 225
  bleeding, 238, 321
  diankuang treatment, 361, 362
  for emptiness, 215
  stress treatment, 320, 321, 324
  whiplash injury treatment, 326, 329
EX-HN-10 *Erjian*, bleeding, 238
EX-HN-15 *Bailao*, 164
EX-HN-37 *Haiquan*, 341
EX-UE-1 *Shixuan*, 335
exaltation, 342

F

fanzao, 97–98
  aetiology, 98–100
fatigue, 173
fear-*kong*, 30–31, 38–39
  see also emotions
fibromyoma case study, 193–196
fire, 30, 35–36, 85, 179
  agitation and, 98–100
  case studies, 91–95, 101–102,
    137–140, 199–200,
    229–232
  diankuang aetiology, 131–133
  emotions and, 85–86
  heart, 91–95, 107–108, 179–183,
    199–200
  insomnia and, 107–108
  liver, 91–95, 183, 199–200
  ministerial fire, 88–90
  phlegm, 137–140, 186–187
  rising, 382–383
  stomach, 91–95, 184, 199–200
  yin fire, 86–88, 99
  see also elements; heat
fire point, 257
'five animal game', 11
fullness-*shi*, 171
  anxiety and, 400
  case study, 298–300
  gall bladder, 298–300, 316
  insomnia and, 106–107, 108–109
  liver, 108
  Yang Qiao Mai, 108–109, 121–123

G

gall bladder, 39–42
  emptiness, 214, 316, 319, 336
  fullness, 298–300, 316
  stagnation, 316, 319
  stress and, 314–317
Gao Lishan, 114–115
GB-1 *Sizhukong*, 137
GB-5 *Xuanlu*, 341
GB-6 *Xuanli*, 338, 341
GB-7 *Benshen*:
  bleeding, 238, 321
  for emptiness, 215
  stress treatment, 319, 321, 322–323
  whiplash injury treatment, 329
GB-8 *Shuaigu*, 334, 342–344, 349
GB-9 *Tianchong*, 334, 336, 342–346,
  348, 349
GB-10 *Fubai*, 335, 346, 347

GB-11 *Touqiaoyin*:
  for psychiatric pathology, 335, 338, 346, 347, 348
  insomnia treatment, 111
GB-12 *Wangu*, 224, 319
GB-13 *Benshen*:
  for psychiatric pathology, 333, 334, 341, 349
    diankuang, 137
  for *qi* stagnation, 179, 197
  insomnia treatment, 111
GB-14 *Yangbai*, 197, 225
GB-15 *Toulinqi*, 336, 340, 342
GB-16 *Muchuang*, 340, 342, 349
GB-17 *Zhengying*, 337, 342–346, 348, 349
GB-18 *Chengling*, 138, 222
  for psychiatric pathology, 335–338, 341–346, 348
GB-19 *Naokong*, 335, 338, 340, 344, 346
GB-20 *Fengchi*, 177
  anxiety treatment, 400, 403
  for emptiness, 215, 224, 225
  for *qi* stagnation, 81, 177, 197, 224, 225, 299–300
  headache treatment, 299–300
  insomnia treatment, 111, 116
  meiheqi treatment, 164, 165
  principal actions, 177
  stress treatment, 319
  zangzao treatment, 156, 157
GB-21 *Jianjing*, 164, 224
  bleeding, 238
  for emptiness, 215
  stress treatment, 319
GB-24 *Riyue*, 214
GB-27 *Wushu*, 194
GB-28 *Weidao*, 194
GB-34 *Yanglingquan*, 41, 177–178
  agitation treatment, 92, 94
  diankuang treatment, 136
  for blood stasis, 193
  for emptiness, 214, 224
  for phlegm, 189
  for *qi* stagnation, 81, 177–178, 197, 224
  for severe psychiatric pathology, 333, 340, 346
  hyperactivity treatment, 393
  meiheqi treatment, 164
  principal actions, 178
  stress treatment, 318, 322, 324
  whiplash injury treatment, 329
GB-37 *Guangming*, 341, 347, 348
GB-40 *Qiuxu*, 214, 319

GB-41 *Zulinqi*:
  agitation treatment, 94
  for chronic disease, 302
  for emptiness, 225
  for *qi* stagnation, 81, 178, 194, 225, 300
  headache treatment, 300
GB-43 *Xiaxi*, 111
GB-44, 111
generalised anxiety disorder, 420–421
  see also anxiety
Guanzi, 9–10, 76
gui points, 136
gui-ghost, 57–58

H

haemorrhage, 189
hallucinations, 341, 347
He point, 258
He Puren, 112
HE-3 *Shaohai*, 137, 258
HE-4 *Lingdao*, 258
  for psychiatric pathology, 341–346
HE-5 *Tongli*, 208–210, 259
  agitation treatment, 93
  anxiety treatment, 230, 231, 400, 405
  bentunqi treatment, 159
  diankuang treatment, 355, 356
  for emptiness, 208–210
  for fire, 200
  for severe psychiatric pathology, 333, 338, 341, 342, 344, 346
  insomnia treatment, 111
  principal actions, 209
HE-6 *Yinxi*, 217–218, 258
  for emptiness, 215, 217–218
  for fire, 185
  insomnia treatment, 119
  meiheqi treatment, 164
  principal actions, 217
  zangzao treatment, 366, 367
HE-7 *Shenmen*, 205–206, 257–258
  agitation treatment, 93
  anxiety treatment, 231, 400, 402, 403, 404
  bentunqi treatment, 159
  diankuang treatment, 137, 138, 355, 361, 362
  for blood stasis, 193
  for emptiness, 205–206, 218, 222, 224, 225
  for fire, 185

for *qi* stagnation/constraint, 201, 224, 225, 228, 229
  for severe psychiatric pathology, 333–336, 341, 345–346, 348–349
  hyperactivity treatment, 392, 393, 394
  insomnia treatment, 111, 115, 116, 117
  meiheqi treatment, 164
  principal actions, 206
  stress treatment, 319
  zangzao treatment, 156, 157
HE-8 *Shaofu*, 181–182, 257
  for heart fire, 181–182
  hyperactivity treatment, 392, 393
  insomnia treatment, 122
  principal actions, 181
HE-9 *Shaochong*, 238, 257
headache, 383
  case studies, 196–199, 224–227, 298–300, 322–324
  see also whiplash injury
heart, 26–27, 35–36
  emptiness, 113, 214, 316, 319
    blood, 348
    case studies, 221–223, 401–402
    in psychiatric pathology, 336, 338
    yin, 215–218
  empty, 7, 294
  fire, 107–108, 179–183
    aetiology, 179
    case studies, 91–95, 199–200
    clinical manifestations, 180
    clinical notes, 180–181
    evolution, 179–180
    treatment, 181–183
  knotted *qi*, 76–77
  stress and, 317, 319
  yin deficiency case study, 119–121
heart points, 255–259
heat, 179–180
  agitation and, 98–100
  hyperactivity and, 386–388, 389–390, 392–393
  in *baihebing*, 152–153
  in *diankuang*, 131–132
  theory of, 85–86
  see also fire
heaven and earth, 53–54
hiccups, 42–43
history taking, 280–281
Hua Tuo, 11, 128
Huainanzi, 127

hun, 52–54, 58–63
  disorders, 341–343
  dreams and, 56
hyperactivity, 339, 385–395
  aetiology, 387–389
  case study, 391
  patterns, 386–387, 389–391
  treatment, 391–395
hysterical paralysis, 380–381

I

illness:
  causes of, 22–23
    emotions, 20–23, 78–79, 90–91
    external and internal factors,
      78–79
    pathogenic processes, 28–30
illusions, 341
incoherent thought, 335
incorrect thought, 336
indifference, 342
insomnia, 103–123
  aetiology, 105–106
  case studies, 112–114, 116–123,
    323–324
  definition, 104
  evaluation, 106–109
    agitated sleep, 108
    initial insomnia, 107–108
    intermittent insomnia, 107
    premature awaking, 108
    total absence of sleep, 108–109
  treatment, 109–123
intelligence, 345
internal alchemy, 13, 16
internal practices, 9–10
Internet, 425–426
irritability, 343
jing, 51, 59–60
  empty, 218–219
  po and, 54–55, 59–60
  zhi and, 67–68
jing point, 257, 258
Jingyui Yaolue, 141, 142, 147–149,
  150–152

K

KI-1 *Yongquan*, 138, 200
  for psychiatric pathology, 333–335,
    340, 343, 346
  hyperactivity treatment, 395
KI-2 *Rangu*, 122, 334, 338

KI-3 *Taixi*, 181–183
  agitation treatment, 92, 93
  anxiety treatment, 400, 402, 403, 404
  baihebing treatment, 162
  bentunqi treatment, 159, 381
  diankuang treatment, 138, 355
  for chronic disease, 302
  for emptiness, 214, 219, 222
  for fire rising, 382–383
  for heart fire, 181–183
  for *qi* stagnation/constraint, 201,
    228, 229
  for severe psychiatric pathology, 336,
    338, 344, 346, 348, 349
    conversion disorders, 380
  insomnia treatment, 111
  meiheqi treatment, 382
  principal actions, 182
  stress treatment, 320
  whiplash injury treatment, 327
  yang reinforcement, 378–379
KI-4 *Dazhong*, 208–209
  agitation treatment, 93
  anxiety treatment, 230, 400, 405
  bentunqi, 159
  diankuang treatment, 138
  for emptiness, 208–209
  for phlegm, 189
  for *qi* stagnation, 178
  for severe psychiatric pathology,
    334–336, 344–346
  principal actions, 209
KI-6 *Zhaohai*, 217–218
  for emptiness, 215, 217–218
  for fire, 185
  insomnia treatment, 109, 111, 119,
    122
  principal actions, 218
  stress treatment, 320
KI-7 *Fuliu*:
  for emptiness, 137, 214
  zangzao treatment, 366, 367
KI-12 *Dahe*, 224, 225
kidney, 26–27, 38–39
  channel, illness of, 377–378
  emptiness, 348
  qi deficiency, hyperactivity and, 387,
    389, 390–391, 394–395
  stress and, 317–318
  yin deficiency, 144–145, 317–318
    case study, 119–121
knotting, 76–77, 90–91
  case study, 116–119
  in *meiheqi*, 154–155
kuang, 125–131, 135–136, 187,
  353–354
  see also diankuang

L

lantern sickness, 100, 191
laughter without reason, 343
Li Dongyuan, 13, 86–88, 98–100, 132
LI-2 *Erjian*, 348
LI-4 *Hegu*, 174–175
  diankuang treatment, 355, 356, 357
  for blood stasis, 44, 193
  for chronic disease, 302
  for phlegm, 189
  for *qi* stagnation, 44, 81, 174–175,
    194, 197, 201, 225,
    299–300
  for severe psychiatric pathology,
    334–335, 339–342,
    344–345
  headache treatment, 299–300
  hyperactivity treatment, 392
  meiheqi treatment, 164
  principal actions, 175
  stress treatment, 320, 321
  whiplash injury treatment, 327, 329
LI-6 *Pianli*, 347
LI-11 *Quchi*, 321
  for emptiness, 136, 137
  for psychiatric pathology, 338, 339,
    342, 345
LI-20 *Yingxiang*, 115, 341, 347
Liji, 5, 18
lingering pathogenic factor (LPF), 388
Lingshu, 23, 142
  'benshen' chapter, 26–28, 54, 63–64
Liu Wansu, 85–86, 131–132
LIV-1 *Dadun*, 349
LIV-2 *Xingjian*, 183
  agitation treatment, 92, 93
  anxiety treatment, 400
  diankuang treatment, 136, 355
  for blood stasis, 193
  for fire, 200
  for liver fire, 183
  for *qi* stagnation, 178
  for severe psychiatric pathology, 341,
    346
  hiccups treatment, 43
  hyperactivity treatment, 392, 393
  insomnia treatment, 111, 122
  meiheqi treatment, 369
LIV-3 *Taichong*, 174–175
  agitation treatment, 92, 94
  anxiety treatment, 231, 400, 405
  baihebing treatment, 162, 163
  for blood stasis, 193
  for chronic disease, 303
  for emptiness, 213, 215
  for phlegm, 189

LIV-3 *Taichong* (*Continued*)
for *qi* stagnation, 81, 174–175, 194, 197, 201, 225, 300
for severe psychiatric pathology, 334, 339–345, 346, 349
headache treatment, 300
hiccups treatment, 43
hyperactivity treatment, 392, 394
insomnia treatment, 111
meiheqi treatment, 164
principal actions, 175
stress treatment, 320, 321, 323, 324
whiplash injury treatment, 327, 329
LIV-5 *Liguo*:
for psychiatric pathology, 335, 341–343, 346, 349
diankuang, 355, 360, 362
for *qi* stagnation, 179
LIV-8 *Ququan*:
for chronic disease, 303
for emptiness, 136, 215
for psychiatric pathology, 341, 342, 346, 349
LIV-13 *Zhangmen*:
bentunqi treatment, 147
for emptiness, 213
for *qi* stagnation, 179, 194
insomnia treatment, 111
LIV-14 *Qimen*:
bentunqi treatment, 147
for *qi* stagnation, 179
insomnia treatment, 116
liver, 26–27, 34–35
anger and, 76
emptiness, 348
of blood, 214–215
fire, 183
case studies, 91–95, 199–200
fullness, 108
qi stagnation, 73, 171–179, 349
aetiology, 171–172
case studies, 193–196, 200–202, 224–227, 298–300, 322–323
clinical manifestations, 172
clinical notes, 173–174
evolution, 172
treatment, 174–179
shuxie function, 74–75
Lower-5, 326
Lower-6, 326
LU-1 *Zhongfu*:
baihebing treatment, 162
for emptiness, 220
for phlegm, 189
for *qi* stagnation, 178
LU-3 *Tianfu*, 220, 221

LU-7 *Lieque*, 208, 210
for emptiness, 208, 210
for phlegm, 189
for *qi* stagnation, 44, 178
principal actions, 210
LU-8 *Ququan*, 395
LU-9 *Taiyuan*:
for emptiness, 178, 220, 347
for phlegm, 189
LU-10 *Yuji*, 44
LU-11 *Shaoshang*, 44, 136
lung, 26–27, 37–38
emptiness, 219–221, 347
knotted *qi*, case study, 161–163
stress and, 317, 319
luo point, 259
on the paired *yang*, 259

M

M-BW-25 *Shiqizhuixia*, 164
M-HN-3 *Yintang*, 399
M-UE-9 *Sifeng*, 392
major depressive episode, 421–422
maniacal psychosis, case study, 357–359
manic depression *see diankuang*
manic episode, 422
manic thought, 334–335
meiheqi, 154–155
aetiology, 154–155
case studies, 163–165, 368–369, 381–382
clinical notes, 155–156
memory disorders, 345–346
metal, 30, 37–38
see also elements
metal point, 258
middle burner weakness, hyperactivity and, 387, 388–389, 390, 394
migraine case studies, 196–199, 224–227, 322–323
mind, 69
zhi as, 68–69
mind-therapy, 261
ministerial fire, 88–90
movement disorders, 339–340
moxibustion-*Jiufa*, 235–236
bentunqi, 148
diankuang, 135, 136
insomnia, 110
MS-1, 110, 242, 321
MS-2, 242, 321
MS-3, 243, 321
MS-5, 110, 242
MS-7, 302

MS-13, 326, 329
MS-14, 326, 329
multiple sclerosis case study, 301–302
mutism, 338

N

N-HN-54 *Anmian*, 324, 360–362, 364, 365
Nanjing, 130, 147
needle, 276–278
negativism, 339–340
Nei Dan, 13, 16
Nei Guan, 14
Neijing, 7–8, 234
bentunqi, 146
diankuang, 128, 129–130, 134–136
emotions, 18, 20–23, 30
fanzao, 97
gall bladder, 40–41
insomnia, 105, 109
meiheqi, 154
needling, 276
yi, 64, 65, 66
yu, 76, 77
zhi, 68
neurosis, 420
neutrality, 286–287
'nourishing understanding with stillness', 5
'nourishment of life', 9
Nucleo Operativo Alcologia (NOA), Milano, 397–398
case studies, 401–406
data collection, 401
evaluation, 401
treatment protocol, 399–401

O

obsessive thought, 335–336
opposite reactions, 342
organs, 24–28
emotions and, 30–31, 34–39
see also specific organs

P

P-3 *Quze*, 258
P-4 *Ximen*, 191, 258
for blood stasis, 191
principal actions, 191

P-5 *Jianshi*, 188, 258
  diankuang treatment, 137, 355, 359,
    361, 362
  for chronic disease, 302
  for emptiness, 213
  for fire, 185
  for obstruction by phlegm, 188
  for *qi* stagnation, 81, 178
  for severe psychiatric pathology, 340
  hyperactivity treatment, 393
  principal actions, 188
  stress treatment, 319
P-6 *Neiguan*, 175–177, 259
  agitation treatment, 93
  anxiety treatment, 400, 405
  diankuang treatment, 355, 356, 360,
    361, 362
  for blood stasis, 193
  for phlegm, 189
  for *qi* stagnation/constraint, 44,
    175–177, 194, 225, 228
  for severe psychiatric pathology, 334,
    341
  insomnia treatment, 111, 112, 113,
    116, 117
  meiheqi treatment, 368, 369
  principal actions, 176
  stress treatment, 320, 323
  yuzheng treatment, 364, 365
  zangzao treatment, 157, 366
P-7 *Daling*, 181–182, 257–258
  diankuang treatment, 136, 138
  for blood stasis, 193
  for heart fire, 181–182
  for *qi* stagnation, 178
  for severe psychiatric pathology,
    333–335, 340, 343, 346
  insomnia treatment, 111, 122
  principal actions, 182
P-8 *Laogong*, 136, 257
P-9 *Zhongchong*, 238, 257, 334, 345
pain, acupuncture effects, 293–294
panic attacks, 150–151, 421
  see also bentunqi
paradoxical emotions, 343
paralysis, hysterical, 380–381
paramnesias, 346
patient–doctor relationship *see* therapeutic relationship
perceptions, distorted, 341
pericardium points, 255–259
persecution delirium, 334
pessimism, 342
phlegm, 29–30, 79–80, 185, 187
  case studies, 80–83, 137–140,
    196–200
  fire, 137–140, 186–187

hyperactivity and, 386–387, 388,
  390, 393
  in *diankuang*, 132–134, 352
  in *meiheqi*, 154–155
  insomnia and, 106
  obstruction by-*tan*, 185–189, 383
    aetiology, 185
    clinical manifestations, 186–187
    clinical notes, 187
    evolution, 186
    treatment, 187–189
  production, 29, 80, 89–90, 185
  stress and, 316
physician as guide, 262–263
pinching-*taici*, 238
plum blossom needle-*Meihauzhen*, 138,
  237
  insomnia treatment, 115–116
po, 52–54, 58–63
  disorders, 338–341
  jing and, 54–55
possession delirium, 334
premenstrual symptoms, 174
projection, 272
prune stone *qi see meiheqi*
pseudoreminiscence, 346
psychic therapeutic method, 261
psychological disorders, 33–34,
  297–298
  conversion disorders, 379–381
  serious pathology, 332–349
  syndromes, 347–349
  see also emotions; *specific disorders*
psychosis, 420
  maniacal, case study, 357–359
pulse, 409–417
  chang-long, 414
  chen-deep, 409–410
  chi-slow, 410
  cu-hurried, 416
  dai-intermittent, 415
  dong-jumping, 416
  duan-short, 414
  fu-floating, 409
  fu-hidden, 416
  ge-like a drum skin, 415
  hong-flooding, 413–414
  hua-slippery, 411
  huan-moderate or slackened, 414
  ji-urgent, 511
  jie-knotted, 415
  jin-tense, 411
  kuo-hollow, 415
  lao-imprisoned or firm, 415–416
  ru-drenched, 413
  ruo-weak, 412–413
  san-scattered, 414

se-choppy, 413
shi guaimai-the ten strange pulses,
  416
shi-full, 413
shuo-rapid, 410
wei-minute, 412
xi-thready, 412
xu-empty, 411–412
xuan-wiry, 411

Q

qi, 3, 19, 51, 233–234, 279–280
  circulation, 10–13, 74–75
  constraint, 73–74, 76–79, 108
    case studies, 196–199, 224–229
  deficiency, 107, 113, 205, 295–296
    kidney, hyperactivity and, 387,
      389, 390–391, 394–395
    spleen, hyperactivity and, 387,
      388–389, 390, 394
    see also emptiness
  movements of, 17, 21
    case study, 43–45
    emotions and, 23–26, 34
    pathogenic processes, 28–30
  of the running piglet *see bentunqi*
  prune stone *see meiheqi*
  setting of therapy and, 279
  stagnation, 21, 73–74, 79, 173,
    338
    case studies, 43–45, 80–83,
      163–165, 193–196,
      200–202, 288–291,
      298–300, 322–323
    in *meiheqi*, 155
    in psychiatric pathology, 338, 349
    liver *qi*, 171–179, 193–196,
      200–202, 298–300
Qi Bo, 129
qigong, 12–13
qing, 17, 19–20
qingyu, 19
qingzhi jibing, 17

R

Ren Mai, 247–251
Ren-1 *Huiyin*, 136
Ren-3 *Zhongji*, 147, 185
Ren-4 *Guanyuan*, 248–249
  agitation treatment, 92, 93, 94
  anxiety treatment, 231, 400, 402,
    404

Ren-4 *Guanyuan* (Continued)
  bentunqi treatment, 147, 159, 160,
    367, 368
  for emptiness, 211, 218, 219, 224,
    225
  for *qi* stagnation, 194, 224, 225, 300
  headache treatment, 300
  insomnia treatment, 119
  meiheqi treatment, 164
  moxibustion and, 236
  principal actions, 248
  zangzao treatment, 156, 157
Ren-5 *Shimen*, 147
Ren-6 *Qihai*, 249
  agitation treatment, 93, 94
  anxiety treatment, 230, 400, 405
  baihebing treatment, 162
  bentunqi treatment, 367, 368
  for chronic disease, 302
  for emptiness, 211, 213
  for *qi* stagnation/constraint, 44, 228,
    229, 299
  headache treatment, 299
  insomnia treatment, 111, 117
  meiheqi treatment, 164
  moxibustion and, 236
  principal actions, 249
  zangzao treatment, 157
Ren-7 *Yinjiao*, 147, 341
Ren-8 *Shenque*, 236
Ren-11 *Jianli*, 111, 364, 365
Ren-12 *Zhongwan*, 249
  agitation treatment, 94
  diankuang treatment, 355, 358, 361
  for emptiness, 211, 212, 222, 225,
    291
  for *qi* stagnation, 194, 225
  hyperactivity treatment, 394
  insomnia treatment, 111, 112, 113,
    116, 120
  moxibustion and, 235
  principal actions, 249
  yuzheng treatment, 364, 365
Ren-13 *Shangwan*, 117, 137
  diankuang treatment, 354–355, 358
Ren-14 *Juque*, 211, 249–250
  anxiety treatment, 399, 402–405
  diankuang treatment, 354, 355
  for *qi* constraint, 228
  principal actions, 249
  yuzheng treatment, 364, 365
Ren-15 *Jiuwei*, 250
  agitation treatment, 92, 93
  diankuang treatment, 354, 355, 358
  for emptiness, 225
  for *qi* constraint, 225, 228
  insomnia treatment, 117
  principal actions, 250

Ren-17 *Shanzhong*, 248, 250
  agitation treatment, 92
  anxiety treatment, 231, 400
  baihebing treatment, 162
  bentunqi treatment, 159, 160
  for emptiness, 211
  for *qi* constraint, 228, 229
  insomnia treatment, 117, 119
  meiheqi treatment, 164
  principal actions, 250
  stress treatment, 319
  zangzao treatment, 156, 157
Ren-18 *Yutang*, 117
Ren-22 *Tiantu*, 251
  meiheqi treatment, 368, 369
  principal actions, 251
Ren-23 *Lianquan*, 338
Ren-24 *Chengqiang*, 136
repetition, 340
restlessness, 97
  see also fanzao

S

sadness-*bei*, 30–31, 37–38
  see also emotions
scalp acupuncture:
  chronic disease, 302
  stress treatment, 321
  whiplash injury treatment,
    326–327
  see also cranial acupuncture
schizophrenia, 125–126, 133
  case studies, 356–357, 359–362
  see also diankuang
sedation, six points of, 114–115
self-punishment, 340
sense perception, 341
setting of therapy, 278–279
Shao Yang, 40
shen, 47–48
  as aspect of physiology, 51
  as extraordinary or transcendent
    aspect, 48–50
  as vitality, 50–51
  calming method, 110–111
  five *shen*, 52
  regulation of, 273–274
  sleep relationship, 103
  tongue diagnosis and, 307–309
shengui, 57
shi guaimai-the ten strange pulses,
  416
shu points, 255
shuxie, 75
  liver function, 74–75

SI-3 *Houxi*:
  for fire, 185
  for psychiatric pathology, 336, 339,
    343
    diankuang, 137
  meiheqi treatment, 164
SI-6 *Yanglao*, 341, 347
SI-7 *Zhizheng*, 185, 259
  for psychiatric pathology, 335,
    337, 341–342, 344, 346,
    348–349
SI-25 *Tianshu*, 44
sight disorder with psychic origin, 380
SJ-5 *Waiguan*, 194
sleep, 103
  agitated, 108
  total absence of, 108–109
  see also insomnia
slow spirit, 335
somatisation disorder, 422–423
SP-1 *Yinbai*, 136, 343
SP-3 *Taibai*, 205, 208
  agitation treatment, 92
  anxiety treatment, 400, 404
  baihebing treatment, 162
  for emptiness, 205, 208, 212, 222,
    225
  for phlegm, 189
  for *qi* stagnation, 178, 194, 225
  for severe psychiatric pathology, 346,
    347, 348, 349
  insomnia treatment, 117
  principal actions, 208
  zangzao treatment, 157
SP-4 *Gongsun*, 175–176
  anxiety treatment, 400, 405
  for emptiness, 224, 225
  for *qi* stagnation/constraint, 44,
    175–176, 224, 225, 228
  insomnia treatment, 111, 117
  principal actions, 176
  stress treatment, 320
SP-6 *Sanyinjiao*, 192–193, 205, 207
  agitation treatment, 93
  anxiety treatment, 231
  bentunqi treatment, 367, 368
  diankuang treatment, 138, 355, 356,
    357
  for blood stasis, 192–193
  for chronic disease, 303
  for emptiness, 205, 207, 215, 218,
    222, 224, 225, 291
  for fire, 185
  for *qi* stagnation/constraint, 194,
    224, 225, 228, 229
  for severe psychiatric pathology, 333,
    335, 337, 342, 344–346
  hyperactivity treatment, 394, 395

insomnia treatment, 111, 116, 119
meiheqi treatment, 164
principal actions, 192, 207
stress treatment, 320, 323
whiplash injury treatment, 327, 329
zangzao treatment, 156, 157,
    366–367
SP-9 *Yinlingquan*, 194, 213, 320
SP-10 *Xuehai*, 192
for blood stasis, 192
for fire, 185
for *qi* stagnation, 178
principal actions, 192
SP-15 *Daheng*, 213
speech disorders, 338
spleen, 26–28, 36–37
emptiness, 113, 212–213, 338,
    347–349
qi deficiency, hyperactivity and, 387,
    388–389, 390, 394
stress and, 317, 320
spreading and draining, 74–75
ST-2 *Sibai*, 44
ST-6 *Jiache*, 136
ST-8 *Touwei*, 299, 334, 341, 349
ST-17 *Ruzhong*, 136
ST-21 *Liangmen*, 184
ST-25 *Tianshu*:
for emptiness, 213
for *qi* stagnation, 194
insomnia treatment, 111
zangzao treatment, 157
ST-29 *Guilai*:
bentunqi treatment, 147
for emptiness, 225
for *qi* stagnation, 194, 225
meiheqi treatment, 164
ST-36 *Zusanli*, 205–207
agitation treatment, 92, 94
anxiety treatment, 231, 400, 402,
    403, 404
baihebing treatment, 162
diankuang treatment, 355, 361, 362
for blood stasis, 193
for chronic disease, 302
for emptiness, 205–207, 222, 225,
    291
for phlegm, 189
for *qi* stagnation, 44, 178, 201, 225,
    299
for severe psychiatric pathology, 334,
    338, 339, 342, 344, 346
headache treatment, 299
hyperactivity treatment, 394
insomnia treatment, 111, 112, 113,
    115, 116, 120
meiheqi treatment, 369

moxibustion and, 236
principal actions, 206
stress treatment, 320, 323
zangzao treatment, 157
ST-37 *Shangjuxu*, 44
for emptiness, 213
insomnia treatment, 111
zangzao treatment, 157
ST-39 *Xiajuxu*, 44, 213
ST-40 *Fenglong*, 188
diankuang treatment, 355, 359, 360,
    362
for chronic disease, 302
for emptiness, 213
for fire, 185
for obstruction by phlegm, 188
for *qi* stagnation, 81, 178
for severe psychiatric pathology, 341,
    346–349
hyperactivity treatment, 393
principal actions, 188
stress treatment, 319, 320
ST-42 *Chongyuang*, 349
ST-44 *Neiting*, 184
agitation treatment, 92, 93, 94
anxiety treatment, 400
for fire, 184, 200
for psychiatric pathology, 339, 341,
    346, 347
for *qi* stagnation, 44, 299
headache treatment, 299
hyperactivity treatment, 392
insomnia treatment, 111, 122
ST-45 *Lidui*, 238
stagnation, 29–30, 173
qi, 21, 73–74, 79, 173
    case studies, 43–45, 80–83, 163–
        165, 193–196, 200–202,
        224–227, 288–291,
        298–300, 322–323
    gall bladder, 316, 319
    in *meiheqi*, 155
    in psychiatric disorders, 338, 349
    liver *qi*, 171–179, 193–196,
        200–202, 224–227,
        298–300
stereotypy, 340
stomach:
fire, 184
    case studies, 91–95, 199–200
stress and, 317
stress, 314
stress syndrome, 314–329
case studies, 322–324
clinical manifestations, 316–318
examination, 318
treatment, 318–322

bleeding, 321
ear therapy, 321
scalp acupuncture, 321
wrist–ankle technique, 322
stuporous condition, 339
stuttering, 338
Sun Simiao, 11, 41, 98, 126–127, 128,
    136
Suwen, 23, 31, 48, 78, 142
sweating, in *bentunqi*, 148–149

T

Tang Zonghai, 144, 149–150
TB-4 *Yangchi*, 114
TB-5 *Waiguan*, 81, 259, 302, 355
TB-6 *Zhigou*, 111, 344
TB-17 *Yifeng*, 341, 348
TB-19 *Luxi*, 341
TB-23 *Sizhukong*, 224
tetanism with psychic origin, 380
therapeutic effects:
immediate effects, 293–294
psychological conditions, 297–298
unexpected effects, 294–297
    psychological effects, 296–297
therapeutic relationship, 271–288
abstention, 284–285
case studies, 288–292
dynamics of, 282–284
empathy, 286
needling, 276–278
neutrality, 286–287
setting and time of therapy, 278–282
shen regulation, 273–274
stumbling blocks, 274–276
thought-*si*, 30–31, 36–37
disorders of, 334–338
see also emotions
time of treatment, 280–282
tiredness, 173
tongue, dark, case study, 91–95
tongue diagnosis, 307–311
coating, 311
colour, 309–310
shape, 310–311
transference, 283–284
trigger finger, 43–45

U

Upper-1, 110, 241
stress treatment, 322, 324
whiplash injury treatment, 327, 329

Upper-4, 326
Upper-5, 110, 241
  stress treatment, 318, 321, 324
  whiplash injury treatment, 326,
     327, 329
Upper-6, 326, 327–328

V

violent behaviour, 340

W

wandering, 341
Wang Bing, 31
Wang Ketang, 100, 358
Wang Leting, 110–111
Wang Qingren, 80, 100
water, 30, 38–39
  see also elements
water point, 258
weeping without reason, 343
whiplash injury, 325–329
  case studies, 327–329
  clinical manifestations, 325–326
  treatment, 326–327
will, disorders of, 344–345
wood, 30, 34–35
  see also elements
wood point, 257
World Wide Web, 425–426
wrist–ankle-Wanhuaizhen technique,
     241, 242
  insomnia treatment, 110
  stress treatment, 322
  whiplash injury, 326
wuqin zhiuxi, 11
wuwei (non-acting), 4–5
wuxing (five elements), 18, 30

X

Xi point, 258
Xunzi, 6, 49

Y

yang, 53–55, 59, 88–89, 213–214
  diankuang etiology, 129–131
  emptiness, 213–214, 348–349
    case study, 221–223
  fullness, 108–109, 121, 121–123
  reinforcement, 378–379
Yang Shangshan, 64
yangsheng, 9–10
yangxing, 11
yawning, 95
  zanzao, 143, 144–145
yi, 63–64
  as an idea, 64–65
  as intent, 64–66
  disorders, 344–345
Yijing, 48, 67
yin, 53–54, 59, 88–89
  agitation yinzao, 98–100
  consumption of, 90–91
  deficiency/emptiness, 107–108, 119,
     379–381
    baihebing, 152–153
    case studies, 119–121, 227–229,
       323–324, 401–402
    heart, 215–218
    kidney, 144–145
    lung, 219–221
    stress and, 317–318, 320
    whiplash injury, 325–326,
       328–329
    zangzao, 143, 144–145
  diankuang aetiology, 129–131
  exhaustion, 114
  fire yinhuo, 86–88, 99

ying point, 257
yu, 74, 78
  emotions and, 76–77
  see also constraint-yu; yuzheng (yu
     syndrome)
yuan point, 257–258
yuanqi, 86–87
yuanwu bilei principle, 373, 376
yuzheng (yu syndrome), 74, 76, 79–80,
     362–365
  case study, 363–365

Z

zangzao, 141–145
  aetiology, 142–144
  case studies, 156–158, 366–367
  clinical notes, 144–145
Zhang Jiebin, 64, 78–79, 90–91, 103,
     104, 106, 128, 133, 272
Zhang Yuansu, 132
Zhang Zhongjing, 76, 98, 130–131,
     141, 142, 151, 154, 264
Zhang Zihe, 31, 265–267
zhi, 63–64
  as emotion, 68–69
  as mind, 68–69
  as will, 67–68
  disorders of, 345–346
  stabilisation method, 110–111
Zhong Meiquan, 115–116
Zhu Danxi, 77, 80, 88–90, 132–133,
     262
Zhu Xi, 53–54
Zhuangzi, 10

Printed and bound by CPI Group (UK) Ltd, Croydon, CR0 4YY

03/10/2024

01040360-0007